NATURAL EARTH:
THE ENGLISH STANDARD REFERENCE
ON HERBAL SUBSTANCES
VOLUME ONE:

THE HERBAL CENTER

OF

HEALING

BY GARY LOCKHART

WITH ARTWORK BY

APRIL BINGHAM

With Green Wishes,

Gary Lockhart

EARTHPULSE PRESS, INC.

ANCHORAGE, ALASKA

Special Note: Earthpulse Press Incorporated (EPI) and the author do not make or imply any medical claims for any of the products it sells or herbal substances described herein. EPI and the author cautions you: Certain of these substances may be dangerous to those not in sound mental or physical health — and others. If you have a medical condition, EPI suggests you contact a licensed medical provider. Medical technology and herbal substances are regulated in the United States by the FDA.

This book is not intended to replace the services of qualified doctors or medical experts. If you have a medical problem, see a doctor or professional according to your choice. Most plants listed in this book have had a tradition of use, but some require great caution. EPI and the author do not specifically recommend any herbs, products or healing techniques, but we do encourage exploring more effective alternative ways of healing

ISBN 1-890693-02-2

©, copyright 1998 by Gary Lockhart

Illustrations April Bingham

First Earthpulse Press Printing

Printed in the United States

Earthpulse Press Incorporated
P.O. Box 201393
Anchorage, AK 99520
http://www.earthpulse.com
voice mail:888.690.1277
fax: 907.696.1277

This book is dedicated to

Arthur Lee Jacobson

As a naturalist, gardener and writer of books on trees,
he shares the adventure of life and love for our green friends.

Contents
AND
List of Illustrations

INTRODUCTION

"The doctors tender of their fame, wisely on me lay all the blame.
We must confess his case was nice; but he would never take advice,
Had he been ruled for ought appears, he might have lived these twenty years.
For when we opened him we found, that all his vital parts were sound."
— Jonathan Swift

In O. Henry's story, "Let Me Feel Your Pulse," a sick man visits doctor after doctor, without success, until he finally meets one very knowledgeable old doctor, who tells him, "Somewhere in these mountains there's a plant growing — a flowering plant that'll cure, and it's about the only thing that will. It's of a kind that's as old as the world; but of late it's powerful scarce and hard to find. You and I will have to hunt it up."

For weeks they hunt in the mountains, but they cannot find the rare herb. When they are about to admit defeat, the sick man realizes that the weeks of climbing and sunshine have healed him. When O. Henry wrote this story in 1909, he must have hoped that it would be his story, for he was very ill, and nobody was able to help him. He needed that rare herb, for he died the next year.

Of course, today, it's not just that the herbs are rare; the information about these herbs is scattered and buried in thousands of old books, indexes and journals.

My search started twenty years ago after I tried to help a friend understand the chemistry of common herbs. It eventually yielded the largest collection of material from medical and scientific literature on herbal medicine ever assembled. I have spent almost all my time during these years, digging through books, indexes and journals to recover whatever I could about this rare, hidden knowledge. Much of this time was spent in the medical and science libraries of the University of Washington, but I also took three 8,000 mile trips and a dozen shorter trips visiting libraries throughout North America. I worked my way through most of the medical and scientific literature from the seventeenth century up to the present. On a good day, I could go through ten feet of old journals.

With diligent work I went through some four miles of journals in about 40 major libraries across the country ranging from the Library of Congress to Stanford. This included most of the material written in the nineteenth century when herbal medicine was more common. Thousands of studies and observations have been published in the past three centuries that are of great interest, but they are lost in the sea of words now gathering dust in the basements of major libraries. Many observations have the ring of truth, but others are doubtful. I have tried to sort out the things that would be of great interest to my readers. I have also tried to summarize ethnobotanical material that might be of interest to researchers. The work has been difficult, but it has yielded thousands of obscure, unindexed bits of information that could not be easily found — until now.

The Herbal Center of Healing is the first of five books covering the use of plants in medicine. The work focuses on the use of herbs for the nervous system, the blood system, and the main organs of the body.

These books are intended to be an encyclopedia of material arranged topically under the subject area. Those who have a medical problem will be able to see most of the herbal material found in medical and scientific literature that has some validity. I found hundreds of surprises in medical literature, which offer help to those suffering from nearly every disorder. Information is also provided on discoveries relating to health on minerals, vitamins and diet.

Only the literature that is deemed "official medical practice" makes its way into the books of medical students. There are thousands of medical, botanical, pharmaceutical, agricultural and chemical journals in which observations about herbs have been made. Some of these observations on herbs are just as revolutionary and worthy of study as the latest technological breakthroughs in medicine, but, since there is little publicity and money to be made, they are largely ignored.

Often there is a contemptuous attitude among medical professionals towards simple treatments. I once had dinner in a small restaurant, where strangers shared tables, for want of a place to sit. The woman at my table was graduating from medical school. When I mentioned that I was writing a chapter on the cures for diabetes, she angrily snapped: "That can't possibly be true. They don't teach us that in medical school!"

In these times, when something is wrong with our heart, kidneys or liver, the tendency is to replace the organ or provide a mechanical substitute. We are no longer practicing healing medicine; we are practicing technology. Richard Bright was famous for his study of kidney disease (Bright's disease) and high blood pressure. In 1813 he wrote to his father: "You must know that surgery is at this moment rising very fast at the expense of medicine – and we must do our best to keep our ground." In our time, the surgeon is the king of the mountain, while the natural healer is lost in the swamp. Often true healers are shut off from grants from the National Institutes of Health, and they become the target of the FDA and the AMA.

I want to thank friends who helped to translate Russian, Ukrainian, Portuguese, Spanish, Danish, Swedish, French and German articles. Thanks to those who answered my queries with letters from South Africa, Indonesia, Spain, France, Germany, Peru, India and Saudi Arabia. Special thanks go to Arthur Lee Jacobson for helping with the botany. Thanks must go to Seth Berholwitz, David Wesley, Doris Jones, Jean Radosevich and Anne Winter for their interest in my work. Special thanks to artist April Bingham.

In most cases I have to use proper botanical names, because common names are inadequate. A dandelion isn't just one plant; it is a collection of some 200 members of the *Taraxacum* genus. Just as we have first, middle, and last names, botanists name plants in the reverse order, so the dandelion is a member of the *Compositae* family, and its genus and species name is *Taraxacum officinale*. Those who grow or gather plants will want the proper identification, for similar plants may not be active. Botanists change these names to reflect new knowledge about family relationships. In some cases I have used the new name with an = sign, followed by the old botanical name, because the old name is better known, but not current.

I have followed the modern trend of replacing clumsy date notations of "Before Christ" and "Anno Domini" with "-" and "+"; milligrams is abbreviated as mgs., and kilograms is often found as kgs., while cc. is cubic centimeters. An extensive bibliography is provided for those who want to study original sources.

These books are not intended to replace the services of qualified doctors or medical experts. If you have a medical problem, see a doctor or professional according to your choice. Most plants listed in this book have had a tradition of use, but some require great caution. I do not specifically recommend any herbs, products or healing techniques, but I do encourage exploring more effective and inexpensive ways of healing.

HEADACHE HERBS

On the 8th [April 8, 1865] I had followed the Army of the Potomac in the rear of Lee. I was suffering very severely with a sick headache, and stopped at a farmhouse at the road some distance in the rear of the main body of the army. I spent the night in bathing my feet in hot water and mustard and mustard plasters on my wrists and the back of my neck, hoping to be cured by morning.... When the officer reached me I was still suffering with the sick headache; but the instant I saw the contents of the [surrender] note [from General Robert E. Lee] I was cured..."

General Ulysses S. Grant

"I'm very brave generally," he went on in a low voice, *"only today I happen to have a headache!"*

Lewis Carroll, The Walrus and the Carpenter

*"Lord, how my head aches! What a head have I!
It beats as it would fall in twenty pieces."*

William Shakespeare, *Romeo and Juliet*

The ancients believed that headaches were caused by evil spirits. The Greeks called these evil entities *keres*. The best way to cure a headache was to cut a hole in the head, so the spirit could escape. This process was called *trepanning*, and ancient skulls have been found all over the world with holes cut in them.

Saint Augustine wrote: "All diseases of Christians are caused by demons." The cure then obviously was a prayer to God, or the intercession of some saint, to release the evil demon. In the sixth century, St. Gregory, the Bishop of Tours, France, told how his headache was cured by touching the railing at the tomb of St. Martin. This resulted in a flood of pilgrims. Pilgrims also traveled to the tomb of St. Julian to cure their headaches.

The Babylonians tried to find a rational explanation for the order of events, by linking the stars to human events. Headaches were the result of bad stars, and there wasn't much you could do about it. People born in the sign of Aries were believed to be especially headache-prone.

Hippocrates tried to explain all problems with the idea that the body was influenced by the four humors. These were influenced by food, water and climate. If you had headaches, you had too much of the wrong humors. By changing the diet or climate, you could change the humors and solve your medical problems.

At some time we all have headaches, but they are much more likely in people who plan and achieve, and are careful and precise. People who 'don't give a damn' are much less likely to suffer from headaches.

Two early US presidents suffered from headaches. Thomas Jefferson was the author of the Declaration of Independence. He also was an inventor, architect, and statesman. He had such problems with headaches that he stated in 1786: "The art of life is the avoiding of pain." General Ulysses S. Grant suffered from headaches all through the American Civil War.

The mechanism of most headaches became clear, with the study of anatomy in the 20th century. Blood vessels are wrapped with muscle strands that relax or constrict to regulate the circulation. The loosening or tightening of these muscular strands regulates the oxygen and nutrient supply. When we are upset about something, we become tense, and the muscular strands constrict. The brain tissue becomes short of oxygen, and it sends out a pain signal. If we eat a dish of ice cream too rapidly, the smooth muscle fibers suddenly constrict and we have a temporary headache. Headaches may also be the result of not enough constriction of the smooth muscle strands.

A doctor discovered that his headaches could be cured by sipping cold water. He tested this discovery by having all of his patients with headaches sip cold water, and the results were plotted against blood pressure. About 60% of the people with low blood pressure were relieved with cold water, but sipping cold water rarely relieved people with high blood pressure. Blood pressure is greater in the sitting rather than lying position, and it is increased by smoking, exercise, and exposure to cold wind. Hot drinks gave some relief to those with high blood pressure.

The pressure caused by moderate constriction of the blood vessels forces lymph through the tissues, and brings nutrition and oxygen. Headaches can be caused by a vasodilator, which makes the vessels too wide. Nitroglycerin is a vasodilator, and this is the reason why it causes 'dynamite headaches.' Angina pain is caused by a lack of blood circulation in clogged blood vessels, and nitroglycerin is an effective remedy in this form of heart pain. The old miners initially got headaches from working with nitroglycerin. When they retired after years of working with it, they developed headaches from not breathing nitroglycerin fumes!

High blood pressure is often a factor in headaches. This can be due to the constriction of the muscular bands around the blood vessels, the kidneys or many other factors. When the blood pressure returns to normal, the headaches go away.

Many old time doctors believed that headaches were due to the liver and they prescribed liver tonics to cure headaches. The enzyme-rich cells of the liver act as a filter for the blood stream, and they break down materials for elimination in the kidneys. There may be some truth to this idea, for one of the strongest liver activators is the green leaf of the common artichoke, which is known for relieving headaches in Italy.

'Intestinal toxemia' was a popular explanation for frequent headaches in the early part of the 20th century. The colon and intestinal tract is populated with gram-positive or gram-negative bacteria. The gram-negative bacteria have an endotoxin in the cell walls, and many people appear to be sensitive to this. Normally we have about 75% gram-negative and about 25% gram-positive bacteria in our intestinal tract. Taking garlic supplements, calcium phosphate salts, castor oil or pantothenic acid can reverse the population. Yogurt and buttermilk are rich sources of gram-positive bacteria, and aid in shifting the population. One study showed that a shift towards gram-positive bacteria resulted in the disappearance of most chronic headaches.

Around 1890, Doctor Alexander Haig popularized his 'uric acid theory'. He suffered from headaches for years, and after keeping a record of his activities, he found that they got worse when he ate large portions of meat. Fish, meat, eggs and coffee generate uric acid. When you eliminate these items, you eliminate the headaches. He added more cheese and beans to the diet to make up for the protein.

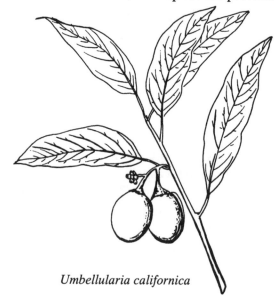

Umbellularia californica

Umbellularia californica is known as the headache tree in California. The wood is valued for ornamental cabinetwork, and insects never attack this tree. It is a popular children's trick to crush a leaf and have someone smell it. The bufotenine in the leaf can cause a severe headache and dizziness. The Indians once used these leaves to cure headaches, because of a constrictive rebound of the smooth muscles. The activity of the leaves must be variable, because the ones in Seattle did not produce headaches when I tried them, but the California trees are said to be very active.

Some Australians have cured headaches by crushing and breathing the headache vine **Clematis glycioides**. The constriction and loosening of the blood vessels provides the cure. Another 'headache flower' is **Daphne genkwa**. The odor of it will give you a headache.

Altering the diet can relieve many headaches. I had a friend who stopped his severe headaches by eliminating coffee from his diet. People with headaches due to constriction of the blood vessels can take niacin. This B vitamin dilates the blood vessels, and large doses leave the face red and flushed. In one study 82% of the people taking niacin reported that their headaches were relieved in an hour.

Calcium salts as dietary supplements were said to be effective in 40 of 48 chronic headaches. Most of these people found permanent relief in three to six weeks. In headaches occurring after meals, 16 of 23 people found relief with calcium supplements.

Could headaches be due to an iodine deficiency? One cure was made by mixing 100 milligrams of potassium iodide with 20 grams of water. A teaspoonful of the iodine mixture is taken every few minutes. This was tried in twenty unselected headaches. In twelve cases potassium iodide gave permanent relief in fifteen to forty-five minutes. Partial relief was obtained in four cases, and it didn't work in another four cases.

Nathaniel Dwight discovered the first 'American cure' for headaches, when he presented his findings to the Hartford Medical Society in 1799. He believed that 'vegetable acids' corrected the 'morbid acid' of the stomach. He found that the malic acid of apple cider was the perfect corrective for a sick headache. His patients drank up to half a pint of apple cider before eating breakfast.

Dr. Dwight found that apple cider cured bilious colic, which he believed had the same cause as headaches: "The cider has been drunk by persons for months together, with entire relief from the colic, who, before they began with the remedy, were subject to paroxysms of it every few weeks." When his patients quit drinking the cider, their problems returned.

There has been little effort to investigate the old headache remedies or study their mode of actions. **Angelica acutiloba** is a popular woman's herb in China. The dry powdered roots turned out to be 1.7 times stronger as an analgesic than aspirin. It is used in China for the same problems that we normally treat with aspirin.

There are at least two herbs that are comparable to aspirin in pain relief. **Dittrichia viscosa** is similar in effect to aspirin, although it doesn't reduce fever. **Scabiosa atropurpurea** has a strong effect on reducing pain and fever. The raw herb is about a third as powerful as refined aspirin.

In the Philippines the sap of **Kibatalia gitingensis** is used to cure stomach disorders, dysentery, worms, and headaches. There is an alkaloid in the tree that antagonizes histamine and prevents histamine contractions. It acts on the serotonin receptors and blocks the painful response that results in the headaches.

A survey of headache remedies in Poland showed that many common herbs were used. The peasants used poultices of horseradish, cabbage or potato peelings. Teas were made of horseradish, cabbage, potatoes, beet roots, garlic, coltsfoot and the linden tree.

Readers of a popular health magazine contributed several tips on how they stopped their headaches. One woman found that taking 25 micrograms of Vitamin B12 could stop headaches with bright shimmering flashes. It took about fifteen minutes for the headache to disappear. Another reader had daily headaches, but stopped them completely in two weeks by taking 500 units of Vitamin E daily.

In the East Indies the leaves of the 'headache tree' **Premna integrifolia** are used to make a tea. In Jamaica and the Caribbean the 'headache weed' is **Hedyosmum nutans**. In North America the 'headache weed' was blue cohosh **Caulophyllum thalictroides**. In Central America, herb vendors sell **Cissampelos tropaeolifolia** under the name of 'aspirina.' The 'headache wood' of Australia is **Scaevola spinescens**. It contains an antagonist of the pain producing chemical 5-hydroxytryptamine. It has also been used for cancer and colitis.

The old Romans drank a tea of **Verbena officinalis** to cure headaches. The active substance is adenosine. Its function has been described as a 'retaliatory metabolit,' remaining in the plasma outside of cells, and helping them to recover when needed. A number of late medieval medical books mention it for curing headaches. Chinese studies show that the plant is synergistic with prostaglandin E2. The prostaglandins regulate cell function.

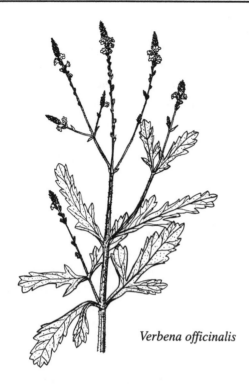

Verbena officinalis

A test of the herb was reported in 1869 in Italy. You don't take the herbal tea when you have a headache, for it doesn't act like aspirin. You drink it in a daily basis when you don't have a headache, and the frequency and severity of the headaches decrease. They are often gone in a few weeks.

Two women had severe headaches coming with the menstrual cycle that lasted up to 36 hours with vomiting and dizziness. The women couldn't stand light, and had to be in a dark room. By drinking verbena tea, made with a half ounce of the herb in nine ounces of water, they were able to reduce and then cure the headaches. Another couple suffered from terrible stress headaches for three years. Often the headaches came before rain. A tea of verbena cured them in a short time.

Cluster headaches are somewhat like short duration migraines. They include intense pain in the same side of the head, dripping nose, blockage of the nasal passages and facial sweating. They may last from 30 minutes to two hours. There may be from 1 to 5 headaches per day.

Thirteen patients with cyclic episodes of cluster headaches had a solution of capsaicin, the hot substance from red pepper, squirted into their noses. The first application produced a painful burning sensation with high nasal flow. By the fifth application, there was little sensation. Seven patients had their headaches completely disappear,

and three had a reduction of 75% of attacks. The remaining three had no help.

Seven other patients had the chronic form, with daily attacks of cluster headaches without interruption for six months or more. The capsaicin treatment cured five and helped the remaining two.

The famous English herbalist Culpepper recommended a tea of yarrow *Achillea millefolium*. In England, wood betony *Stachys officinalis* was said to cure the most obstinate headache known. John Floyer, the doctor to King Charles II wrote: "The juice of ground ivy *Hedera helix* snuffed up the nose out of a spoon taketh away the greatest pain that is."

Among the American Indians, we find that the Apaches used the root of *Lycium andersonii*, the Omahas used the roots of *Physalis lanceolata* and in Nevada the cure was the roots of *Mirabilis alipes = Hermidium alipes*. The early settlers got their remedies from the Indians and passed on the information. In New England a tea of the trailing arbutus *Epigaea repens* was once used to cure 'liverish-digestive headaches.' A tea of *Berberis vulgaris* was once considered to be an unsurpassed remedy for headaches and neuralgia. Mexicans drank a tea of marigolds *Tagetes lucida* for headaches.

The Bushmen of South Africa use *Heinsia jasminiflora*. The Zhosa tribe of South Africa used *Ocotea bullata*. In Zaire a tea of *Pterotaberna inconspicua* leaves is used. It contains 0.3% methuenine, which is a powerful antihistamine. In central Africa headaches are treated with a tea of *Warburgia salutaris* or *W. ugandensis*.

The seeds of *Vitex rotundifolia* are widely used in Asia. In Nepal, *Cerastium fontanum* is used, and in China the flower buds of *Magnolia biondii*. In Korea a tea of the boiled roots of the *Chrysanthemum cinerariifolium* is said to be a sure headache cure. Australians drink a tea of *Melaleuca quinquenervia*. In Java headaches are treated with the roots of *Bidens chinensis*. One of the best known headache cures of the Amazon was a tea of *Fittonia albivenis*.

The first Spanish explorer of the American Southwest was Coronado. He was seeking the seven cities of gold, which his interpreters assured him were always just a short journey away. Of course, the Indian tribes were glad to get rid of him, and everyone told him that with another two weeks journey into the desert, he would find what he was seeking. In 1540 his biographer Pedro de Castenado wrote: "Granted they didn't find the gold, but at least they found a place in which to search for it."

On May 4th, 1563 Coronado was stationed on the Pacific side of Costa Rica. He wrote to his superior, "In this province [Quipo, Costa Rica] we have found a spice called chiro, of which I have sent a sample to you from this village, so that you could experience it. We have all used it, and found it good for headaches. It seems to us tasty, but I don't know if it caused me to lose my taste for good things. Brahman is again bringing a little of it."

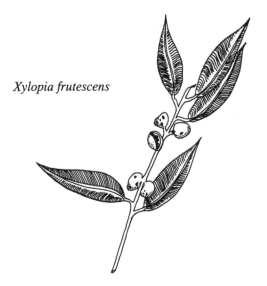

Xylopia frutescens

The identity was not given but chiro could be **uliana caryophylata** or the black palm **Bactris**

minor, which has a delicious fruit known as ciro. The mystery spice is almost certainly ***Xylopia frutescens***. It is known as Malaqueto chico, and the grains are used as a pepper substitute.

Coronado might have made billions by setting up a monopoly to import chiro. He could have spread word that the secret headache cure makes people live long and increases their virility. But green gold and yellow gold don't have the same attraction, and Coronado missed his golden opportunity to becomes rich and provide a service.

Before trying any or all of these cures, we should be prepared to deal with our emotional problems. Charles Darwin was so troubled with a bad headache, that he nearly didn't marry his fiancee Emma Wedgwood. The closer the wedding, the worse his headaches got.

A woman went to her doctor complaining of intense, persistent headaches. He gave her drugs, but there was no change. When she returned, he sent her to a gynecologist. Next she went to a specialist in internal diseases, and then to a neurologist, but the headaches persisted. Then she went to naturopathic doctors and chiropractors, but without result.

Months later she returned to her original doctor and they sat down and had a long talk. She had been newly married and her mother had moved in with her. The mother was a domineering and overbearing woman, whom none of the other children could stand. When the mother was placed in a home, the daughter's headaches ceased, and her life returned to normal.

✧ ✧ ✧

MIGRAINE HEADACHES

The general sight did not appear affected; but when I looked at any particular object it seemed as if something brown, and more or less opaque, was interposed between my eyes and it, so that I saw it indistinctly, or sometimes not at all. Most generally it seemed to be exactly in the middle of the object, while my sight, comprehending all around it, was as distinct and clear as usual; in consequence of which, if I wished to see anything, I was obliged to look on one side. After it had continued a few moments, the upper or lower edge appeared bounded by an edging of light of a zigzag shape.

– Caleb Parry 1825

The word migraine, comes from the Greek words 'hemi-crania,' meaning 'half-head.' Through the centuries the word was chopped down to micrania, and it finally became 'migraine.' It refers to the fact that the headaches only occur on one side of the head.

The beginnings of a migraine headache are marked with 'fortification spectra.' These are visual signs, which include showers of sparks, balls of fire, and zigzag lines. Colors may include flashes of purple, black or mixtures of color like a rainbow. The zigzag nature of certain paintings makes the artwork seem alive with motion, and it resembles a migraine. Artists like William Blake, and Saint Hildegard seem to have included migraine figures in their artwork.

The earliest descriptions of migraines appear on the clay tablets of the ancient East. A Sumerian poem reads: "The sick-eyed says not 'I am sick-eyed.' The sick-headed says not 'I am sick headed.'" Another cuneiform tablet reads: "The head throbs, when pain smites the eyes and vision is dimmed."

Many times the person gets premonitory symptoms of migraines in his or her dreams. One person had dreams of storms, volcanic eruptions and fires before his attacks. Another person dreamed of a white figure with great beauty that appeared from the right and then disappeared. The next day his migraine headache would start.

Mental states seem to be able to kick off an attack of migraine. Sir John Herschel found that he could get a migraine attack, by picturing in his mind the visual phenomena of the disorder. Another person could get migraines just by looking at zigzag wallpaper.

The English novelist George Eliot had migraines. And she would feel 'dangerously well' before her attacks. Stress often acts as a trigger, and the person begins to see sparkles of snow or rings of flashing silver. The ache begins to grow around your eyes, and you seek darkness. Loud noises are as disruptive as gun shots at close range. Waves of nausea and vomiting come over the sufferer, and the attack lasts from three to twenty-four hours, but the person can remain sick for several days. Studies show that about 15% of all men and 25% of women suffer from migraine headaches at one time or another.

The Swedish botanist Carolus Linnaeus suffered from migraines, and prior to an attack, he would notice someone walking alongside of him. Once he entered a lecture room to teach a class, but he saw someone standing at the lectern. Thinking that he arrived too early, he left, only to realize that he was looking at a spectral illusion of himself. This is a common manifestation of migraines in Scandinavian countries, and it is called 'nautoscopic hallucinations.' People also call them 'doppelgangers' and they are responsible for a whole class of ghost stories.

Migraines have been the domain of the famous, for Alfred Nobel, Alexander Graham Bell, George Bernard Shaw, Woodrow Wilson and Thomas Jefferson suffered from them. Sigmund Freud had migraine attacks, and he did not find an answer through psychoanalysis. It might have been a response to stress, for although he was famous, he wasn't well liked by professionals, and he was never given a full professorship in Vienna.

Charles Darwin often suffered from migraines. When his father died, he was so ill, that he was unable to attend the funeral.Migraines must have been hereditary in his family, for three of his children suffered from them.

During the early part of the nineteenth century the Swedish chemist Jons Jakob Berzelius laid the groundwork for modern chemistry. He devised Latin symbols for the elements and combined the atomic weights with a chart of electrical charges. His book *Larebok I Keon* [Foundation of Chemistry] was translated into all European languages, and was largely responsible for the spread of basic chemical knowledge. From the age of 23, he was tortured by migraine headaches, which he believed followed the cycles of the moon. In earlier life, they were irregular, but now they came twice a month, on the days of the new and full moon. During these days he accepted no social invitations, but stayed home in a darkened room.

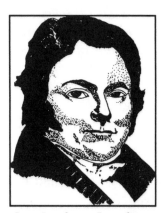

Jöns Jacob von Berzelius

He was able to cure his migraines by going to the mineral springs at Carlsbad, Czechoslovakia for treatment. When the migraines returned, he made artificial Carlsbad mineral water, and by drinking it he remained free of migraines. Could migraines be due to a mineral imbalance in the body?

Carlsbad has 17 mineral springs, and they may not all be identical. An analysis done by the German Apothecary Society in 1879 is probably close to the formula used by Berzelius.The springs contain traces of lithium, manganese and iodine. The prominent salts are 0.24% Na_2SO_4; 0.13% of Na_2CO_3; 0.10% of $NaCl$; 0.03% of $CaCO_3$ and 0.02% of $MgCO_3$.

In 1887 a German doctor reported that he had a cure. When he felt the migraine coming on, he put a half or whole teaspoonful of salt in a glass of water and drank it.If done at the very beginning, this completely stopped it. If done when the migraine started, the attack would stop in about half an hour.

In 1923 a London doctor had migraine patients take a soluble form of calcium as soon as they felt a migraine headache coming on. He found that 18 of 20 patients had their migraines stopped by taking calcium tablets. The trick is to chew the tablets to get the calcium into the blood stream at once. A friend of mine tried taking a gram of calcium gluconate immediately before her migraines. She told me that the tablets turned what would have been a severe migraine, which would have disabled her for a day, into an ordinary headache, which left in a few hours.

A Washington woman wrote in 1925, "Calcium lactate works wonders with me; without it, I always counted on a full day of severe headache, following the appearance of the typical visual hallucinations. Now a dose of calcium lactate gives relief from practically all the nerve-racking pain and difficulties I used to have to expect as the usual things. On several occasions I have made long drives in the car shortly after the beginning of the scintillations. Before the use of calcium, I would not have dared to have attempted this. I experience a double relief – that of the physical agony and that of the mental worry and dread incident of the attack. I carry it with me at all times; I never want to be without it."

In 1888 a French doctor reversed an astigmatic lens on his own glasses, and got a migraine headache. He found that many cases of migraines could be cured, by getting the proper glasses. Seeing an eye doctor is a good step in helping yourself.

A woman was unable to find relief from her migraine headaches. Then she developed ulcerative collitis, and her doctor gave her supplements of **Lactobacillus acidophilus** hoping to alter the bacterial flora of her intestinal tract, and cure the collitis. It did improve the collitis, and unexpectedly her migraines disappeared. The doctor tried giving the friendly bacteria to ten persons with migraines, who weren't helped by other means. There was marked improvement in eight persons when capsules were taken three times a day.

Migraines are also triggered by foods. The complex phenols that make up the coloring of red wine trigger migraines, but other forms of alcohol do not trigger migraines. Some foods known to produce the headaches are cow's milk, eggs, chocolate, oranges, and wheat. The foods that migraine sufferers must avoid are cheese, chocolate, and red wine.

There is an old theory that migraines are due to a poorly functioning liver, which doesn't break down impurities in the blood. A test was made of the liver function theory by giving twelve men with migraines a gram of the amino acid methionine and multiple B vitamins. The average number of migraines went from 4.3 per month to 1.5. In one instance a 59 year old man went from ten migraines a month to only one. Only one person in the study wasn't helped.

Henry Leclerc was a well-known French doctor who did numerous studies on medicinal herbs. He began to treat migraines and trigeminal neuralgia with a strong tea or tablets of powdered chamomile *Matricaria recutita*. A cup of strong tea or tablets of 3-5 grams of chamomile are taken at meals. There is normally a marked reduction in pain by the end of the day, and in a few days the problem is essentially cured. It is said to be a long term preventive, but no studies have been done.

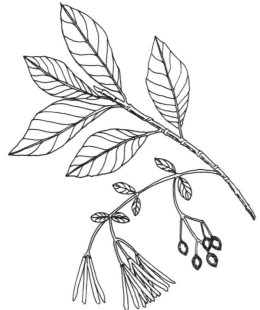

Chionanthus virginicus

A young woman suffering from migraines was an astrologer. She reasoned that Jupiter was the ruler of the liver, and on the dates she suffered from migraines, her natal Jupiter was affecting her. She looked up the 'Jupiter herbs' in an astrology herb book and took a tincture of the fringe tree *Chionanthus virginicus*. This cured her migraines and those of her mother. When she published a letter in a popular health magazine, another reader wrote to say that the herb eliminated her headaches.

The root bark of the tree has long been used as a liver stimulant.

Father Sebastian Knapp became famous for his book *My Water Cure*. He treated all illnesses with special baths and herbs. His ideas evolved into modern naturopathic medicine. He had migraine sufferers chew 6-8 juniper berries *Juniperus communis* per day and take baths.

In the Ayurvedic medicine of India and the Unnani Tibb medicine of the Arabs, ginger is used for migraines and cluster headaches. At the very beginning, about 500 mgs. of powdered ginger *Zingiber officinale* is mixed with water and drunk. It begins to be effective in about 30 minutes, and it is taken as often as needed. One woman found that this worked fairly well, so she included fresh ginger in her diet daily. The intensity and frequency of migraines decreased. In India, ginger was mixed with equal parts of *Withania somnifera*. Sixty grams taken daily for three weeks were said to be a cure.

Many doctors still use ergot alkaloids to constrict the blood vessels in migraines. It constricts blood vessels all over the body, with considerable side effects. It was first used by doctors for migraines in 1925.

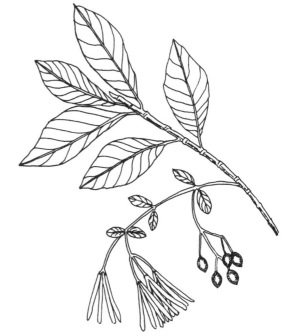

Tanacetum parthenium

Two centuries ago John Hill wrote in his herb book: "The mother of the late Sir William Bowyer told me that during the first half of her life, she suffered from terrible and constant headaches fixed in one small part of the cranium, raging to distraction." Then the woman discovered that a tea made of two handfuls of feverfew *Tanacetum parthenium* with boiling water was able to cure her migraines. Richard Brook noted in his herbal in 1772: "In the worst headache, this herb exceeds whatever else is known."

The old remedy was basically forgotten until a miner who had been a long-time sufferer cured himself by chewing several leaves of feverfew daily. He told his success to the wife of the chief medical officer of Britain's National Coal Board. She tried the treatment and in two weeks she was free from migraines. Her husband told this to Dr. Steward Johnson of the London Migraine Clinic. He began by giving ten patients feverfew leaves. Three were cured, and seven had less frequent migraines.

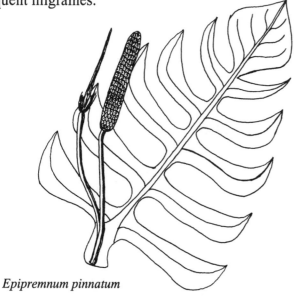

Epipremnum pinnatum

Feverfew has recently become well known in England for helping migraine headaches. A survey of 300 users showed that 72% had fewer headaches. When the remedy was compared to a placebo, there were five cases of vomiting and 34 cases of nausea in the feverfew group. In the placebo group there were 21 cases of vomiting and 95 cases of nausea. It is now known that the parthenolide in the herb provides the cure. Some varieties of the herb don't have this, and they don't work. The amounts of freeze dried leaves taken vary from 50 milligrams to 2 grams a day.

Tablets of *Pueraria tuberosa* proved to be an effective migraine treatment in China. Volunteers

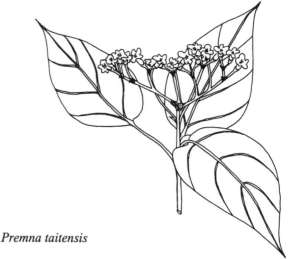

Premna taitensis

took 500 mg. tablets, three times daily. The herb has cerebral vasodilator effects, which help to normalize circulation in the head. Within two weeks, 83% reported that they were markedly improved, or had no more migraines.

One of the most interesting migraine remedies began on the island of Lomaloma, in the South Pacific. A Hungarian traveler married a native woman and settled on the island. He suffered constantly from migraines, and his wife insisted that the islanders had remedies, which would cure him. During a period of two years, Mr. Vessey took 55 different native remedies, but only four of them gave him temporary relief. He suspected that the natives were trying to poison him, so he had them take everything first, and he took careful notes on all the plants. At long last, four cups of a tea made from a mixture of *Premna taitensis* and *Epipremnum pinnatum = E. vitiensis* permanently cured his migraines.

His wife named the medicine "Tonga" and bundles of the barks were sent to England in 1882. There was a great deal of interest in learning the identity of the medicine, and botanists figured out the plants. Sufferers used a ball of chopped bark with netting around it. This was soaked in water and drank as a pleasant tasting tea before meals. One ball of the bark would generally provide a cure. In its first medical test, six of a group of eight migraine sufferers were permanently cured. The remedy was sold in Holland until about 1960, but it seems to have been forgotten in recent times. Some doctors used it in the United States until 1925, but it finally vanished from the medical scene.

☆ ☆ ☆

ORIGINS OF MENTAL PROBLEMS

One should with diligence take note of the spirit of man, of which there are really two, that are inborn. For this is indeed true that man is in the image of God, and thereby has a godly spirit in him, but on the other hand, man is also an animal, and as such has an animal spirit. These spirits then are two antagonists, and yet the one must soften the other. Now therefore, it is necessary to recognize these two spirits, from which the true spirit of mankind is derived, in distinction to that of the animal spirit. This is the reason for this book, the title of which is "Of The Lunatics."

Die Lunatici, Paracelsus

Mental problems are generally categorized into four areas. Affective disorders cover depression, anxiety, and manic depressive problems. Anxiety disorders cover the phobias, panic attacks and unreasonable fears. These often happen to shy people, when faced with some sort of psychological trigger. Schizophrenia is what most call real mental illness. The dementias are generally late life disorders, such as losing rationality and Alzheimer's disease.

In Biblical times, people accepted the theory that mental illness was caused by demons. When Jesus cast out the demons, the mentally ill were cured. This view of mental illness gradually broke down in the 18th and 19th centuries. There was a series of notorious 'exorcisms' in which leaders of the church tried to drive out the demons and cure the patients. These public failures gradually produced a more rational attitude towards mental illness.

Five centuries before the time of Christ, Herodotus wrote his history, and talked about the beliefs of the Scythians. The Greek king Scylas went through the Bacchic mysteries. The Scythians stated: "Our god has seized your king who raves like us, and is maddened by the influence." Were psychoactive mushrooms or plants part of this sacred ritual?

Plato wrote in the Timaeus: "Even if they knew it wouldn't understand reason, and even if it did share in the perception of reason, there is no natural instinct to pay heed to any of them, but they would be bewitched in part by images and phantasms. To guard against this, God devised and constructed the form of the liver, which he placed in that part's abode."

Plato's idea that the liver protects against mental illness might have some basis in fact. The enzymes of the liver break down toxic products in the blood. It may be that abnormal chemicals in the blood stream disturb the functioning of the brain. If the liver doesn't break them down in a reasonable length of time, the brain is affected.

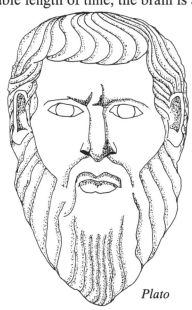

Plato

It is known that an excess of amphetamines creates symptoms clinically identical, to those of schizophrenia. There is a theory that one of the causes of mental illness is phenylethylamine, an amphetamine-like chemical in excessive amounts. One study found that 40% of the mentally ill had abnormal liver function. Could any of the liver-strengthening herbs help the mentally ill? The liver is the richest source of B vitamins in the body, and these vitamins work with the liver enzymes as co-factors. Some cases of mental illness can be helped with magadoses of B vitamins, and this is partial evidence that liver-active factors may help mental illness.

In 1929, researchers at the University of Wisconsin, tried to find out if an increase in brain circulation, would aid mentally ill patients. They used a hospital respirator, and had their patients breathe a mixture of 15% carbon dioxide and 85% oxygen. Then this was increased to a 40:60 ratio for the next ten to twenty minutes.

The results of this therapy with mental patients were dramatic. One patient, who had been mute for six years, began to carry on a normal conversation. The silly expressions of severely ill patients disappeared, and they began telling about families and jobs, which they had years before. When the respirator was removed, the patients carried on normal conversations lasting from two to twenty-five minutes. Then their voices became less audible, and the normal eye movements ceased. The twisted facial expressions returned, and they re-entered the world of the mentally ill.

The experiments raise the question of whether mental illness is actually a starvation of the brain for oxygen and nutrients. The high proportion of carbon dioxide is a powerful capillary dilator, and one wonders if continued therapy would provide long-term benefits. Ladislas Meduna worked with carbon dioxide therapy for many years in the Chicago area. He obtained good results in psychosis (disorders such as schizophrenia), but poor results in neurosis (anxiety disorders and fears). With the coming of the tranquilizers, and new drugs his research was ignored by other workers.

Why does shock therapy work for some patients? One suggestion is that shock stimulates the oxygen consumption of the brain. There is a relationship between the thyroid, the adrenal cortex, the respiratory enzymes of the cells, and oxygen consumption of the brain.

Thyroxin, the hormone put out by the thyroid gland, is an active stimulant of oxygen consumption. In one experiment, doctors gave 24 mental patients, four milligrams per day of the sodium salt of thyroxin. Four of thirteen schizophrenics recovered and three were improved. Three of five psychoneurotic patients recovered. Although some needed shock treatment, 21 out of 24 patients showed improvement.

Could minerals help insanity? In 1905 a French doctor reported that he diluted seawater to the same salt content as the blood. Then he injected 100 cc. of seawater into the blood every five days, for two months. His sixteen cases included epilepsy, schizophrenia and senile dementia. He reported that everyone was improved in digestion, condition and appetite. There were several cures of depression and mania.

Another theory of mental illness relates the misfunctioning mind to a streptococcus infection. In 1914 Edward Rosenow discovered the streptococcus that causes rheumatic fevers. As an expert bacteriologist, he cultured bacteria from mentally ill patients and injected them into mice and monkeys. The monkeys and mice developed bizarre behavior. They dashed about, threatening to attack, and apparently saw and heard strange noises.

Rosenow isolated an alpha streptococcus bacterium from a mentally ill woman. He injected it into two rabbits, and they dashed about in extreme excitement, apparently seeing imaginary enemies.

A test was made of the streptococcus theory by a skin test. A streptococcal preparation causes local inflammation, if the immune system recognizes streptococci bacteria. In severe schizophrenia 91% reacted, but in mild schizophrenia 80% reacted. In epilepsy with convulsions, 73% reacted to streptococcus, but in mild cases 42% reacted to the preparation.

A teacher developed epilepsy and couldn't work because of numerous seizures. When he had a decayed tooth pulled, the bacteria on it produced seizures in rabbits. The removal of the tooth stopped all seizures for nine years.

A group of 57 schizophrenics received a weekly shot of a streptococcal preparation to build up immunity. They weren't helped after ten weeks. This doesn't disprove the bacterial toxin theory; it may mean that the bacteria cause a reaction that persists after they are removed. It could mean that different ways of neutralizing them would have to be employed.

In 1930, a study of 200 patients with suicidal tendencies and manic depressive psychosis was published in Germany. Researchers measured three different aspects of blood pressure phenomenon: a reduction of pulse rate, diastolic (filling) pressure, and vasomotor ration (the ratio of the oscillation of the humeral artery to the radial artery). When corrected, this resulted in a disappearance of depression, suicidal, and manic depressive tendencies. The action of 'tranquilizers' on the mentally ill is generally believed to make them 'tranquil,' but most tranquilizers lower blood pressure. That may be far more important than tranquillity.

Most of us will never enter a mental institution, but many normal people suffer from anxieties, phobias and obsessions, which are generally known as neuroses. An Arkansas doctor had a neurotic patient whom he treated with bromides, chloral, and sedatives without effect. A fellow doctor practiced old time botanical medicine. He gave the man black cohosh *Cimicifuga racemosa*, which relieved the symptoms, and surprised the first doctor.

A Chinese formula, which was described in the Chin Kuei Yao Lueh in -115, was recently tested. It is a mixture of *Ziziphus zizyphus, Poria cocos, Ligusticum chuanxiong, Anemarrhena asphodeloides,* and *Glycyrrhiza uralensis.* The extract worked well in treating people with anxiety and insomnia. It decreased hyperactivity, improved the mood and alleviated other symptoms of anxiety.

The parahippocampal gyrus is a region of the brain, which mediates panic, anxiety and vigilance. When sodium lactate is taken, people become more susceptible to panic disorders. This causes a marked difference between the blood flow between the right and left sides of the brain.

When we are anxious, the levels of lactate salt rise in the body. Anxiety is marked by 'stage fright,' 'lumps in the throat,' palpitation, and shakiness. People with anxiety problems were asked to rate themselves on an anxiety scoring. The group was split and half drank a solution of sodium lactate, and the others got a placebo. At a level of five mg/kg., the anxiety scores improved from an average of 30 to 55 after drinking the solution.

This led to the idea that giving patients a sodium lactate solution in a neutral setting could treat anxiety. Twice a week 33 people took a lactate solution, and within three weeks their anxiety scores fell by about half. As their bodies adjusted to the high levels of sodium lactate, they no longer reacted with anxiety, when it happened naturally. This is a simple way of dealing with phobic disorders, which plague so many normal people.

Phobias are altered reactions to common situations. One of Freud's disciples, Otto Fenichel noted the connection between phobias, dizziness and motion sickness. The inner ear is our organ of balance, and when it is not quite normal, we are likely to suffer from phobias. After an ear infection, a two-year-old child was suddenly unable to walk and at the same time developed a fear of the dark. Sinus infection can aggravate the inner ear system and bring on phobic behavior.

Harold Levinson worked with treating dyslexia with motion sickness remedies. Then he extended his experiments to include phobias. We begin to understand that some of the old remedies, which worked on the inner ear and controlled motion sickness, might help overcome phobias. The doctor who used black cohosh *Cimicifuga racemosa* to clear up a neurotic patinent was using an old remedy for tinnitis; which is noise in the inner ear. Motion sickness remedies such as ginger, thyme, and *Silybum marianum* might help phobias.

A study was done of a native psychiatry practitioner of Tanzania. Abedi practiced divination to reveal the source of the mental problems of people coming to him. Every person was asked five basic questions. "Have you committed adultery? Did you steal? Did you borrow money and not repay it? Was there a quarrel with anyone? Have you fought with anyone?" If the person answered yes, the next step was to clear up that wrong.

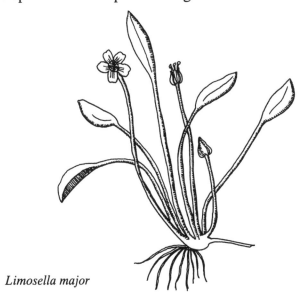

Limosella major

Abedi then tried to find if the illness was either due to natural causes or witchcraft. He began by treating the patient with emetics. His main herb was *Limosella major*, which often put people to sleep, right after it was given. It proved to be a strong tranquilizer, which doubled the barbiturate sleeping time of mice.

When the health care system of the Cameroons collapsed with an economic slump, nobody could afford western medicine. Street medicine flourished and Adam Fokounang became famous for his treatment of mental illness. In a dream, his late father revealed the herbal secrets of treating mental illness, so he opened a clinic in the town of Foumban. He began by purging patients with powdered *Lavigeria macrocarpa*. Then he squirted *Polyscias fulva* up their nose to wash the brain. Then a heather plant *Agauria salicifolia* was taken like snuff to induce sneezing which helps to stabilize the memory. He had treated 60 mentally ill people and 56 of them were on the road to recovery. The theories are different, but the results are good.

In our search for the origins of mental states we should not forget vitamin deficiencies. As early as 1905 doctors found that pernicious anemia patients had psychotic states. This is caused by a lack of Vitamin B12. A lack of this vitamin may cause paranoia, irritability, panic and phobic disorders. A deficiency can cause 'bi-polar disorders', which are now treated by lithium.

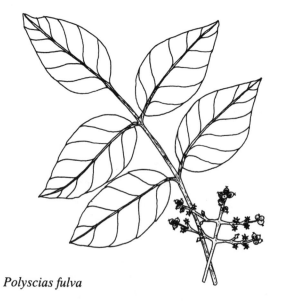

Polyscias fulva

An eleven year-old girl was expelled from a girl's camp. She heard voices and claimed that other children were planning to attack her. The doctor planned on putting her on the drug trifluoperazine, but the girl refused to take anything but vitamins. So the doctor gave her 75 micrograms of B12 a day, intending to secretly substitute the drug after a few weeks. The delusions and hallucinations ceased. The mother remarked: "It's like having a different child in the house. I used to dread her coming in, but now it's a happy home."

 ✿ ✿ ✿

MENTAL ILLNESS HERBS

Madness cometh sometime of passions of the soul, as of business and of great thoughts and of too great study and of dread. Sometimes it is of the biting of a mad dog, or some other venomous beast; sometimes of melancholy meats, and sometimes of drink or strong wine. And as the causes be diverse, the tokens and signs be diverse. For some cry and leap and hurt and wound themselves in privy and secret places. The medicine of them is that they be bound, that they hurt not themselves and other men. And namely such shall be refreshed, and comforted and withdrawn from cause and matter of dread and busy thoughts. And they must be gladdened with instruments of music and some deal be occupied.

The Encyclopedia of the Clergyman Bartholomew 13th century

It is of some interest to the study of history, when we learn that Adolf Hitler spent time in a mental institution after WWI. Yet, we cannot say that mental illness leads to dangerous behavior, or that we ourselves are not mentally ill. In the late 1950s a series of sensational newspaper reports dealt with children who had been confined to mental institutions because their behavior was 'strange,' yet these children turned out to be perfectly normal. Once they were categorized as unusual and confined, nobody was willing to let them out, and they were confined for many years.

This brings to mind that piece of dialogue from *Alice in Wonderland:* "Oh there's nothing you can do about that," said the cat, "here everyone is mad. I'm mad, You're mad."

"But how do you know that I'm mad?" asked Alice.

"But you must be," said the cat, "otherwise you wouldn't be here."

If you listened to the following monologue, would you confine this person? " The devil knows well enough how to construct his arguments. He delivers himself with a grave and yet with a shrill voice. Nor does he use circumlocutions and beat about the bush, but excels in forcible statements and quick rejoinders. The devil's manner of opening a debate is pleasant enough, but he soon urges things so peremptorily that the respondent in a short time knows how to acquit himself." The person writing these words was Martin Luther! Many saints and religious leaders have had experiences on the edge of sanity, and some were well over the edge.

There are several landmarks in the treatment of mental aberrations. Sigmund Freud sought a way of treating neurosis by talking out problems, while lying on a couch. He dealt with sexually repressed people, who were unable to express their thoughts. At the time, great stigma was attached to divorce, and a lack of expression and counseling led to a neurotic population. Psychiatrists have accomplished very few cures with the mentally ill. They might succeed only after years of effort and great expense. The statement, "Neurotics build castles in the sky, psychotics live in them, and psychiatrists collect the rent," has its own truth.

The modern revolution in treating the mentally ill began in 1952 when Doctor Henri Laborit used a new antihistamine to treat patients before surgery. This drug was used to block histamine release, which could cause life-threatening shock. It made patients sleepy, and they experienced no fear about surgery. When chlorpromazine was given to psychiatric patients, it calmed them down, and many of them were able to lead normal lives. It led to a whole series of new drugs.

The center of the ancient Chinese civilization was the wind-swept Yellow River. These people believed that the wind brought disease and mental illness. Their name for mental illness was 'chung feng', meaning 'overwhelmed by the wind.' They used herbs, which they believed could counter the effects of the wind.

In ancient times, one of the few available ways to treating the mentally ill was by using the narcotic mandrake *Mandragora officinarum*. It contains hyoscyamine, which paralyzes the voluntary muscles and puts patients to sleep. It was a way of sedating restless patients, but in some cases it acted on the problem. In 1875 an English doctor published a report on treating the mentally ill with hyoscyamine. In one instance a patient was convinced that the doctors were secretly shampooing him during the night, and sending electrical currents through wires in his pillow. After a single treatment with hyoscyamine, his delusions were gone.

The first article on an herbal cure for mental illness was published in 1723. The doctor was using about a gram of a tincture of camphor per day. The main source of camphor is the ***Cinnamomum camphora*** tree of Southeast Asia.

A 19 year-old woman slept little, moaned and talked wildly. For nine months doctors bled, vomited and purged her without results. She took two grams of camphor tincture each day. In three weeks she recovered the normal use of her reason.

A 17 year-old man became silly and stupid. He went days without sleeping and began to attack people. He became well in six weeks with camphor. A textile merchant's wife became erratic and uttered terrible oaths during church services. She had the best medical help, but after six months she wasn't improved. After four days of camphor tincture, she was greatly improved. These reports suggest that the strange medical disorder known as "Tourette's syndrome," which is marked by involuntary shouts or curses, may be helped by camphor.

Around the year 1800, several articles were written on the cure of insanity by the hedge hyssop ***Gratiola officinalis***. The plant was known as "Gratia Dei," meaning "The Grace of God." It is a member of the scrophulariaceae family, of which some members have neurosedative action. In older medicine the plant was taken in amounts of about 15 grams to cause laxative, vomiting, and diuretic effects. Generally the root was powdered, but the top of the plant was used as well.

Baron Kostizewsky of Vienna claimed good results in treating the insane and other doctors tried it. Several became interested after hearing of successful cases. Dr. Lebrecht Lentin treated three mentally ill people using 620 milligrams of the powdered herb taken morning and night. All three were said to have become normal, and Lentin was greatly pleased with the herb.

The nervous system is a curious mass of nerve 'wiring' joined by chemical links. At the junctions of the nerves, a chemical carries the impulse to the next nerve, and the chemical itself is broken down, or the nerve would literally become a 'short circuit.' We can think of mental illness as being due to 'defective insulation,' and 'short circuits,' between the nerves. The inability to sort out a single train of thought, and the multiplicity of impressions, would seem to argue that some forms of mental illness are 'short circuits' of the brain.

The alteration of the levels of neurotransmitters may reduce mentally deranged behavior. In 1889 a British doctor reported that he was treating a powerful man who was singing, shouting, gesticulating, talking wildly and seeing illusions. The man didn't respond to any of the remedies then in use. The doctor injected him with 11 mgs. of pilocarpine. This comes from the Brazilian herb jaborandi ***Pilocarpus*** species, which was used for other disorders at this time. After the man had undergone profuse salivation and sweating, he became perfectly calm and rational.

Similar results are reported with the acetylcholinesterase inhibitor physostigmine. This alkaloid comes from an African tree and was used as a truth poison in Africa. Injections of 0.5 mg. doses of physostigmine were given every five minutes until 1.5 to 3 mgs. had been taken. Three female psychiatric patients switched from wild maniacal behavior to fairly normal behavior. What we call mania, may be an increase of noradrenaline and dopamine, and the herbs that reduce it, can enable people to live a normal life.

In 1819 Dr. Sutliffe published a short article on the use of ground ivy ***Hedera helix*** to treat mania. A wineglass of the juice of the plant was taken twice a day. No case studies are given, but the doctor claimed many cases of success over a twenty-year period of usage.

Lecithin is a yellow-brown fatty substance found in egg yokes and the tissues of plants. When manic-depressives were given 30 grams of lecithin, there was a marked improvement in mental symptoms. When they stopped taking lecithin, the symptoms of mania came back.

There are a number of interesting notes on herbs used to treat mental illness. Some of these herbs have been tested and the active biochemicals are known. Other herbs are totally unknown. In the little country of Dahomey in Western Africa a soldier went AWOL and had to be locked up in a local prison. He became mentally ill, and a village priest called on him, and gave him an herb, which restored his reason. The case came to the attention of Doctor Lepeyssonie of the Dahomey Whydah hospital. He called on the priest repeatedly, until he learned that the secret herb for mental illness was *Sabicea calycina*. This plant comes from the *Menispermaceae* family of plants, from which curare, fish poisons and sweeteners are derived.

Rats were given surgical lesions of the brain, which made them 'mentally ill.' They became emotional, hyperactive with aggressive biting tendencies and extreme difficulty in handling. The rage reaction of the rats lasts for about two weeks and they can be used to test possible mental drugs.

One group of rats was given the common mental illness drug chlorpromazine. The other group was given 10 mgs per 100 grams of weight of a 10% alcoholic extract of *Luffa tuberosa*. The alcohol was evaporated and the residue made into a water solution. Fifteen minutes after the rats received the extract of the cucumber family, their violent rage left. The herb was about as effective as chlorpromazine.

A study has been done of the herbs used by the Sotho tribe of South Africa. *Rauvolfia vomitora* is used as a sedative in neuro-psychotic conditions. The leaves of I*ndigofera tristoides* are used in great sorrow. In insanity, epilepsy and hysteria, the leaves of H*eteromorpha arborescens* = *H. trifoliata* are mixed with *Cussonia paniculata* and boiled for 15 minutes. A Sotho herbalist remarked:"It proves efficacious in cases where orthodox medicine has failed."

India has a long history of using herbs and metal preparations known as bhasmas. In northern India a species of millet known as koda *Paspalum scrobiculatum* is grown for food. An alcoholic extract of the husk of millet was used at a mental hospital on 37 schizophrenics and three manic-depressives who had been treated with western drugs and failed to respond. Sixteen patients completely recovered or were greatly improved, but 12 had little or no change. The extract produced tremors in the fingers, but these disappeared, when the extract stopped.

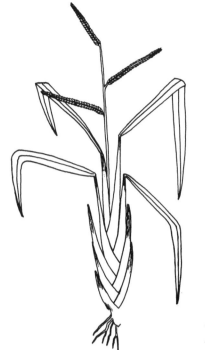

Paspalum scrobiculatum Koda

Acorus calamus is a swamp plant, which has a wide reputation as a brain medicine in India. It is also found around many lakes in the United States. When an extract was given to 28 patients with anxiety neurosis, six were considered cured, and 11 showed an improvement of 50% or more in three weeks. When a high dosage of the herb was given to 75 schizophrenics, seven showed a 75% improvement and 16 showed a 50% improvement. These figures are not sensational, but they show that a common plant could aid in treating a difficult disorder.

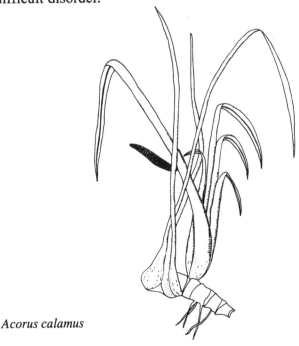

Acorus calamus

One of the best known herbs in India is ***Bacopa monnieri***. It was known as a "medhya rasayana" herb, having rejuvenative and calming effects. It is not a tranquilizer, and it does not appear to directly influence the brain. It does stimulate the adrenal glands and reduces stress.

The herb was first investigated in 1960 for cases of nervous breakdown and anxiety disorders. A group of people with high anxiety scores took two doses of a syrup representing 12 grams of the dry herb. Nervousness, heart palpitation, insomnia, headaches, lack of concentration and other factors were rated on a numerical scale. After four weeks the anxiety scores dropped from 53 to 35. The patients noted better mental performance and a slight gain in weight.

Bacopa monnieri

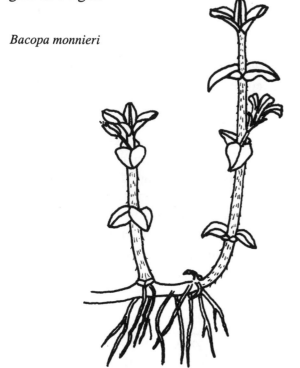

There is an old theory that mental disorders result from blood toxins, which are not eliminated by the liver and the kidneys. If we could stimulate these organs, we could eliminate the toxin. A 56-year-old woman was disoriented and suffering from hallucinations. Her breath was fetid and the urine was scant with albumin. She drank a tea of ***Orthosiphon stamineus***, which is a powerful kidney tea. In two weeks she was calm enough, that she could visit with her family. In three weeks she was almost normal.

A 60 year-old woman suffered from manic-depressive states. She could go from great excitement to depression, and shout: "You want to kill me." After being given a tea of ***Orthosiphon***, her mental state improved and she became calm and rational. In five weeks the woman became quite normal. It was not the only therapy the doctors were using, but it seems to have made the critical difference in healing.

There are other plants that should be investigated. There is a woolly clublike plant growing in the Himalayas known as ***Saussurea gossypiphora***. It is used in Tibet for 'infective condition of the brain.' Mental illness has also been treated in India with the bark of the shrub ***Alstonia venenata***. It is claimed to elevate the mood.

Another plant which deserves investigation, is Thomas Willis' seventeenth century specific for madness, which was the red pimpernel ***Anagallis arvensis***. The herb shows tranquilizing properties, but it was somewhat toxic in rat tests. The Chickasaw Indians called mental illness "lyagamaca abeka" (little peoples disease). They treated it with the roots of the huckleberry ***Vaccinium*** species. In the 17th century, the French treated the insane with the roots of the common fern ***Polypodium vulgare***. The roots are known to contain an insect molting hormone, which acts somewhat like an anabolic steroid. In Zimbabwe, insanity is treated with the leaves and stems of ***Ansellia humilis***.

The famous Arab doctor Rhazi once met a madman while leading a group of his pupils. The man stared at Rhazi.

When Rhazi returned he ordered a decoction of dodder ***Cuscuta*** species. This is a remedy for mental illness in the herbal of Dioscorides. Asked why he was taking it, he replied, "Birds of a feather flock together. The madman must have seen something of himself in me!"

☆☆☆

SCHIZOPHRENIA

A madman is a sick man whose brain is suffering, just as a gouty patient is one who suffers in his hands and feet. One can have gout in the brain, just as in the feet. I am sorry to think that Hippocrates prescribed asses' blood for madness, and still more sorry that the Ladies Manual *says that madness can be cured by contracting the itch. There are funny remedies which seem to have been invented by the patients themselves.*

– Francois Voltaire

In ancient times all those who were mentally ill were considered 'mad.' With the coming of the twentieth century, we sorted disease into various classifications. The German professor Emil Kraepelin named the condition of confusion and hallucinations "dementia praecox."

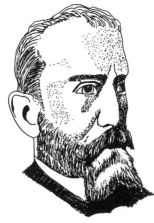

Eugene Bleuler

The Swiss psychoanalyst Eugene Bleuler named it "schizophrenia." With whatever name we call it, it is one of the most difficult illnesses to cure.

Scott Fitzgerald, the great writer of the early 20th century, was fortunate enough to marry his childhood sweetheart Zelda. After a few years she came down with schizophrenia. In desperation, he traveled all over Europe to see the famous psychotherapists, who were unable to give her any help. Fitzgerald eventually came to believe that some mysterious poison in the body attacks the cells of the brain, for he was unable to find a cure.

The Greeks had a cure for schizophrenia, which dates back to a legend a thousand years before the time of Christ. Proteas, the king of Argos, had three daughters, who became mentally ill, and imagined themselves to be cows. Melampus was a Greek shepherd who noticed that sick goats ate hellebore. He told the king that he would cure his daughters, in exchange for a third of the kingdom. When everyone else failed, Melampus got his chance. He cured the daughters with hellebore treatments, and then married the most beautiful one.

There was a town along the Turkish coast called Anticyra, where patients came for hundreds of miles to take baths, massages and herbal treatments for mental problems. We say, "You're crazy," but in ancient Greece they said, "You ought to go to Anticyra." At Anticyra, black hellebore **Helleborus niger** grew in abundance, and was used to treat mental illness.

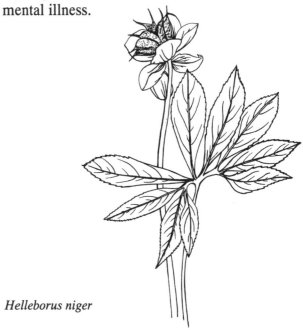

Helleborus niger

The treatments were said to have cured the popular Roman leader Druses of epilepsy. The philosopher Careades went to Anticyra for training, before holding a strenuous series of debates. He reasoned that if hellebore made mad men sane, then hellebore would give sane men extra mental powers. He won his series of debates, and began a new fad. The legend that hellebore sharpened the mind became popular, and before tackling difficult books, students took 'smart pills' of hellebore.

In the late 19th century, several doctors tried to revive the hellebore treatment. It produces nausea and vomiting, and proved to be too toxic for safe use.

Around 1920 Bernard Asher began wondering if the vomiting reflex was really the means of producing the hellebore cure. The vomiting reflex comes from a particular part of the brain that controls vomiting. Could the stimulation of this part of the brain, be a cure for schizophrenia?

It is difficult to get a mentally ill person to take something by mouth, particularly if it causes vomiting, so Doctor Asher used small injections of apomorphine to induce vomiting. Among his many cases was a 22-year-old doctor's daughter who had delusions, confused speech and ideas of sin. Her father took her to the best European doctors who used sedatives and hormones, but gave her no help at all. When she was given apomorphine to induce vomiting and laxatives to purge the bowels, she was completely cured in one week.

In 1919, the 24 year old daughter of a high European government official spent three years in a mental hospital in Vienna, after being diagnosed as schizophrenic. She was kept sedated with narcotics to control her behavior, but Doctor Asher gave her emetics, hydrotherapy and made sure that she got exercise. In four months she was completely cured. During the next 15 years, she taught at a girl's school and worked as a painter. Dozens of similar cases are listed in Bernard Asher's books, but they seem to have made no impression on the mental health community. We like to use sedatives and tranquilizers, but we think of vomiting as a repulsive therapy.

The use of apomorphine as an antischizophrenic agent has been revived in recent years, but without any attempts to duplicate Asher's treatment. The general theory of schizophrenia is that excess dopamine in the brain results in too many signals. The delicate mechanisms of the brain are blocked and many signals are sent, instead of a single rational line of thought. When three milligrams of apomorphine was injected to reduce the neurotransmitter dopamine, nine out of 18 schizophrenics had a 20-50% reduction in symptoms. It takes about 0.1 mg/kg injected subcutaneously, to produce vomiting in about five minutes.

In early American medicine, lobelia was the sovereign herb of Thomsonian medicine, because it produced vomiting. Would it work on schizophrenia? A test was done in Italy with small doses, which didn't induce vomiting. The patients were particularly benefited three hours after taking it, but there was no long-term benefit. The doctors regarded it as an interesting start for a difficult condition.

There are other observations, which might increase the success of curing the mentally ill. Dr. Wagner Jauregg was a pioneer in the use of malarial fever, for treating paralysis. He noted a number of cases in which high-prolonged fever had cured schizophrenia, and remarked that this fact was like a pot of gold on the road, which nobody was picking up. There has been some work done on this, but in many cases the cure was temporary.

The mental illness called schizophrenia, can be a variety of other conditions. The vitamin deficiency, which we call pellagra, creates a condition much like schizophrenia. During the past century some ten conditions have been separated from true schizophrenia. These include a B12 deficiency, an allergic reaction to wheat, temporal lobe epilepsy, and Kleinfelter's syndrome. A few schizophrenic cases respond to manganese supplements, and manganese deficiency must be added to the list of causes. An examination of cases of true schizophrenia shows that 50% are histapenic, i.e. they have low levels of blood histamine and high levels of copper. Another 20% are histadelic; i.e. they have high levels of histamine and normal levels of copper. The remainder has normal levels of copper and histamine, but they secrete an unusual chemical in the urine.

Some schizophrenia seems to be due to wheat gluten. These are 'celiac patients,' who react to wheat gluten. Some people have allergies to gluten, and when they eliminate it entirely, they began to improve. The gluten produces paranoid, repetitious behavior.

Some cases of schizophrenia could be due to viral attacks. About 1% of humans suffer from the disorder at some time in their lives. Half of these suffer as a long-term problem, and the rest have single or multiple episodes. We all know about the 'bag ladies,' and the mumbling incoherent old men. We know that many cases of schizophrenia followed the great 1918 epidemic of flu.

The one vitamin that seems to benefit schizophrenia is Vitamin B6. Fifteen schizophrenics were unable to work for years, and no occupational programs worked. They were given 50 milligrams of B6 both morning and evening. After six weeks, eight patients had some subjective improvement. By ten weeks, most patients were willing to talk about themselves and their condition. After three months, most were able to participate in a vocational program.

The early traders brought camphor as a medicinal agent to Europe from Southeast Asia. It is quite toxic, and in high doses produces artificial epileptic attacks. In 1851 Doctor Szekeres treated the mentally ill by giving them 620 mgs. of camphor, and increased this by 300 mgs. per day until the patients developed epileptic attacks. When the patient awoke from the attacks, his reason was said to return.

In the early 1930s Dr. Ladislas Meduna pondered over the strange fact, that if you had schizophrenia, and then had epileptic attacks, you would generally get well. In epilepsy, there was a great proliferation of the glia cells of the brain, but in schizophrenia, there was a general absence of functional glia cells. He began his research by trying to produce a series of artificial attacks in laboratory animals.

Meduna found that an injection of camphor and oil was the least toxic, and produced the desired epileptic convulsions. In 1934 he was allowed to experiment on a catatonic patient who had been in a stupor for four years. Seventeen days and five camphor injections later, the patient got out of bed, dressed himself and asked how long he had been in the mental hospital. When he was told that he had been in a catatonic stupor for four years,

the patient refused to believe it. Meduna found that his first five patients recovered, and then 13 of the next 26 recovered or were greatly improved.

In China the alkaloid coriamyrtin from *Coriaria sinica* has been used in the same way to produce convulsions. Several Chinese mental clinics give injections of this herb for schizophrenia.

Prolonged fasting can modify the body's metabolism in a way that no other therapy can do. It is seldom used in mental health, but it was used in Russia. At the Gannushkin Institute for Schizophrenics, it is the main therapy for the treatment of mental illness. More than 8,000 patients have gone through the 30 day fasting program with a cure rate of about two-thirds.

By the third day of the fast, hunger diminishes, and there is little appetite by the fifth day. There is plenty of water, daily massages, counseling, and exercise, but no food. The patients must stop smoking and drink at least a liter of water each day. During the first week, patients experience a coated tongue and acidosis, then the tongue clears and the skin color improves. By the third week the mind begins to clear.

Patients often lose up to a quarter of their body weight. During the first days after the fast, they get fruit juice. By the third day they are eating yogurt and applesauce, and then they are introduced to regular foods. Butter milk and salads are used to ease to transition to a normal diet. The fast produces up to 70% improvements and half of these are long-term cures.

In *King Lear*, William Shakespeare wrote about 'poor mad Tom.' Tom lived alone in a cave, he was naked with his hair in knots, and he stuck things in his arms and ate cow dung. He said things like: "Suum, mun, hey no nonny, Dophin my boy, my boy, sessa! Let him trot by." When I see a woman mumbling with her bags on the street, or an incoherent man gesturing irrationally, I wonder why we are not using the discoveries of the past.

✵ ✵ ✵

THE TRANQUILIZER STORY

A foolish extravagant spirit, full of forms, figures, shapes, objects, ideas, apprehensions, motions, and revolutions. These are begot in the ventricle of memory, nourished in the womb of pia mater.
— *Love's Labor Lost* William Shakespeare

Hamlet: Ay, marry, why was he sent into England?
Clown: Why, because 'a was mad. 'A shall recover his wits there; or, if 'a do not, 'tis no great matter there.
Hamlet: Why?
Clown: Twill not be seen in him there. There the men are as mad as he.
— *Hamlet* William Shakespeare

The Greek classical epic known as the *Iliad* and the *Odyssey* is the story of the Trojan War and the events surrounding it. At the end of the war, Troy is in ashes, as the Greeks get their revenge. The survivors gather together to walk back to what seems to be an uncertain future. Menelaus, who is skilled in the magic of the Egyptians, gathers together medicines and herbs and mixes a magic potion called a nepenthe, which makes the fighters forget their pain and sorrows and gives them such a feeling of euphoria, that the tragedy they have just gone through means nothing to them.

Linnaeus remembered the story of the magic potion that abolished sorrows and cares when he named a genus of plants **Nepenthes**. These pitcher plants do not have any known tranquilizing activity, but one species is known to have pain-reducing activity.

Aldous Huxley got the story of the magic 'soma' from the old Hindu legends of India. He pictured a magic kingdom of peace and tranquillity in *After Many Summers Dies the Swan*. Nobody has any cares or worries in this kingdom where everyone takes their daily dose of soma. The story concludes when an army from a neighboring kingdom marches in and takes over the land with no opposition from the tranquilized inhabitants.

The era of tranquilizers began in the early part of this century when a family in Patna, India, used a mysterious drug to cure insanity. A rich philanthropist in Delhi purchased the 'pagal-ka-dawa' [madman's medicine] for a high price and allowed it to be distributed to poor people without charge. A mixture of ground roots, black pepper and rock salt was taken for three weeks.

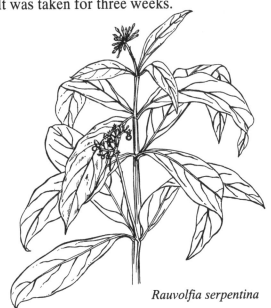

Rauvolfia serpentina

In 1931 Ram Nath Chopra, the director of the Calcutta School of Tropical Medicine, began to investigate the herb. **Rauvolfia serpentina** had marked blood pressure lowering effects and reduced nervous excitation. The plant was mentioned in the old Ayurvedic textbooks of India for a variety of uses, but its usage in mental illness was unknown. The herb is a small shrub, which grows in the lower elevations of the Himalayan Mountains.

Mohandas Gandhi was known to have chewed the roots of the plant during his long struggle with

Table 1. *Effects of various herbs on the number of spontaneous activities of animals during a 15 minute period. (Reduced to a baseline number of 200).*

Plant	One hour later	Four hours later	
Centranthus ruber	100	75	
Passiflora incarnata	120	150	
Tilia petiolaris (flowers)	60	100	
Valeriana officinalis (roots)	75	125	
Voacanga africana	.50	100	

Centranthus ruber

British authorities over the independence of India. The first western studies of the plant began in 1948, and by the 1960s the era of tranquilizers burst on modern medicine. People flocked to doctors to get prescriptions for tranquilizers.

This is not the only herb used for insanity in India. In Behar, the root of **Desmodium latifolium** is considered a specific for insanity. Another insanity herb is mentioned in the hymns of the Atharava Veda: "Head diseases attack evil of the eyes, of the body; and all that kushtha relieves [*Costus speciosus*] verily – a divine virility."

Before the tranquilizer era, herbs having a sedative action and preventing jerky movements of the muscles were called antispasmodics. Valerian, used in India for epilepsy, hysteria and in perfumes, is the best known herb of this class.

Valerian was used for treating shell shock in WWI with the result that the price tripled by 1918. The fresh juice has a strong sedative action, but the dry plant is relatively inactive. Care must be taken to make an active lasting preparation. Valerian sedates the nerves, but it does not affect the heart. The most active member and the most unpleasant smelling is the **Valeriana latifolia** of Japan.

Contrary to the statements in other herb books, the drug Valium is not based on the biochemicals of Valerian. In 1957 Dr. Leon Sternback was working at the Hoffman La Roche laboratories in New Jersey. He was cleaning up his lab bench after a long series of unsuccessful tests, when he found a chemical that he had forgotten. It tasted bitter and he decided to try it. After some more modification it was trademarked Valium. Valium, **Valeriana**, **Tilia** species and **Passiflora caerulea** seem to stimulate the same receptors in the brain.

Nardostachys grandiflora = N. jatamansi is a member of the valerian family from the Himalayan mountains. It was once valued for expensive perfumes and was the ingredient of the perfume that Mary was said to have wiped the feet of Jesus with. When an extract of the root was given to hostile and aggressive rhesus monkeys at a level of 100 mg/kg. it resulted in a 75% reduction in excitement and aggressive hostility. There was an 80% increase in sociability and contentment. An extract of the plant calms hyperactive children. It works very well initially, but the effects wear off in a few weeks.

Nardostachys grandifloia

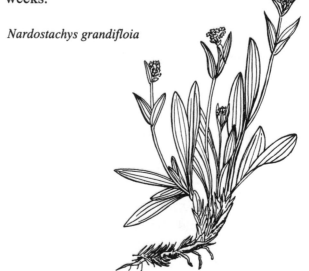

Researchers in India have shown that an alcoholic extract of the sedge **Cyperus rotundus** is a good tranquilizer. It relaxes the smooth muscles, and provides protection from vomiting, itching and pain. It has low toxicity and high activity.

A study was done in France on the herbs which have possible tranquilizing effects. The study includes a number of herbs used in sleeping treatments. The researchers measured the number of spontaneous activities of animals during 15 minutes, and reduced this to a baseline number of 200. This number was measured one hour after taking the herb and then four hours later. The dosage of the plants was varied, and the more active plants were studied. (See Table 1.)

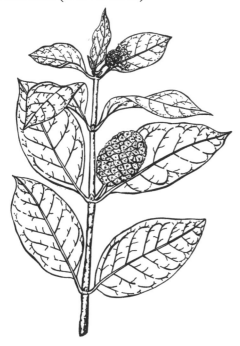

Morinda citrifolia is a small tree which grows in Viet Nam and across the Pacific islands to Hawaii. Doctor Van Dang Ho brought attention to this herb when he found that people taking the herb were exceptionally calm and unflustered. It was popular to use a tea of the yellow branches and roots for pregnant woman. The tree has about the same tranquilizing activity as *Rauvolfia*, but it appears to act through different mechanisms. It is an excellent blood pressure lowering agent, and is useful in mental conditions.

In 1769 when Captain James Cook landed in Tahiti, the natives offered him kava to drink. This herb is either *Piper methysticum* or *P. wichmannii*. The herb is calming and mentally stimulating. The pupils dilate, and the perceptions are altered. Kava was tested in Germany against a placebo. The patients receiving the real kava had significant stress reduction after a week of treatment.

There are two major chemotypes of the kava plant. One type has strong antibacterial chemicals, and it is used to treat urinary and fungal infections. The other type has stronger muscle relaxing ability, and it is used as a tranquilizer.

Ocotea glaziovii is an extremely rare tree growing in the Amazon basin, and only a few specimens are known. The extract is named 'glazlovine,' and its action is similar to Valium. It improves learning in unconditioned rats and counteracts ulcers. It is active when taken by mouth, but unlike Valium, does not cause drowsiness. An awareness of a valuable agent in this tree should make us conscious of the importance of saving the endangered flora of our planet. Nearly 100,000 species grow in the Amazon, and during the dry season miles and miles of the forest are burned to support marginal farming operations.

An extract known as "placon" in Italy comes from the common coltsfoot *Tussilago farfara*. It has been used to treat emotional disorders in Italy. It calms nervousness due to illness, and helps headaches and buzzing in the ears. It was used for insomnia and neuropsychiatric states. Mental patients had good results from taking 20-30 drops of the extract.

A sedative and tranquilizing mixture of *Eschscholtzia california* and *Corydalis cava* has been studied in Germany. Both of the plants belong to the poppy family and are rich in isoquinoline alkaloids. The roots of both plants are high in alkaloids. The alkaloids of *Eschscholtzia californica* are only active in a preparation when extracted with alcohol at a temperature of 80 C. The two herbs have a synergistic effect and are strong sleep modifiers.

Asarone from *Acorus calamus* resembles part of the reserpine molecule, but it acts in a different way. An alcoholic extract of the roots of the *Geranium macrorrhizum* proved to be one of the most active tranquilizers in a screening of Bulgarian medicinal plants. It has hypotensive activity and decreases spontaneous motor activity in mice. *Seseli sibiricum* is a member of the *Umbelliferae* family growing in the Himalayan mountains. It is used in Kashmir for treating psychic disturbances.

✿✿✿

EPILEPTIC HERBS

Feodor Dostoyevsky

"All you, healthy people do not even suspect what happiness is, that happiness which we epileptics experience during the second before the attack. In his Koran, Mohammed assures us that he saw Paradise and was inside. All clever fools are convinced that he is simply a liar and fraud. Oh no! He is not lying! He really was in Paradise during an attack of epilepsy, from which he suffered as I do. I do not know whether this bliss lasts seconds, hours, or months, yet take my word, I would not exchange it for all the joys, which life can give."

–Feodor Dostoyevsky (describing his experiences with epilepsy. His characters Prince Myshkin in *The Idiot* and Kirillov in *Demons* suffer from it.

The sudden convulsive seizure, the foaming of the mouth and falling to the ground unconscious, has a deep effect on others. In primitive times, people believed epilepsy was either a seizure by the gods, or by the devils. The Hebrews accepted the latter explanation. In Matthew's Gospel 17:14, a man comes to Jesus complaining about his son falling into the fire and water. Jesus casts the devil out of him, and he is cured of epilepsy.

The Babylonians blamed epilepsy on the demon Labashu, and the Hindus blamed it on possession of the goddess Grahi. In northern Africa, the Arabs blamed it on possession by jinn's. In Wales, epilepsy was known as the 'rod of Christ,' with the belief that the person was being punished by God.

During the Medieval era when the *Malleus Maleficarum* (Hammer of Witches) became the textbook of the inquisition, many innocent people lost their lives. The inquisitors usually didn't persecute the epileptics, but they turned their attention to the suspected persons associated with them, who used the dark forces to make them have epileptic fits.

Hippocrates called epilepsy 'the sacred disease.' There was also a belief that epilepsy was part of a sacred calling from God. The pythoness that served as the priestess of Apollo was considered lucky, if she suffered from epilepsy. A 13th century book on the rules governing Christian hermits, *Aneren Ruele,* says that it is good for an anchoress [female hermit] to have the falling sickness.

Epilepsy was associated with the moon in ancient times, and many of the remedies were taken at the time of the full moon. The disorder was also known as 'morbus lunaticus,' 'interlunis,' and 'astralis.' This belief was destroyed in 1854, by a French study showing that in 42,000 attacks, epilepsy had no connection with any phase of the moon.

In 1891 Louis Pasteur treated two epileptics for rabies. They were cured, and had no more attacks. He mentioned this fact to another doctor, who sent over a patient who had severe epileptic attacks for 12 years. The man took six days of rabies shots and was cured. Pasteur's chance discovery could help those who don't receive help from other sources.

The first real study of the old epileptic remedies was published in the *Encyclographie de Medicine* in 1852. Doctor Herpin tried copper ammonia, valerianic acid salts, wormwood, hyoscyamus, *Selinum palustre*, and boiled mole flesh, which had a good reputation among farmers in France. He published a statistical table, but he found that the only effective remedy was zinc oxide. Doctor Gaubium, who learned about it from a charlatan, had introduced it into French medicine. He gave epileptics 370 mgs. of zinc oxide daily, and cured 28 of 42 cases.

The zinc cure was tried once in the United States. A doctor was assigned to a home for the disabled and mentally retarded. He gave the epileptics in the home 62 mgs. of zinc lactate three times a day. He found that the spasms came less frequently, and they were milder. Some patients would go up to four months without epileptic fits.

William Gowers wrote a book on epilepsy and convulsive diseases. He remarked that zinc deserved to be tried as a remedy. He had tried various forms of zinc, but he liked zinc oxide best because it had less irritation. In a case of his, a man suffered twice a month from epileptic fits for eleven years. When he took 300 mgs. of zinc oxide twice a day, he went for two months without an attack. Then he had an attack, and the dose was doubled. He had no further attacks for a long period of time.

A tremendous amount of unusual lore on the cure of epilepsy exists. Every animal, distasteful thing or legend has been invoked to cure it. St. Hildegard of Birgen soaked agates in water at the time of the full moon, and cooked the patient's food with agates. Jade was worn by the Greeks and Romans to prevent epilepsy. Emeralds were believed to prevent epileptic attacks.

Through much of recorded history, there were essentially six popular plants used to treat epilepsy. The Bower manuscript was found in Chinese Turkestan and dates some 300 years before the time of Christ. It contains a hymn written in Sanskrit praising the virtues of garlic. The plant was often used to treat epilepsy, but it is probably valueless for the condition.

There is a tremendous amount of lore on the use of mistletoe. Medieval legend told how King David was herding sheep, when he saw a woman collapse. He prayed to God and an angel appeared. He was told that mistletoe worn on the right hand would cure the problem. At least 16 books and pamphlets were published in earlier times on the use of mistletoe to cure epilepsy. But it had to be growing on a special tree, and it had to be cut with a special knife on a holy day. There is no evidence that it did anything.

James Frazer explained the real reason for the use of mistletoe in The Golden Bough: "As mistletoe cannot fall to the ground because it is rooted on the branch of a tree high above the earth, it seems to follow as a necessary consequence, that an epileptic patient cannot possibly fall down in a fit, as long as he carried a piece of mistletoe in his pocket, or a decoction of mistletoe in his stomach."

The roots and seeds of the peony were also highly popular. Galen contributed to this legend by telling the story of a boy, who when wearing the root, was free of seizures, but when he took it off, he had an attack. There is a chemical in the roots of the peony named paenoflorigenone that blocks the twitch responses of muscles. It can only be obtained from a cold water extract, for hot water decomposes it.

Paeonia officialis–peony

There are several mentions of *Paeonia officinalis* in older medical literature. In one instance a nine-year-old child had convulsions for weeks, and three doctors were unable to do anything. Then Aunt Polly came, with some dried 'piney' root in her pocket. She grated half a teaspoonful of the dried root and made it into a tea. After the first cup, the convulsions ceased.

The elder *Sambucus* species has a history of fighting evil and controlling epilepsy, but its value hasn't been scientifically explored. In 1855 a study was done on five incurable cases of epilepsy. The outer bark was discarded, and the inner bark was infused in water for 48 hours. When taken while fasting it produced vomiting and purging. All five cases were claimed to have been cured.

Fabius Columna introduced Valerian as an epileptic remedy in the 16th century in an attempt to cure himself. His claims led to many people using the herb, but it seems to have been ineffective.

There are several nutritional factors which may reduce or eliminate epileptic attacks. About a third of epileptic children have low levels of manganese in their blood. Manganese is linked to neurological disorders in rats. When a 12-year-old boy with uncontrollable seizures was given 20 mgs. of manganese daily, he had fewer seizures and his speech and learning improved. Other experiments show that supplements of folic acid and Vitamin D can reduce the frequency of seizures.

During the years of 1951-4, a considerable number of babies in the United States suffered from seizures. It turned out that palm oil had been used in place of coconut oil in a popular formula. It had almost no Vitamin B6 and this resulted in epileptic seizures. About one out of ten epileptics are said to be helped by Vitamin B6 supplements.

Boron is a trace mineral and exactly what it does in the body is unknown. Corn farmers know from the streaks on the leaves, that their crop needs extra boron in the fertilizer. There are about 30 articles in medical literature on the use of boron to reduce or eliminate seizures. In 1881 an English doctor treated a 17-year-old boy. Bromides could no longer control the attacks and the severe seizures make it impossible for him to work. He was given about a gram of borax three times a day. In two months his attacks ceased, and he was able to return to work.

A French study was done in 1920 using boron potassium tartrate. The effect on epilepsy was marked within a week after taking the supplement. The time interval between attacks gradually progressed. Studies using borax show that 10% of epileptics have a good effect and 20% more have some effect. Large amounts of borax may cause eczema, red plaques on the skin and hair loss.

Medical literature contains numerous accounts of plants used to cure epilepsy. *Capparis coriacea* was brought to Peru to control epilepsy, but a test wasn't promising. People came from all over France and England to take the *Galium mollugo* cure for epilepsy on Hermitage Mountain near Tournon, France, in 1862. There seemed to be valid claims for this plant and Linnaeus listed it in his Materia Medica in 1772 as an epilepsy cure. The crowds faded away when an official French test on eight people failed, and it was quietly forgotten.

There are quite a few herbs for which individual accounts of cures exist. Naboru Muramoto tells of a man with a history of 22 years of epileptic attacks. When he drank a tea of day lily *Hemerocallis thunbergi* or *H. dumortieri* for 60 days his seizures ended. John Jesselyn was the first major writer of the early legends and lore of New England. He said that the Indians used the sycamore *Platanus occidentalis* as an infallible cure for the falling sickness.

The first epileptic remedy of America to be studied was the cow parsnip *Heracleum maximum*. A New England well digger became sick in 1773. His doctor tried camphor, valerian, bleeding and alkalies, but they didn't work. His neighbor advised him to try cow parsnip, because it cured his wife. Each day 8-12 grams of the pulverized roots and an infusion of the leaves were taken. In a short time he had no more fits.

His doctor tried this on five epileptics and cured three of them. He noted that in cases where it worked, the patients were often flatulent. He believed that the cure was due to a healthful tone of the bowls. He remarked that he had never cured an epileptic, before he tried this.

Heracleum maximum

There are accounts in literature of the use of *Clematis cirrhosa*, which postponed attacks for up to three months after taking the herb. The patent medicine known as Bartlett's epileptic remedy was made from *Zizia aurea*.

In Jamaica 'fit weed' is *Eryngium foetidum*. Scientists tested it on picrotoxin convulsions in rats and found that it eliminated the convulsions. French scientists discovered that the roots of **Cnestis ferruginea** from the Ivory Coast of Africa have strong antiepileptic activity. In 1821 Dr. Salvatori of St. Petersburg, Russia, reported that he had great results in treating epilepsy, with the leaves and flowers of *Campanula graminifolia* = *Edraianthus graminifolius*.

A woman who suffered from frequent epileptic attacks was free for up to nine months after drinking a tea of peach roots. In another instance a woman had epileptic attacks for 20 years and went to numerous doctors. The only thing that helped her, was a tea of the bark of peach tree roots. She drank a small cup of the tea three times a day, which eliminated her attacks.

In 1883 an American doctor was treating an epidemic of skin disease with chaulmoogra oil and burdock seeds. He happened to treat a man with a skin disorder and epilepsy. After taking an alcoholic extract of burdock seeds ***Arctium lappa*** three times a day before meals, his epileptic fits stopped.

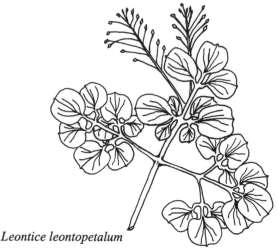

Leontice leontopetalum

In Lebanon, ***Leontice leontopetalum*** is pounded up and a teaspoonful of the juice is taken three times a day. It is supposed to produce small convulsions every two to three minutes. After the first three days, the pulp is taken and this is said to result in a cure for epilepsy within a year. The plant has a number of unusual alkaloids, but I know of no clinical trials.

In India, ***Marsilea vestita*** is a small water fern that floats on the surface of ponds and lakes. The leaves contain about 0.06% marsiline, which produces sleep and affects the nerves. Dr. Ashima Chatterjee claims that a test on 2,000 epileptics showed a cure rate of 30%, a control rate of 60% and 7% had no results at all.

Another story worthy of investigation comes from South Africa. An epileptic had spent all of his money on cures, but grew steadily worse. As a last resort, he tried the native remedy by boiling a handful of leaves of ***Exomis axyroides*** in milk. A tablespoonful was taken three times a day after meals, and soon the epilepsy disappeared. Care must be taken, because a tea of the weed produces a stupor.

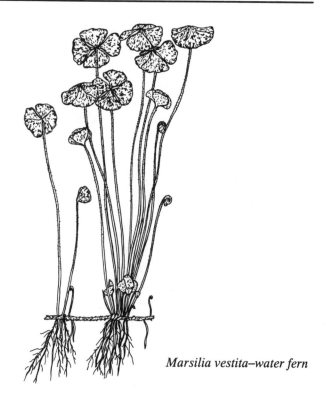

Marsilia vestita–water fern

Chinese scientists found that the root of ***Cynanchum otophyllum*** is a safe effective anticonvulsant in experimental seizures. It elevates the 5-hydroxytryptamine content of the brain. The herb increases the acetylcholine in the cerebral hemispheres and brain stem. In doing this, its actions are similar to several modern drugs.

Japanese researchers tested an old compound formula known as 'Saiko-keishi-to' on epileptic patients who did not respond to modern drugs, or to each of the nine herbs when used separately, The compound was composed of ginseng, scutellaria, pinellia, licorice, ginger, peony, ginger, cinnamon, bupleuri roots and ziziphus fruit. When tested on 24 epileptics with uncontrollable seizures, it completely controlled six and improved 13.

One of the strange remedies which may have some effect is smelling jasmine. The smell of jasmine increases the amount of dopamine in the brain. One doctor treated a woman by having her smell jasmine and stare at a silvered bracelet each time she had a seizure. After eight days of conditioning, she simply looked at the bracelet and had a strong memory of jasmine. Soon, all she had to do was stare at her bracelet, whenever she felt a seizure coming on.

✵ ✵ ✵

PARKINSON'S DISEASE

"People plagued by gout, so that the mouth is distorted and the limbs tremble [Parkinson's disease] and is pulled together in the limbs, should powder celery seeds and add a third of that amount of rue to it, and a little less nutmeg powder than rue, and less cloves than nutmeg, and less saxifrage than cloves. Make a powder out of these ingredients and gout will go away, because this is the best remedy against gout."

– St. Hildegard of Birgen Twelfth century

Leonardo da Vinci described certain people "Who owe their trembling limbs such as the head or the hands without permission of the soul; which soul with all its power cannot prevent these limbs from trembling." Since Parkinson's disease normally affects an older population, it must have been uncommon during this era, due to the short average span of life. A smaller population had little chance of living to an age where it is common.

James Parkinson was a founding member of the Geological Society of London, and he wrote a book titled *Organic Remains of a Former World*. In 1794 he wrote an anonymous booklet called *Revolution with Blood Shed or Reformation Preferable to Revolt*. Both the French Revolution and the revolution in the United States probably influenced his thinking. He advocated progressive taxation, abolishing the game laws, religious freedom, and free labor unions. For England, which was based on class privileges, this was truly revolutionary.

He is not remembered for what was truly revolutionary and worthwhile, but for his 1817 paper on "The Shaking Palsy." He defined this strange disease as "involuntary tremulous motion, with lessened muscular power, in parts not in action and even when supported; with a propensity to bend the trunk forwards, and to pass from a walking to a running pace, the senses and intellects being uninjured."

Parkinson called this new form of palsy "paralysis agitans." He noted that it occurs most commonly after the age of 50, and that it was marked by both muscular rigidity and slowness of movement. His work was forgotten, until the great French physiologist Jean Charcot drew attention to it. He called the disorder "La maladie de Parkinson" and since that time it has been known as "Parkinson's disease."

In the western Pacific islands of Guam and Rota in the Marianas, there used to be a common form of Parkinson dementia. Doctors tried to isolate a virus or a heredity factor, but they were unsuccessful. After 1955 the problem gradually ceased to exist except in a few older people. The problem turned out to be eating the seeds of the false sago palm *Cycas circinalis*, which was used in foods and traditional medicine. The palm had an unusual amino acid. When the components were separated and fed to monkeys, they developed muscle weakness, tremor and a loss of aggressive behavior. They developed a blank stare and long periods of immobility. When the animals were treated with an oral antiparkinson drug, they began to show normal behavior.

The disorder was traced to a lack of the neurotransmitter dopamine in the brain. A dark pigmented area deep in the brain known as the 'substantia nigra' needs dopamine to operate. Dopamine may become depleted by the tranquilizer reserpine, and this produces Parkinson-like symptoms.

The leaves of the common house plant *Tradescantia spathacea* have purple patches, which are rich in dopamine. This plant has been widely used in folk medicine in Cuba, but it cannot be used in Parkinson's disease, because the dopamine is not in a chemical form, that can be absorbed into the brain.

Most beans have some dopamine, and broad beans *Vicia faba* and velvet beans *Mucuna pruriens* contain therapeutically active levels of this chemical. A large helping of these beans (about 250 grams) ought to be able to control the shaking, but nobody wants to eat a large helping of beans three meals a day. A cultivar of broad beans known as WH 305 contains about 3 milligrams of dopamine per gram of beans. It could be used as a dietary therapy.

The bean species have been investigated for their content of L-dopa. The richest is ***Mucuna pruriens*** *var.* ***utilis*** of Mexico, which contains 5%, but ***M. aterrima*** of Florida contain 4.3% of L-dopa. These are wild plants, and it would take some work in order to cultivate them for the chemical.

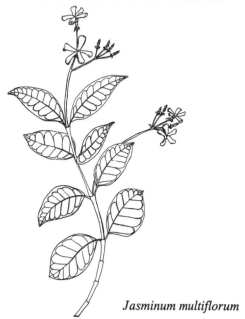

Jasminum multiflorum

Jasminum multiflorum is another herb which may have an effect on the disorder. It has been used by nursing mothers in south India to dry up the milk supply. What it seems to do, is increase the dopamine supply of the brain, which in turn sends a signal to the breasts to dry up the milk. Tests with mice prove that merely smelling the flowers decreases milk, and bandaging the breasts with jasmine in contact with the skin exerts a marked suppressive effect.

The disorder appears comparatively late in literature, and there is little advice in folk medicine. There is an Indian tribal remedy made by mixing 60 grams of ***Gymnema sylvestre*** with 25 grams of dry ginger. Four grams are taken twice a day for two weeks. The treatment is repeated for two weeks each months.

In Ayurvedic medicine, Parkinson's disease was known as 'kampavata' caused by a vata imbalance. It was treated with ***Withania somnifera***, the fruit of ***Hyoscyamus reticulatus*** and the root of ***Sida cordifolia***.

The first help for the disease was ***Datura stramonium***, which was recommended in 1797 for relief in mania, epilepsy and fevers. This is a dangerous herb, and even a small dose will produce mental disorder that may last for days. It does diminish the rigidity, dries up the excessive saliva, and improves the general mental condition. The side effects are blurring of vision and dry mouth with occasional dizziness.

Around 1930 Ivan Raeff of Chipka, Bulgaria, became known for his success in treating Parkinson's disease with belladonna root ***Atropa belladonna***. His treatment involved herbs, diet, exercise and sleep. Patients received four packages with instructions. These were belladonna roots, charcoal pills of bread dough, nutmegs and calamus roots. He achieved fame throughout Europe and a special hospital was set up in Rome to use his treatment. The results of using the complete root were superior to high dosage atropine.

The traditional form of Japanese medicine evolved from Chinese sources into what became known as Kampo medicine. Only a handful of doctors practice this medicine today, because the inroads of western medicine were so strong. The bark of the magnolia tree ***Magnolia hypoleuca*** contains substances that resemble curare. A trial was made of this in Parkinson's disease, and it proved to be able to treat the tremor and muscular rigidity.

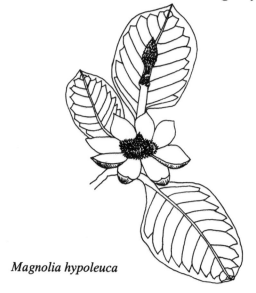

Magnolia hypoleuca

In 1887 Doctor McCartney published his remedy for Parkinson's disease. He made a tincture of the pulverized inner bark of the Ohio buckeye *Aesculus glabra*. He covered the ground bark with alcohol, and left it standing for two weeks. Then he gave his patients a teaspoonful every two to three hours. He wrote that the muscles were now completely controlled by the will. He does not give information on whether this controlled or cured the shaking over a long-term period.

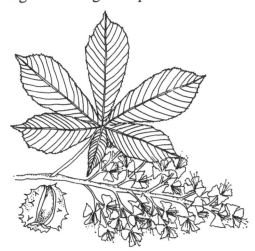

Aesculus glabra

There is some nutritional help for sufferers of Parkinson's disease. A group of sufferers began by taking a gram of the amino acid methionine each day and built up gradually over three weeks to a dosage of five grams while continuing to take standard medication. After two months they were evaluated. Six people had little improvement, but seven were definitely improved. They were able to move better and felt better with improved sleep. Drooling and tremor did not improve.

A recent experiment showed that supplements of Vitamins C and E reduce the severity of the symptoms. After four weeks, 13 out of 15 people showed some improvement. The idea here was that these vitamins blocked the action of free radicals, which are reactive chemicals. They affect the brain cells that produce dopamine.

When Vitamin B1 came on the market, it was tried for a variety of things. A woman with Parkinson's disease was unable to walk. She could only whisper, constantly drooled and had urinary incontinence. Using only thiamin supplements, she was able to stop drooling in six weeks, and in three months she was able to walk. The marked tremor in her hands was now insignificant. She was still improved three years later. The amount of the vitamin was not stated.

Another study showed that Vitamin B6 could produce dramatic improvement in about 20% of the cases. The two studies on this used anywhere from 50 to 350 mgs.

A French study on the use of magnesium chloride was published in 1930. This mineral salt had major effects on shaking nerves. In one case a 69 year old man had trembling writing which was almost impossible to read. He took 1.2 grams of magnesium chloride and gradually raised this to 3 grams a day. In ten days there was less shaking, and in a month, his hands were calm most of the time.

A 50-year-old man contacted cerebral meningitis in 1918. Five years later, his Parkinson's disease became more severe, and there was trembling and difficulty in speaking. After five weeks of magnesium chloride therapy, the shaking was much less, his memory returned, and he was able to speak much more easily.

The great flu epidemic of 1917-8 left in its wake many people suffering from tremor, rigidity, and drooling. The medical journals of the time had many articles on postencephalitic Parkinson's disease. These reports suggest that some cases could be due to unknown viral infections of the brain. If we develop ways of combating these infections, we may be able to help the 25,000 cases of Parkinson's disease that appear in the United States each year.

✡ ✡ ✡

NERVE DISORDERS

I will adore my Father, my God, and my supporter.
Who placed throughout my head, the soul of my reason.
And made for my perception, my seven faculties.
Of fire, and earth, and water, and air, and mist, and flowers,
And the southerly wind, as it were seven senses of reasons,
For my father to impel me: With the first I shall be animated,
With the second I shall touch, with the third I shall cry out,
With the fourth I shall taste, With the fifth I shall see,
With the sixth I shall hear, With the seventh I shall smell.
— "The Macrocosm" by Taliesin A sixth century Welsh poet.

In 1871 a letter published in *The Practical Farmer* read, "I have known so many men and women afflicted with nervousness, so that when they stretched out their hands, they shook like aspen leaves on a windy day. By moderate use of the blanched stocks of celery and leaves as a salad, they became as strong and steady as other people."

The writer goes on to say that fear and nervousness would vanish by moderate use of celery.

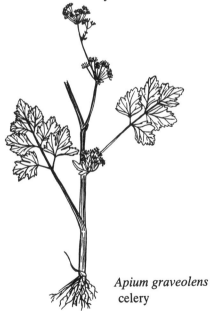

Apium graveolens
celery

It seems unbelievable that a common vegetable can control nervous problems, but it is even more of a surprise to learn that the common celery *Apium graveolens* is used in south China as a treatment of epilepsy. Chinese pharmacologists investigated and found that celery has two anticonvulsive compounds that protected laboratory animals against electroshock. It may be that some varieties of celery are effective and others are worthless. The Chinese work is a surprising confirmation of an observation published a century before.

There is an old French proverb: "Sage [*Salvia officinalis*] helps the nerves, and by its powerful might, palsy is cured and fever put to flight." It is difficult to evaluate the value of sage, because it has received no study. The English herbalist John Hill believed that red sage was particularly good for shaking hands. This sage had reddish leaves and is propagated by cuttings. John Wesley, the Methodist founder, was afflicted by palsy and wrote: "The use of sage tea has fully answered my expectation: My hand is as steady as it was at fifteen."

Henri Leclerc was a French doctor who specialized in the use of herbs. On one occasion, he recommended a wash of sweet clover *Melilotus* species to treat an attack of conjunctivitis.

The woman misunderstood and drank a tea of bird's foot trefoil *Lotus corniculatus*. Her heart palpitations and nervous troubles vanished.

Experiments done in India turned up an exceptionally active antispasmodic plant. Nerve fibers were isolated and placed in a nutrient bath, and barium chloride was used to produce spasms. Then a dozen extracts of Ayurvedic plants known for their use in nerve disorders were introduced. The narcotic plant *Atropa belladonna* prevented spasms.

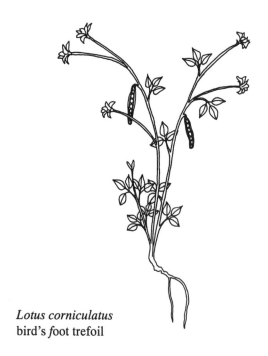

Lotus corniculatus
bird's foot trefoil

A solution of the stems of the Deodar cedar *Cedrus deodara* was much stronger and more lasting than any other herb. Even after the solution was replaced, the nerves still refused to react to spasm causing agents. This tree makes up the bulk of the forests on the lower slopes of the Himalayas and is grown in many North American cities. The sesquiterpenoids have to be dissolved in alcohol. The problem is that they are poorly absorbed into the body. If better-absorbed derivatives could be prepared, this might be an extremely valuable medicine.

Among the herbs known to control shaking or trembling is dodder *Cuscuta europaea* growing on thyme in England, although this has received no investigation. The maidenhair fern *Adiantum pedatum* is said to stop the shaking of palsy. *Cimicifuga racemosa* is known to control muscle twitching. When the muscles of the eye twitch repeatedly, painting the area with a fluid extract of black cohosh can control it.

One of the first articles to appear in medical literature on black cohosh *Cimicifuga racemosa* appeared in 1831. A four-year-old boy was affected by chorea or what was called St. Vitus's dance. The boy was in constant motion, and an old herb woman came to help him. The boy was given a teaspoonful of the powdered root of black cohosh for three mornings, and then the cycle was skipped, and repeated. The boy was cured.

A 19 year-old woman suffered from constant irregular motion in her left side. She had involuntary jerky motions and couldn't walk or support herself. She took a teaspoonful three times a day before meals. After five days she was able to walk, speak and sleep fairly well. In two weeks she was essentially normal.

Muscular twitching and convulsions occur when magnesium levels are low in the blood. Normally the blood contains 2-3 mgs. of magnesium per 100 cc. of blood. When additional magnesium is given by mouth, twitching and convulsions disappear. High levels of magnesium make people drowsy and unresponsive. Magnesium supplements can be used as a sleeping pill. Mystagmus, which is the twitching of the eyes, can often be controlled with magnesium supplements.

In 1968 Miromichi Matsui was planning on using five tons of roasted coffee beans in his laboratory for research, when a typhoon struck Japan. The basement where the beans were stored was flooded and he didn't want to throw them away. He constructed a large box and filled it with fermented coffee beans. He found that by adding the pineapple enzyme bromelain to the fermenting coffee beans he could control the smell. After twenty minutes of soaking he felt very relaxed, and soon he had friends waiting in line to take coffee bean baths. Several people claimed that it relieved the symptoms of Raynaud's disease, which usually comes from vibrations, such as using chain saws.

Some 20% of people who take antipsychotic medication develop involuntary twitches, jerks and grimaces. When 16 people were given high doses of Vitamin E, the involuntary movements decreased for nine. Only one of the 12 placed on placeboes showed any improvement. It worked better in younger patients. The vitamin is believed to protect key areas of the brain from free radicals.

When neuroleptic drugs are taken for a prolonged period of time, patients develop a condition known as tardive dyskinesis. The drugs bind manganese and make it unavailable to the enzymes. After an analysis of hair in these people showed that manganese levels were only half of normal, a supplement of 10 mgs. twice a day cured the tremors.

Myasthenia gravis is a rare disease in which the muscles simply cease to respond to nerve impulses. The most common outward manifestation of the disorder is an inability to keep the eyelids open. In 1943 Emanuel Josophson published a report stating that the disorder was essentially a manganese deficiency. He treated myasthenia gravis patients with 50 mgs. of manganese three times a day and added Vitamin E. There was long lasting relief from the disorder.

In one instance a 26-year-old woman suffered from double vision and dropping eyelids. It took great effort to force her eyes wide open. Walking upstairs gave her severe pains in her legs, and chewing hard food made her jaws feel extremely tired. After taking 30 mgs. of manganese three times a day, there was marked improvement in two days. This was briefly increased to 150 mgs. three times a day. It took six months before she could open her eyes normally, and two years for her lips to become normal. The strength of her jaws and limbs began to improve.

Emanuel Josephson believed that the treatment could benefit several other disorders. In 1958 he treated a man with Parkinson's disease. The man was completely paralyzed, and was able to swallow food with extreme difficulty. After manganese and supportive treatment were used, he was able to feed himself and walk with a walker in six weeks. Since manganese can cause nerve damage, it is important to seek medical help when considering such a treatment.

Multiple sclerosis is another degenerative nerve disease marked by patchy demyelination and hardening of nerve tissues. In 1839 the first description of the disorder was made in Jean Cruveilhier's *Anatomie Pathologique de Corps Humian*. It seems to be an autoimmune disorder in which the immune system cells attack the nerve coating by mistake. Ninety percent of MS patients show primary aggression against the myelin sheathing of the nerves.

A New Zealand doctor found that several of his MS patients reported a remission of the disease after being stung by bees. These curious reports provide some hope for sufferers of the disorder.

The early vitamin researcher Edward Mellanby suggested that MS was the result of a Vitamin A deficiency. He found that rats fed on diets low in Vitamin A showed that same type of nerve and spinal cord degeneration.

He believed that MS could be stopped in the early stages with high amounts of Vitamin A, and slowed with a good diet and plenty of Vitamin A in the latter stages.

The first hint that multiple sclerosis might have some nutritional basis came from a study in Norway. There is very little MS along the edges of the country, where salt spray from the sea adds minerals. In the inland areas, where there is little selenium, the frequency of MS is much higher. Selenium deficiency was a real problem for sheep farmers, on the south island of New Zealand. It also causes Keshan disease in China, and an extra milligram a week, caused a remarkable drop in death rate from heart disorders.

People with MS have a slow descent towards blindness, paralysis and an inability to care for their most basic needs. During the 1930s, experiments showed that deficiency diets caused nerve problems resembling MS. When dried alfalfa and cold pressed wheat germ oil were added to the diets of rabbits with symptoms similar to MS, they received no help. When green alfalfa and wheat germ oil were added, they were protected. The rabbit experiments may not bear a close relationship to the human condition, however.

One patient remarked to her doctor that she did better when she drank orange juice and ate liver. The doctor tried a diet of four glasses of orange juice daily with Vitamin C supplements and 2 cc. of liver extract given by injection twice a week. The diet produced physical improvement, but the speech was slow to improve.

Both Vitamins B1 and B12 are essential components of myelin, and the degeneration of this coating may be due to a B12 deficiency. Fourteen MS patients were selected to receive an injection of liver extract and 150 mgs. of thiamin. At this time Vitamin B12 was not available.

A 43-year-old woman was developing severe symptoms of MS. With injections she recovered and gave birth to a child two years later. If she failed to take the injections, the symptoms returned. As she got older, the injections enabled her to do normal housework.

The study showed that patients treated early

responded quickly, but advanced patients responded slowly. Some factor in the liver extract was remyelinating the nerves. Most patients had help, and some were able to live a normal life.

Doctor Simon Stone had the idea that since beriberi was caused by a lack of thiamin and it created the same condition as MS, it might be useful. He noted that other experiments showed that a lack of B6 caused demyelinizaiton of the nerves. He injected the combination of thiamin and B6 into the spinal fluid for greater effectiveness. About 50 mgs. of each vitamin is mixed with 8-10 cc. of spinal fluid and reinjected. Vitamin E is taken by mouth to complete the treatment.

All nine cases of MS showed good improvement with this treatment. In one case the vision was limited to light and darkness. After two spinal injections a week apart, the patient was able to recognize large objects, perceive some colors and distinguish large letters. Another patient was unable to flex his thigh or extend his leg. A year after two injections he was able to walk around with a cane.

In the six worst cases with incoordination and spasticity, there was great improvement in four cases. The therapy cleared up much of the spasticity, gave them better bladder control, and enabled them to walk. There was a transient burning sensation, but no unpleasant reactions. The improvements lasted for years.

Severely affected children with Sydenham's cholera required 2-3 injections. These children were in a state of continuous motion for weeks before treatment, and many required feeding and protective bed rest. A third of the cases had great relief from the treatment.

The English actor Roger MacDougall got steadily worse with MS. In his case the problem seems to have been an allergy to wheat and cereal grains. When he eliminated all flour, oats, rye and barley together with sugar and animal fat, he began getting better. Eventually he was able to lead a fairly normal life.

There are a number of herbs which have value for multiple sclerosis patients. Ten French patients tried an injection of a solution from *Ginkgo biloba*. The results were a sustained improvement in five of the patients. The others had transient results or little improvement.

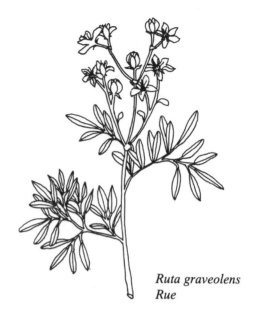

Ruta graveolens
Rue

A tea of the leaves and seeds of rue *Ruta graveolens* seemed to be valuable for helping the body to adjust. As the outer coating of the nerves (myelin) is stripped off, the channels through which potassium enters the nerves are uncovered. Rue helps to correct the current flow in the potassium channels.

Blocking the effects of the overactive immune system could overcome the disorder. The mint known as *Lycopus europaeus* contains something which blocks autoimmune disorders. It was once used in diabetes and Graves' disease, which are autoimmune disorders.

The colchicine in *Colchicum autumnale* reduces the actions of the white blood cells known as macrophages, which destroy myelin. Colchicine acts on the cytoskeleton of the cells and interferes with the assembly of the three proteins into microtubules. These act like the steel girders that make up the frame of buildings and the cells are built around them.

Twenty-five people suffering from MS took 1.8 mgs. of colchicine by mouth for 14

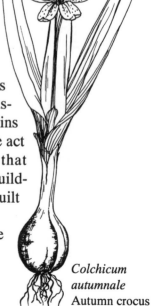

Colchicum autumnale
Autumn crocus

months. Five people had problems tolerating it, and they dropped out. Fifteen people did not get worse and some got better. The improvement was minor, but it was appreciated. It is possible that taking colchicine in the early stages may enable sufferers to lead a fairly normal and productive life. It doesn't cure the disorder, but generally it doesn't get worse.

A combination of fatty acids and colchicine is more beneficial. A test was made on six patients with evening primrose oil and colchicine. Four improved, and two didn't respond. Two became almost normal. One person returned to work after being unemployed for eight years.

Bell's palsy is a nerve disorder in which the facial nerves fail to operate, and the muscles become paralyzed. This may be caused by exposure to cold weather in which the constriction of the blood vessels impairs the nerves. The disorder has been treated in India by injections of Vitamin B12.

A 44-year-old woman suffered from Bell's palsy for one and a half years. The upper and lower part of her face was paralyzed on the left side. She received injections of 0.5 milligrams of B12 for ten days with remarkable improvement. After five injections she was nearly normal.

A 40-year-old man had right-sided facial paralysis for four years. He couldn't close his right eye, and food would collect in the right side of his mouth. He had to use his fingers to clear it out. He was given daily injections of a milligram of B12 for ten days. Each day he massaged his face and exercised the muscle in front of a mirror. In a short time, his facial movements became almost normal.

In 1868 Guillaume Duchenne described progressive muscular dystrophy. The children suffered from weakness, and increasing fatigue. There were spasms in the muscles and the legs began to shake, while the arms slowly became useless. In 1884 Wilhelm Erb did a microscopic examination of the muscles. He found a difference between adults and children, but the results were the same.

In 1930, researchers showed that a diet deficient in Vitamin E produced muscular dystrophy. By 1940 they showed that a deficiency of Vitamin B6 produced the same results. When MD was treated with vitamins E, B6 and selenium, a few patients were helped, but the overall results were disappointing.

Since the muscle proteins were degenerating, doctors tried treating the disorder with amino acids. Glycine, methionine, and cystein produced temporary help in many patients, but there was no permanent benefit.

Three herbs show some benefit in muscular dystrophy. Licorice increases muscle strength, but unless it is processed, it also increases blood pressure. A tincture of the roots of *Aristolochia fangchi* shows benefits in treating both muscular dystrophy and Alzheimer's disease, by inhibiting the enzyme that breaks down acetylcholine. The rishi mushroom *Ganoderma capens* and *G. japonicus* has uracil and uridine which help the disorder.

Anaerobic bacteria in punctured food cans produce botulism toxin. In 1967 an experiment using chickens showed progressive muscular dystrophy using the toxin. The nerve junctions of the muscles are paralyzed. They are unable to release acetylcholine, and they waste away.

It is known that tetanus toxin and botulinus toxin create a condition much like muscular dystrophy. Tetanus has been successfully treated with *Lobelia inflata* and *Ericameria laricifolia* = *Haplopappus laricifolia.* Could these herbs become a useful treatment for MD?

✧✧✧

PARALYSIS

"Hermodicus of Lampsacus, having been paralyzed, the body was cured by God. After incubation, he was ordered by him to bring into the sacred place a stone as large as he could. He brought that one which is lying in front of the Abaton."

"A man having the fingers of his hand, except one, paralyzed came to supplicate God. Seeing the tablets in the temple, he disbelieved the cures indicated, and ridiculed the inscriptions. When he went to sleep he saw a vision. It seemed to him that he was playing dice, and as he was about to throw one of them, the god appeared, seized the hand and stretched out the fingers. When the God left him, he thought that he bent them up and stretched them out one by one. When all were straightened the God asked him if he still disbelieved the inscription. He replied, "No!"

– Inscription on the Greek temple of Asclepius at Epidaurus excavated in 1883. People slept in the temple and got a dream healing.

The Lewis and Clark expedition of 1803 was the beginning of the vision of a country that stretched from the Atlantic to the Pacific Ocean. During the expedition, William Clark saw an Indian chief who had lost the use of his limbs for the past three years, but was otherwise normal. Clark remarked: "One of our hunters mentioned that he had known persons in similar situations restored by violent sweats. At the request of the patient, we permitted the remedy to be applied. For this purpose a hole about four feet deep and three feet in diameter was dug in the earth, and heated well by a large fire at the bottom of it. The fire was then taken out, and an arch formed over the hole by means of willow poles and covered with several blankets, so as to make a perfect awning. With a jug of water we sprinkled the bottom, and sides of the hole so as to keep up as hot a steam as he could bear. After remaining twenty minutes in this situation, he was taken out, immediately plunged twice into cold water, and brought back to the hole, where he resumed the vapor bath. During all this time he

William Clark

drank copiously a strong infusion of horsemint *Monarda punctata*. This operation was performed yesterday, and this morning he walked about, and is nearly free from pain."

The next day their fame spread, and another paralyzed Indian arrived in a canoe. After a day of sweating and plunging into cold water he was able to use his arms, and he felt better than he had for months. The next day he received another sweating, and the paralyzed man was able to move one of his legs, and some of his toes and fingers.

The heat treatment of paralysis was popular during the 1920s. During this time doctors used malaria or sodoku, a rat-bite fever organism, to produce a high temperature in hopes of curing 'dementia paralytica.' The invention of diathermy used radio waves to heat the body and produce an artificial fever. A clinical trial showed a 24% cure and a 26% improvement, during a course of 12 treatments lasting up to two hours. It was a technological adaptation of the old sweating treatment, once used as a curative.

The vetch *Lathyrus sativus* is a relative of the common pea. It produces small pea pods, which are fairly good eating. The vetch is used as a famine food; i.e. when there is nothing else to eat, they are gathered and eaten. In 1671 the Duke of Wurtemburg issued an edict forbidding the use of vetches as food. In 1786 the peasants around Florence, Italy, were ordered not to use vetches for food, as they might become paralyzed by them. It was said: "Even the swine [who ate vetches] became pitiable monsters, and grew fat lying on the ground, not able to rise."

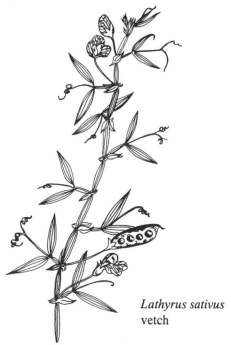

Lathyrus sativus
vetch

The British administrators of India were puzzled by recurring epidemics of 'dal' poisoning. During times of famine, peasants picked the vetches growing wild and ate them. Nothing generally happened for several weeks, but after two to three months the back muscles of the legs become sore, and suddenly the men became paralyzed in the legs. The problem rarely affects women, but whole villages of men were known to walk with sticks for support. The paralysis can be felt coming on, and if the eating of vetches is stopped, there is no danger. Since vetches produce large amounts of food, the toxic chemical has been studied and less toxic vetches have been bred.

There are several tribal remedies in India, which deal with paralysis, possibly due to dal poisoning in cattle. The whole plant of *Amaranthus spinosus* is cut and fed. Cattle are also fed a mixture of 250 grams of *Convolvulus microphyllus* and ten grams of black pepper in 250 mls. of water. They are given this for seven to ten days.

Another curious form of paralysis is caused by the 'tullidora' *Karwinskia humboldtiana*. In 1916 a Mexican army unit mistook these berries for edible capulon berries *Prunus serotina*. Two days after eating the berries, paralysis of the lower limbs began and spread out over the body.

Dr. Castillo Najera treated 106 patients in the military hospital at Guaymas in Sonora. Some Maya soldiers claimed that the cure was a tea of the roots, but it had to be taken during the first days of paralysis. Najera tried this without results, but more than ten days had elapsed since the men had been poisoned. He wrote a memoir of his experience titled: *A Contribution to the Study of Toxic Paralysis.*

In the summer of 1921, Franklin D. Roosevelt went swimming in the Bay of Fundy. The next morning he awoke with a peculiar feeling in his legs. A day later he was unable to stand up when he tried to get out of bed. The diagnosis was polio, and he was afraid that his hoped for political career was in ruins. When he became president in 1932, it was the height of the depression, and few people knew that the president's legs were paralyzed. His powerful voice reassured the nation that things would improve and everything was being taken care of.

In 1825 Alexander Manson wrote *Medical Researches on the Effects of Iodine.* He remarked that the success of iodine in reducing the enlarged thyroid led him to think that iodine would reduce the fluids pressing on the brain and spinal cord. Manson gave as examples of his therapy 25 cases of paralysis. A newer generation of doctors tried potassium iodide, which was easier on the patients. They had the same results in polio paralysis.

A 19 year-old man was paralyzed with polio. Manson began with ten drops of iodine in water on April 4, 1821. In two days the man could move his right arm a little, and in another three days, he could raise it up to his head. By April 10 he could bend his left leg a little and hold his urine. By April 16 he was able to feed himself with the left hand. The iodine was now increased to 30 drops a day. By May 7 he could walk a little, and he was discharged as cured on August 7.

Some vitamins are of service in polio paralysis. Ergot makes the nerve tissue in the spinal cords of animals degenerate. Vitamins B1 and B2 prevent this degeneration, and Vitamin A is a strong preventive. One animal was unable to stand, but after three weeks of Vitamin A therapy, it was able to stand.

In the days before vaccine tamed diphtheria, the aftereffect was often temporary paralysis in children. In 1939 a German study was published in which part of a group of children were given Vitamin B1 and the others were used as a control. Those who took thiamin had paralytic symptoms that lasted an average of 30 days, but in the other group they lasted for 49 days. Diphtheria produces a toxin that is apparently blocked by the vitamin.

A 70 year-old woman was treated for muscle dysfunction of polio with immunosuppressive drugs. She didn't respond, but when she was given 1,600 units of Vitamin E, she nearly recovered completely, except for some residual muscle weakness.

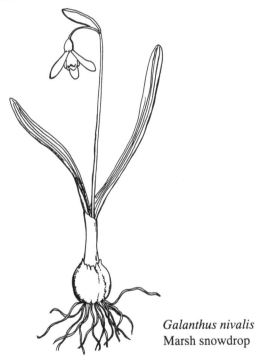

Galanthus nivalis
Marsh snowdrop

With the advent of the polio vaccine, paralysis due to the polio virus is now uncommon. One of the few treatments found to be useful was the flowers of the marsh snowdrop *Galanthus nivalis*. This beautiful flower was originally used in Bulgaria to help polio patients repair damaged nerves. The alkaloid has a prolonged activity, and it augments the nervous reflexes of the central nervous system. About ten flowers make a single dose, which amounts to about 20 mgs. of the alkaloid. The flowers may be ordered from seed catalogues, but in any quantity they are quite toxic.

Another aid in helping polio paralysis, were the leaves of the birch *Betula pendula*. Eleven of 14 people suffering from polio paralysis had positive changes. They didn't recover fully, but they had better muscular control.

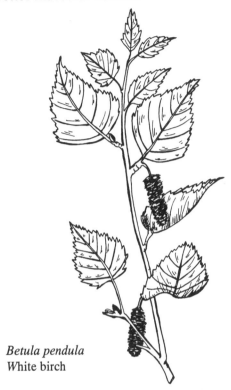

Betula pendula
White birch

With the discovery by French doctors that magnesium chloride was able to control nervous shaking, it was only natural that it be tried in polio. Doctor Auguste Neveu wrote: Therapeutic *Treatment of Infectious Diseases by Magnesium Chloride — Poliomyelitis*. With the summer polio epidemics paralyzing thousands of children, he believed that every household should keep 20 grams of magnesium chloride handy. At the first appearance of a sore throat and stiff feeling in the back of the neck, mix this with water and drink it. Tablets of magnesium gluconate should have some effect, but the salt form of magnesium is probably the most effective.

Neveu advocated mixing the 20 grams in a liter of water (1000 cc.). This makes a gram of magnesium chloride in 50 ccs. of water. A four-year old boy came down with polio and his left leg was paralyzed. He was given 80 cc. to drink at three-hour intervals. When he woke up the next morning, the fever and paralysis were gone.

A 47 year-old woman was completely paralyzed in the lower right leg and lumbar region. After

12 days of magnesium therapy she was completely cured. A two-year-old girl wasn't able to stand or move his right arm after an attack of polio. She was given 60 ccs. of magnesium chloride solution every four hours. Her legs regained movement, but her right shoulder remained paralyzed.

A 19 year-old woman had her left leg paralyzed by a polio attack, and it began to atrophy four months later. She was given 125 cc. of the solution every six hours and after 15 days there was a marked improvement of the paralyzed leg. In a few months she was able to walk with a limp and ride a bicycle.

The poison that we know as strychnine comes from the nuts of the **Strychnos nux-vomica** tree. In India and Malaysia, it was used to tip arrows and poison fish. It was imported to Germany under the name of 'drahenaigen' [crow poison]. It gained fame from several murder trials and the 'strychnine panic' of 1852. There were rumors that a beer company imported large quantities of strychnine to make beer bitterer. Consumption of beer took a nose-dive, until the rumor died.

The muscles of the body are made in pairs which pull against each other. One muscle pulls and the other one relaxes. Strychnine contracts both sets of muscles at once. It is used in small amounts to exercise the muscles in some cases of functional paralysis. It does not provide a cure, but it does prevent the muscles from degenerating any more.

Curare, the famous arrow poison of South America, blocks the transmission of nerve impulses across the junctions, so that acetylcholine cannot carry the nerve impulse. Rat nerves were suspended in a nutrient bath, and blocked with curare, while various amino acids were added. Several amino acids increased the blockage, but glutamic acid unblocked the nerve. The level at which it unlocked the curare is equivalent to six grams for a 120-pound person. Could this be applied to other forms of paralysis?

Brazilian Indians in an area known as Raudal de Jerijerimo on the Rio Apaporis, suffer from a peculiar form of leg paralysis. They scrape the bark off of the branches of *Pagamea coriacea* and boil it into a tea and drink it for two to three weeks. Drinking the tea stimulates the nerves, and often the paralysis disappears.

Another herb growing in northern Brazil used in paralysis is *Liriosma ovata*. It is used in nervous diseases, rheumatism and paralysis. It has a good effect in jerky muscular motions, and is a constituent of the tonic Esthenol. It is known under several common names, but the most popular name is 'muira puama."

In 1882 Doctor Keith wrote enthusiastic articles on the tincture of oats. He claimed to have been paralyzed for four years, and after taking a concentrated tincture of oats, four times a day, his paralysis was cured in three weeks. He sold the tincture, which resulted in believers and unbelievers. Fresh oats is known to contain active physiological principles, but as oats age, the activity drops.

The late Utah herbal doctor John Christopher believed that nerves could be repaired. He told the story of two boys playing with a gun. A bullet severed the spinal cord of one boy, and he was rushed to the children's hospital at Salt Lake City. Before he left, his mother gave him a spoonful of cayenne pepper to control the bleeding. The doctors told the parents that their son would never be able to walk or have normal bowel or urinary control again. His mother was a believer in herbs and she gave him large amounts of Doctor Christopher's lower bowel tonic and nerve formula. Two weeks later, the boy was able to control his bowls. Six weeks later he was able to wiggle his toes, and eventually he was walking and acting perfectly normal. The power to regenerate nerves might be far greater for an eight-year-old boy, than for someone who is older, but a study of the herbs in the tonics should be of interest.

Christopher's nerve tonic was composed of a mixture of black cohosh – *Cimicifuga racemosa*, cayenne pepper– *Capsicum annuum*, hops– *Humulus lupulus*, lady's slipper– *Cypripedium pubescens*, lobelia– *Lobelia inflata*, scullcap– *Scutellaria lateriflora*, valerian root– *Valeriana officinalis*, wood betony– *Stachys betonica* and mistletoe- *Viscum album*. It was usually taken in "oo" capsules of finely powered herbs several times a day.

There is a study which indicates that the herbs having strong granulating agents, such as comfrey or eucalyptus, could help nerves regenerate. Rats were anesthetized, and their sciatic nerves were crushed. Five grams of allantoin from comfrey were added to a liter of water, and this was used for drinking water. The rats were sacrificed, and the regeneration of the sciatic nerve was studied under a microscope. Allantoin increased healthy tissue, and aided in the removal of dead tissue. There was a 30% improvement in healing rate, and a significant difference in appearance under a microscope.

The Asian plant *Hygrophilia erecta* contains long chain alcohols, which are strong nerve growth stimulants. It might aid in spinal cord injuries in stimulating the damaged nerves into regenerating. Wheat germ oil had a 28-carbon alcohol known as octacosanol, which serves as a nerve growth factors. Experiments on mice show, that if their body is rich in Vitamin E when injured, they are less likely to have spinal cord damage. The experiments suggest that in major accidents, the first treatment should be Vitamin E. It stimulates healing, and might prevent paralysis.

A 27 year-old man had an accident in a freight elevator. His spine was broken, and he was completely paralyzed. Soon he was deteriorating and was covered with large bedsores. He was removed from the hospital, and placed under the care of a private doctor. Each day he was injected with 500 mgs of Vitamin C and 50 mgs of thiamin. He also took B and C vitamins by mouth.

In a week there was a striking improvement, and the bedsores started to heal. After another week of injections he could wiggle his toes. In two months the patient was able to control his bowels. The doctor does not finish his story by waiting another year to report this. He is clearly surprised that the injections of high dosage vitamins are improving a once hopeless patient.

In an age marked with mechanical gadgetry, we have poured millions of dollars into sophisticated equipment to help the handicapped. We have not bothered to investigate centuries of observations, which indicate that in some cases nerves can regenerate and carry impulses. Studies of natural products could bring hope to the paralyzed.

THE MYSTERY OF PAIN

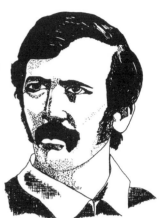

"He caught me by the shoulder as he sprang, and we both came to the ground together. The shock produced a stupor, similar to that which seems to be felt by a mouse, after the first shake of the cat. It caused a sort of dreaminess in which there was no sense of pain, nor feeling of terror, though quite conscious of all that was happening. It was like what patients partially under the influence of chloroform describe who see all the operation, but feel not the knife. This peculiar state is probably produced in all animals killed by the carnivora, and if so, is a merciful provision by our benevolent Creator for lessening the pain of death."
– David Livingstone on his experience of being attacked by a lion

Aristotle defined pain as the opposite of pleasure. The Greek poet Homer defined pain as the arrows shot by the gods. Many societies had the idea that pain was either sent by the gods or the devils. Pain comes from the Latin word 'poena' meaning 'punishment.'

Pain is an old subject of theology and the prophet Jeremiah spoke of God sending "fire into my bones." The prophet Isaiah spoke of "a man of pains acquainted with sorrows." The early Christians put great emphasis on the idea that the death of Jesus was an act of supreme pain. John Milton wrote in *Paradise Lost*: "Pain is perfect misery, the worst of evils, and if excessive, overturns all patience."

Pain evokes fear, which in turn evokes self-protection. If we did not have pain, would we be able to survive? There are a handful of cases in which children were born without pain receptors. These children fail to show the fear and self-care that comes to us naturally. They might put their hands on a hot stove and hold it there, until the muscles are burned so badly that they are almost useless. If they break a bone they ignore it, and it can become damaged so badly, that healing becomes impossible. If they bite their tongue while eating, they don't feet anything, so they may bite all the way through.

When dogs are raised in isolation, they show aberrant reactions to pain. They repeatedly poked their noses into flaming matches and sniffed at it, as long as it was present. They endured pinpricks with little evidence of pain. Pavlov found that if he gave food to dogs after shocking them, the dogs developed a new reaction. After a shock, the dogs salivated, wagged their tails, and turned eagerly towards the food dish.

Nature defends itself with pain, and we learn quickly to leave nettles or poison ivy alone. The Australian stinging tree known as ***Laportea moroides*** is perhaps the most painful plant known. The Chinese call it the 'dog-bite-man-tree,' and contact means a day of severe pain. People have been known to commit suicide, because they cannot stand the pain of the tree.

Bees produce pain by injecting histamine into the sting. Wasps produce much more pain with peptides known as kinins. Ants with formic acid venoms are described as 'sharp stinging' pain. Some African and South American ant stings are excruciatingly painful. Catfish, weaverfish, and stonefish spines produce severe pain, which is not relieved with morphine.

The pains of the body are equally baffling, because we can't fully describe them. Virginia Woolf wrote of her headaches: "Let a sufferer try to describe a pain in the head, to a doctor and language runs at once dry."

We describe pain as 'itching, burning, or tearing,' but this isn't quite it. The pain of ulcers comes from acid in the stomach, but hunger pains are the contractions of an empty stomach.

Pain is a baffling mystery within medical literature. Researchers have tried to produce measurable standard units of pain in humans and rats only to be baffled with the inconsistencies, which made their experiments less useful. Just when they thought they had a standard unit of pain produced by tail pinching, the next group of rats wouldn't react the way they expected.

Researchers have been equally baffled with hypnosis and acupuncture analgesia. Major operations have been done under hypnosis, but other attempts have produced scared patients fleeing from the operating room. After President Nixon's visit to China, acupuncture was in vogue. It was theorized that acupuncture analgesia released endogenous opioides within the brain. Crying is said to reduce pain. Pain reduces pain, which is why the old time doctors induced a second pain, such as a painful blister to take away the attention from the affected area.

In one Swedish experiment, a jet injector used for shots had no mechanical contact with the body. Volunteers were given stopwatches and a series of five shots. They asked to grade the intensity of pain from 0-5, and the duration of pain with a stopwatch. The more acid the solution, the greater the pain. Malignant tumors with low pH values (acid) produce extreme pain, but those with normal pH are generally painless. Potassium has a pronounced pain-producing effect. Scorpion stings are extremely painful, and it floods the body with potassium. The greatest level of pain was produced with distilled water! The doctors theorized that solutions which changed the osmotic pressure of cells, caused pain.

In recent years a controversial concept of pain has emerged. Pain is created in the brain, from the patterns of impulses transmitted from the site of the stimulus. These theorists believe that there are no pain nerve endings or specific nerve pathways for pain.

During WWII badly wounded men were studied for their sensations of pain. Less that half of the badly wounded men had severe pain. Most of those reporting severe pain had penetrating abdominal wounds and compound fractures of the long bones. Just mentioning to the soldiers that they were severely wounded, or that they needed morphine was enough to make them feel severe pain. Because of its side effects, morphine was avoided, unless the men asked for relief from the pain.

There are some strange ways of relieving pain. In 1875 a Philadelphia dentist discovered that by causing his patients to breathe rapidly for a few minutes, the sense of pain was reduced enough, to enable him to extract teeth without causing any discomfort. After two to five minutes of rapid breathing, teeth can be pulled without anesthesia for about a minute, and pain is greatly reduced for about five minutes!

Many ancient doctors compressed the carotid artery in the neck, which cuts off the circulation to the brain. About two-thirds of all people can be anesthetized for five to fifteen minutes in this way.

The prophet Amos spoke of "the wine of the condemned." Passages in the Talmud speak of the practice of easing the pain of death and torture, by stupefying the sufferers. The "wine mingled with myrrh" offered to Jesus, was a narcotic draught intended to make death painless.

Myrrh is the sap of the ***Commiphora myrrha*** tree. A test was made to see if myrrh had analgesic effects. When rats were put on a hot plate, they began licking their paws after 14 seconds. When they were given extracts of myrrh, they began licking their paws after 19 seconds. Myrrh had a significant effect in blocking pain. These effects are believed to be due to influencing the same receptors that morphine inhibits.

During the middle ages knowledge of the "spongia somnifera," or soporific sponge was passed from surgeon to surgeon. The ingredients of this sponge was a mixture of opium, mulberry juice, hemlock, mandrake leaves, lettuce and water hemlock. The sponge was applied to the nose of the person to be narcotized. After the operation, the patient was revived with another sponge dipped in vinegar or fenugreek.

The narcotic sponge was studied in France in 1927, but it didn't work very well. Maybe the herbs were inferior, or the solutions were too weak, but it seems likely, that the sponge never did work.

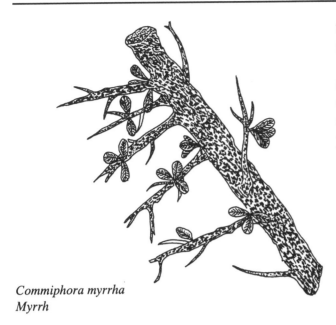

Commiphora myrrha
Myrrh

Even back in the 17th century the great surgeon Ambroise Pare spoke of the 'spongia somnifera, which had been formerly used.'

Modern pain relief began in 1800 when Sir Humphry Davy breathed nitrous oxide. He had an inflamed tooth, and after several breaths of nitrous oxide the pain vanished. In 1806 ether poured into a saucer was used to the control the pain of Lady Byam Martin. She relieved her asthma attacks this way for many years, but doctors ignored her. In 1844 Horace Wells inhaled nitrous oxide gas and had a tooth extracted while under its influence. With this demonstration, the use of anesthesia spread throughout the medical profession.

Although several herbs like the opium poppy control pain, they do not always work well. In 1867 the *Lancet* printed a letter from a man who recovered from a serious illness. He offered £2,000 to anyone who could discover a mode of permanently and completely extinguishing pain, in all cases during the next year. He must have suffered a lot of pain, for this was a huge sum of money for his time. He kept his money as well, and he could probably still keep it today, although we have made major advances in pain control.

It must be one of the most miserable experiences in existence, to suffer long-term chronic pain. You look entirely normal, and your friends treat you normally, but life is a hell of suffering. One way that some people can gain relief is by taking a 250 mg. tablet of the amino acid d-phenylalanine three times a day. One in three persons receive significant pain relief.

At the time of childbirth doctors used to make a cut known as an episiotomy to widen the birth canal. While this aided birth, it produced pain and discomfort in healing. Women were given either a placebo or bromelain tablets (an enzyme of pineapple). In the group that took a placebo, 70% needed pain killing medication stronger than aspirin. In the group that took bromelain, 28% of the women needed a similar painkiller. The women rated bromelain as an excellent medicine 78% of the time, but the placebo was rated as an excellent medicine only 18% of the time.

In 1874 Professor Hermann Kolbe perfected his process, which enabled the large-scale production of aspirin. The new drug was competing with many other remedies, and was slow to become popular. Our most popular painkiller today is aspirin, which is about one-fiftieth as active as morphine. The maximum effect of aspirin on pain comes at about 600 mgs., so more aspirin is not more effective. It works on moderate, but not on severe pain.

Aspirin is one of the many drugs known as analgesics. These have mild pain relief without putting the body to sleep. Twelve herbal remedies known for analgesia in the area of Sao Paulo, Brazil, were tested. The only one to have significant effects in both tests used was the bark of ***Serjania communis***.

Brazilian scientists tested an alcoholic extract of ***Phyllanthus corcovadensis***, which was used as a folk remedy for kidney and bladder stones. These conditions cause a great deal of pain. Using a mouse tail flick test, they proved that the extract was highly effective in reducing the pain response. The herbal extract can be taken either orally or by injection.

In South Africa, chewing the leaves of ***Mesembryanthemum tortuosum*** treats general pain. This has a strong narcotic effect due to the mesembrine, and is used for stomach pain and toothache. Children are given the leaves to help them to sleep.

The herb 'tormentil' ***Potentilla anglica*** was named because it was a painkiller. A powder or poultice of the roots was applied for the toothache. The leaves of ***Glaucium flavum*** contain glaucine, a good substitute for codeine. The mignonette ***Reseda odorata*** was once in great demand for pain and swelling. The bioflavanoids of ***Prunus spinosa*** reduce the response to pain causing histamine. We have forgotten about these old herbs, and it is time to take another look.

☆☆☆

NEURALGIA

Neuralgia is a general term for pain in the nerves of the body. When it affects the fifth pair of facial nerves with shooting pains we call it 'tic douloureux' or 'trigeminal neuralgia.' If it affects the main nerve leading to the foot, it is called sciatica. Although I have written about the neuralgias as separate entities, anything which cures one, may cure the other. Doctors have a difficult time in treating the neuralgias, and as a last resort they may cut the nerves, or inject alcohol into them to deaden them.

Headaches and migraines are related to the problems of neuralgia. The word 'neuritis' means 'an itching of the nerves'. During the 19th century, doctors used the word 'neurasthenia,' which meant 'nerve weakness.' This was almost always applied to women. Today we use the words 'fatigue,' and possibly 'depression' to describe this. A century ago a woman's place was in the home, with a large family. This meant that many women did not get enough exercise, and a good diet. As a result they complained to doctors, who diagnosed them as 'neurasthenics.'

'Causalgia' is another forgotten word, which applies to amputations, or wounds in which nerves are damaged. It was first used in the American Civil War of 1861-65, to describe nerve pain after the wounds had healed.

The neuralgias have a direct relationship to external influences, and many people, particularly those with arthritis, are storm sensitive. Doctor Weir Mitchell did studies on the sensitivity of these people more than 100 years ago. He found that major storms had a 'neurological belt,' which extended about 150 miles in front of the main storm activity. This is believed to be due mainly to barometric pressure drop, but changes in the electrical fields influence people as well. Desert sandstorms are particularly noted for their high positive ion content, and for their abilities to make people irritable and give them headaches. On the other hand, the negative ion belt following storms provides a feeling of peace and comfort.

While on an expedition towards the North Pole, Captain Robert Catlin noticed the effects of the northern lights on neuralgias. When the northern lights are active, people with amputated limbs suffer more from phantom pains. The rest of us are more restless at these times, and times of high solar activity, seem to be marked with more wars. A sudden outburst of the northern lights makes the fish more restless, and it's a good time to catch them.

The absence of Vitamin B1 results in pain. Two patients with painful neuritis were given injections of 10 mgs. of thiamin. This didn't help, but when it was increased to 100 mgs every other day, there was marked relief of pain. In seven of nine patients with severe pain, thiamin gave them complete relief in one day to two weeks. Two patients were partially relieved.

The herbs used in treating neuralgia and their modes of action are little known. The leaves of the common artichoke **Cynara scolymus** came into medical use in the 1830s as a treatment for arthritis and gout. It was discovered that the preparation was useful in treating neuralgic problems. A drachm tincture, taken three times a day, relieved long-standing cases of sciatica. By 1960 Italian pharmacists had isolated the active agent from the artichoke and were selling it in tablets. It proved to be useful in a variety of disorders.

In Cuba and the Caribbean islands, neuralgias are treated with bitter broom *Parthenium hysterophorus*. When morphine failed to control the pain Dr. Antonio Esperon gave two people with severe neuralgias an extract of the plant. Several doses of a sixth of a gram of 'parthenin' given at hour intervals resulted in complete disappearance of the pain. The preparation worked well in facial and malarial neuralgias. This plant is of considerable interest to allergists, becauses it produces skin rashes, and it causes problems in cattle where is grows. That should make us cautious in using it.

The mixture of tree barks known as 'Tonga' is a powerful remedy in neuralgias. A ball of the two tree barks is steeped in cold water for 20 minutes and the tea is drunk. It usually cures the neuralgia by the second or third day. The pain might return ten days later, but a few additional cups of the pleasant tea will remove it permanently.

In 1887 Dr. A. Sacconi of Edwardsville, Illinois, wrote: "I have used Tongaline in many cases of facial neuralgia, also neuralgia of the nervous trigeminus and of nervous headache, have frequent opportunities to do so through my position as county physician of Madison County, Illinois. I must frankly acknowledge that whenever I resorted to tongaline the patients obtained instant relief, and was thus able to save the county further care and expense."

A 20 year-old woman suffered from severe neuralgia for ten days in the temples and under the eyes. She had about five attacks a day lasting from one to two hours each, but after drinking three glasses of tonga tea, she was cured in three days. An 18-year-old woman suffered from toothache and neuralgia of the lower jaw. The extract of tonga cured the neuralgia in 24 hours, but the toothache remained. A 40-year-old man suffered for months with spasms of pain in his forehead. Drinking tonga cured him in three days.

Tonga appears to have little toxicity, for larger amounts produced only a slight drowsiness. The amount used is small and the cure is rapid. The herbal mixture of the barks of *Premna taitensis* and *Epipremnum pinnatum = E. vitiensis* have been forgotten and their chemistry ignored.

Yellow jessamine *Gelsemium sempervirens*

was used by many 19th century doctors for neuralgia. In one case a 16-year-old girl had severely painful headaches and got no help from the traditional therapies. She was given ten drops of a fluid extract of *Gelsemium* every three hours in a small glass of water. After the first dose she was entirely free from pain.

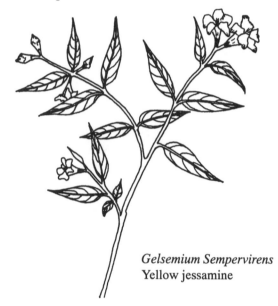

Gelsemium Sempervirens
Yellow jessamine

American pharmacists prepared a tincture of yellow jessamine by mixing two ounces of the powdered roots with a pint of strong alcohol. The normal dose was 5-10 drops of the tincture. It sometimes produced dim vision, and extreme prostration. It was often used for strong stabbing pains. Overdoses were dangerous and the herb is no longer used.

A woman suffered from grinding, shooting pains in the teeth, jaws and temples. The dentist said that nothing could be done, but eating brought on the pain, and left her in misery. She took ten drops of the tincture three times a day. She got relief on the first day, and steady improvement over the next three weeks.

A 32-year-old man had severe pain in the lower jaw. He took five drops of yellow jessamine tincture every three hours. Soon there was complete relief of pain. The bitter alkaloid, which relieves the pain, is gelsemin. The maximum safe dose of this herb is considered to be 25 mgs. of the dry powdered root three times a day.

Neuralgias that have lasted for years may yield to castor oil. This was discovered around 1890 when Professor Carl Gussenbauer of Vienna, Austria, gave a patient castor oil prior to surgery. The neuralgia disappeared, and the surgery was unnecessary. The oil is not any more disagreeable than fish oil. It can be given in capsules so that you don't taste it at all. It is curious to note that a few drops of castor oil taken daily for a week, often relieves cases of severe itching, and when taken for a longer period of time, clears up skin disorders.

It usually takes from 15 to 30 grams to treat the neuralgias each day. This dosage has a laxative effect at first, which wears off, and then the neuralgia pains begin to disappear. It is theorized that the castor oil turns into an altered form of prostaglandin, which does not cause pain. Several prostaglandins (cell regulator chemicals) are formed from oils and are implicated in menstrual pain and headaches.

A 37 year-old man suffered from neuralgia on the right side of his face for five years. He couldn't stand the pain, and asked for surgical relief. He took one to two ounces of castor oil, with a little anise oil added to it, and taken at breakfast. At first it acted as a laxative, but this passed in a few days. He was cured in a week.

Dengue fever is a mosquito carried disease, which may cause severe after pains. A European lady living in India contacted dengue. Four weeks later, she had neuralgia in the upper arms and legs. The muscles were swollen and extremely painful when touched. Heat, massage, wintergreen liniment, guaiacum and aspirin were tried without result. The disorder resembled gout, and as a last resort, a wine with colchicum from the autumn crocus was drunk. This provided quick relief from the pain.

A 30-year-old woman suffered from pain in the middle right finger. The pain was so severe that the neighbors were disturbed by her screams. She had no progress with current medicine, but began taking colchicum wine three times a day. On the following day the pain was less, and in a few days it was gone.

A 56-year-old man suffered from extreme pain in the area of the forehead and left eye. During attacks, it felt like a nail was being driven into his head, and he would bellow with pain. Colchicum wine relieved him in three days.

Elderberries come from a small tree growing in hedgerows and in pastures. In Europe wine growers used them to color white wine so it could be sold for more money. There was a law in Portugal during 1756–1833, that any wine grower having elderberry bushes on his land, could have his land confiscated by the government and be "transported for life." The problem of adulterated wine must have been real, if these restrictions were in effect.

In 1899 Dr. Alois Epstein of Prague, Czechoslovakia had a 51 year old American under his care for trigeminal neuralgia. The patient heard that sailors cured rheumatic pain by getting drunk on a brand of dark red Oporto wine. The patient drank half a liter of wine, and this cured his neuralgia completely. He gave several bottles to Dr. Epstein, who promptly cured a case of sciatica. In the next five years Epstein cured 28 cases of neuralgia, with the remainder of his wine. When his stock ran out, he couldn't find any more wine that cured neuralgia.

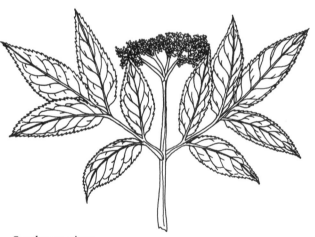

Sambucus nigra
Black elderberry

In 1908 he found another cheap brand that cured neuralgia. He came to the conclusion, that the curative wine was cheap white wine, colored with something to make it red and thus sell for more money. Eventually he found that it was the juice of black and red elderberries ***Sambucus nigra*** and ***S. racemosa***, that colored the wine. He made an artificial port by mixing 18% alcohol with 20% elderberry juice, and with the mixture, he cured a difficult case of neuralgia.

By 1914 he studied 48 cases. The juice would cure early cases in a few minutes, and long standing cases in three to five days. For trigeminal neuralgia, he would give the juice of about 20 grams of the berries for five days. The summer of 1913 was very wet and the berries were inert.

His claims were tested at a Prague hospital on 60 cases. The effects were fast, when the juice was mixed with wine. Neuralgia pains weren't cured if they were due to tuberculosis or other disorders.

A 25-year-old woman was suffering from sciatica. The hospital treatments weren't working, so she was given 25 grams of elderberry juice with ten grams of port wine. The pain ceased almost immediately. Day by day it would return, but less and less until she was completely cured in three weeks. Other patients were treated with morphine and belladonna to relieve their pain, but only elderberry juice permanently took away the pain. It should be added that the roots of ***Sambucus chinensis*** were used in China for pain and numbness.

Facial neuralgia is said to be cured by a tincture of ***Spigelia anthelmia*** if the neuralgia is on the left side of the face. A tincture of ***Prunus spinosa*** is said to cure neuralgia on the right side of the face. The idea is unlikely, but it is possible that both plants are useful in facial neuralgia.

In 1931 the pitcher plant ***Sarracenia purpurea*** was found to relieve the pain of neuralgia. One injection would provide permanent relief of pain for a long time. Initially, the pain would increase, and then it would disappear for a long time. It was tested against Novocain, which provided short-term pain relief only.

Ammonium chloride and ammonium sulfate were isolated from the pitcher plant, and it was believed that these were the active ingredients. However they didn't provide long-term pain relief.

One of the most unusual remedies for the cure of the neuralgias is putting a pinch of powdered salt into the nose on the affected side. One minute the person is suffering from intense pain, the next minute, they are free from pain.

A 59-year-old woman suffered from severe pain around the left eye. A pinch of table salt was applied to the left nostril, and the pain and tenderness disappeared instantly. When the doctor told her that it was only table salt, the patient was astonished.

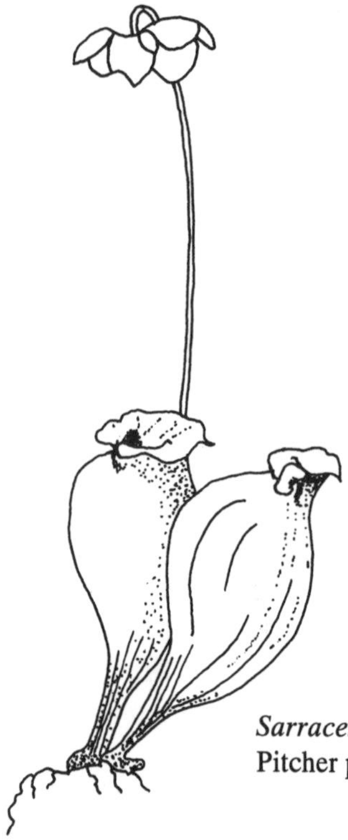

Sarracenia purpurea
Pitcher plant

A 50 year-old woman suffered from severe facial neuralgia, and she tried many remedies without success. The pain was so severe, that she was rarely able to sleep. A pinch of table salt up the nose resulted in instant disappearance of pain from the temples. Both the pain and tenderness disappeared.

A little salt in the nose cured neuralgia following herpes and facial erysipelas. It cured frontal headaches. In some cases of bronchial asthma, there was complete relief. The asthma kept returning, but each time it was used there was more complete relief. Eventually the bronchial asthma disappeared by using only salt.

☆☆☆

TRIGEMINAL NEURALGIA

"Johannes Laurent Bausch had suffered for four years from a harassing sharp, shooting pain in his right maxilla. The pain varied in intensity. It was less at times; at other times it retreated deep into the tissues, or even completely disappeared. However, on the fifth of November 1664, the pain grew so intense that our beloved master became bedridden. Suddenly, like a lightning-flash, the pain penetrated his jaws and his brain. He was almost unable to speak, and was incapable to taking any solid food. Scurvy complicated the neuralgia."
    – A eulogy to the founder of the Imperial Leopoldina Academy of Natural Sciences at Nuremberg

The old medical writers spoke of seven pairs of cranial nerves, for they were unable to do the precise anatomical work needed to differentiate the nerves. In 1778, Samuel Soemmering found that there were 12 pairs of nerves, exiting through the openings at the base of the brain. It took a long time for his classification to be recognized in medicine, but eventually it was added to the textbooks. Generations of doctors said to themselves, "On old Olympus towering tops, a fat armed German viewed some hops." What they were remembering was: "olfactory, optic, oculomotor, trochlear, trigeminal, abducent, facial, acoustic, glossopharyngeal, vagus, spinal accessory, and hypoglossal nerves."

The trigeminal or fifth nerve has three branches, which run from the upper part of the ear to above the eyes; to the nose through the upper cheeks, and through the lower cheeks to the jaw. This nerve transmits the sensation of the face. Unlike other parts of the body, these nerves are subject to greater extremes of cold and hot, so perhaps they have a reason for misbehaving.

Electric shock-like pains, usually restricted to the trigeminal nerves characterize trigeminal neuralgia. It is curious that 60% of the sufferers are women, and the majority have problems on the right side of the face.

In his famous *Canon of Medicine,* ibn Sina Avicenna (+980-1037) mentions the disease of 'leqvet,' which affects the face and teeth. Most of his description covers facial paralysis, but he does mention that another sign of the disease is pain in the face with convulsions on one side. He recommends hot baths, resting in a dark room and wine.

The first true description published by a doctor was in +1677. John Locke examined the wife of the English ambassador to France, and wrote a description to four doctors, asking for their advice. He describes Lady Ambassadise as being in a fit of such virulent and exquisite torment, that it forced her to such cries and shrieks, as you would expect from one upon the rack. The fits came on like a flash of fire on the right side, with convulsive motions. These 'fits' began sometimes by opening her mouth, or touching her gums. Doctor Locke treated her with purges, and applied a 'blistering plaster' to her neck, and it seemed to do her some good.

The first cure to be discovered for the disorder was written up in an 1822 book by Benjamin Hutchinson. He treated 30 cases with ferrous car-

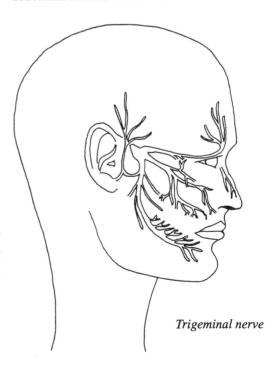

Trigeminal nerve

bonate in four-gram doses twice daily. His cure was ignored for over a hundred years, until a doctor dug up the book in a library, and read some of the letters written by the suffering patients. Iron carbonate brings relief in about half of all cases, and it usually lasts for years. Relief generally comes in eight to ten days, and even if it doesn't cure the problem, it brings enough relief, so that sufferers can eat and carry on normal activities without experiencing unbearable pain. The mineral is taken with the meals, to avoid intestinal upset. This large amount of iron borders on the toxic level, but it did not seem to harm anyone.

A modern study of the old remedy was done on 91 people. Twenty-four had major improvement, and ten were benefited. However, the other 57 didn't obtain much help.

Medical literature contains several remedies which worked for one sufferer, but were not tried on a group of people. Castor oil as a remedy was discovered by Carl Gussenbauer. He gave a patient castor oil as a laxative before surgery to clean out the intestinal tract. The patient reported that it cured his trigeminal neuralgia.

A further report on castor oil in 1902 indicates that it may permanently relieve the pain. An ounce is taken before each breakfast, and in three to four days the pain begins to disappear, and it produces a cure. One doctor gave his patient injections of iodides, bromides, morphine and chloroform. Nothing controlled the pain, until he took castor oil. Then it stopped for a long time.

A 74 year old man had trigeminal neuralgia for seven years. The act of speaking and swallowing began to cause him great pain. Mucus collected in his mouth and swallowing was impossible. This greatly disturbed the man, and made sleep difficult. His doctor gave him pilocarpine to dissolve the thick mucus, and he began to sweat and salivate profusely. The symptoms of trigeminal neuralgia left, and with further treatments the man was cured. Pilocarpine is the alkaloid of a common Brazilian herb, known as jaborandi.

In 1912 a French doctor published a report on the use of *Chelidonium majus* in treating the disorder after he was unsuccessful in treating it with *Thuja*. He tried adding five drops of greater celandine juice to a glass of water, and had the sufferers drink the water whenever thirsty. It reduced the pain and suffering to manageable levels within a week and cured the disorder.

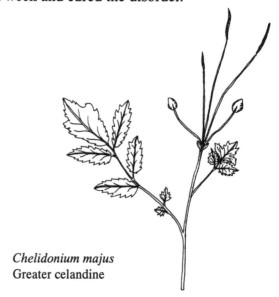

Chelidonium majus
Greater celandine

A 43 year-old woman had excruciating pain when she brushed or combed her hair on the right side. She tried drinking 30-60 grams of *Aloe vera* juice daily. In two weeks her pain diminished significantly. Then she went on a two-week trip in which she did not take the juice and the pain returned. When she resumed taking the juice the pain disappeared. She drank the juice for six months, and the neuralgia was cured.

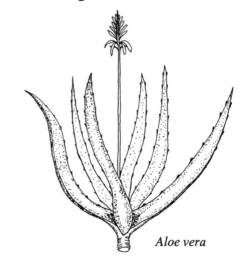

Aloe vera

There are few poultice type remedies for trigeminal neuralgia, because the pain is so intense that people are afraid of triggering it by touch. Ice has been applied to deaden the nerves and stop the pain. A poultice of well-bruised laurel leaves *Laurus nobilis* was applied to the face for about 15 minutes until it is slightly red. This results in a particular smell on the breath and taste on the tongue. Applications of laurel poultices are said to be helpful, and often permanently remove the affliction.

Perhaps the best treatment discovered for neuralgias and trigeminal neuralgia was discussed in the medical literature back in 1854. Doctor Lecointe found that high doses of German camomile *Matricaria recutita* over a period of a few days would permanently remove most neuralgias and reduce the frequency of migraines. Another French doctor confirmed his results in 1923 by successfully treating trigeminal neuralgia and migraines. The remedy was taking three to five grams of the powdered flowers daily or mixing 100 grams of the herb in boiling water and drinking it.

Generally four grams of powdered German chamomile are taken every three hours during waking hours. In one case a 60 year-old man suffering from severe facial pain, noted that the pain was almost gone by the second day, and by the third day he was cured. A 50 year-old woman suffered from facial pain for ten years. After drinking three cups of strong chamomile tea each day, her neuralgia diminished in intensity by the third day. In six weeks, she was completely free of pain. Another woman had neuralgia with migraine headaches. After taking German chamomile her pain began diminishing the same day. In four days the neuralgia was gone, and the migraines became rare. She found that she could stop migraines, by drinking strong chamomile tea before they developed.

During WWI workers in an English airplane factory complained that their faces were getting numb. An investigation revealed that the solvent they were inhaling at work was at fault. One of the men had the idea that older people subject to trigeminal neuralgia should inhale trichlorethylene, and this was quite successful in relieving the pain. The problem is that the solvent damages the liver, so its use was discontinued. In our time, doctors discovered that about 60% of the sufferers have satisfactory pain relief by taking a gram of the drug carbamazepine a day.

In 1939 an attempt was made to treat trigeminal neuralgia with injection of Vitamin B1. From 30 to 100 mgs. of B1 was supplemented with fish liver oil and Vitamin D. The injections were given every day, and no attempt was made to treat this by mouth. Within three months 7 of 11 people became symptom free and 2 were improved.

In 1951 when Vitamin B12 became available in quantity, it was discovered that high doses of the vitamin frequently brought long-term relief from the pain of trigeminal neuralgia. The vitamin is so active that 30 micrograms taken over a period of a few days cures anemia. When 1,000 micrograms (1 milligram) was given by injection two to three times a week over a period of four to eight weeks, it cured the condition. In the first study nine out of 13 cases were completely relieved, and the other four cases had moderate relief from severe pain. It should work by mouth was well, but in many people, the vitamin is poorly absorbed from the intestinal tract. Many cases had long-term remission of pain, but other people needed to take it on a daily basis to remain free from pain.

Dentists occasionally see a painful condition known as TMJ or Temporomandibular Joint Disorder. The pain is so severe that surgery and nerve crushing is often done. It seems that TMJ is another version of trigeminal neuralgia. The simple therapies used to treat the neuralgias should bring relief to sufferers of this disorder as well.

SCIATICA

"These diseases occur at all ages, but are more frequent in middle age. In sciatica, there is pain in either or both hips; the latter is called 'double sciatica.' There is a feeling of heaviness and difficulty in moving about; and sometimes there is numbness and irritation of the skin, sometimes with severe pricking and burning pain. This gives the patient the feeling of an animal's sharp movements. The pain begins in the hip and moves into the side and the buttocks. It can pass into the knee from the hip and the ankle down into the foot."

Caerius Aurelianus +5th century.

The word sciatica is derived from the Greek word for hip-joint. Sciatica is a syndrome characterized by pain, radiating from the back into the buttocks, along the sciatic nerve. This is the nerve which ultimately controls the movements of the legs, feet, and toes. It is the manifestations of this syndrome that create such a problem with low back pain.

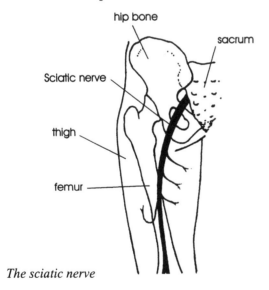

The sciatic nerve

The cause of sciatica can be purely physical. In 1932 an operation was performed on a man who had a skiing accident resulting in intractable low back pain. A small projection of the cartilage had pressed against the nerve. There is no physical cause for the majority of cases, and operations will do nothing to solve the problem of low back pain.

There is some evidence that the problem of sciatica is related to the the ability of the nerve to stretch. If you have sciatica and lie flat, then when your legs are lifted, there may be pain or tension, if you try to keep the legs straight.

One of the ways sciatica is treated is to anesthetize the person and then flex the leg, stretching the nerve. It takes about ten days of stretching for the problem to be solved. Since it is known that low back pain can be cured or helped by doing sit-ups, it is probably of great benefit to do toe touching exercises, so these will stretch the nerve.

Local applications are rare in the treatment of trigeminal neuralgia, but they were common in treating sciatica. French doctors were said to have obtained good results with an ointment of **Veratrum viride** mixed in lard. A poultice of **Iberis amara** also relieved sciatic pain. A poultice of powdered sulfur was also applied. The pain was usually speedily cured. The next day the urine would smell of hydrogen sulfide.

A patient who was treated in an Algerian hospital discovered one of the odder treatments of sciatica. Doctors injected him with salt solutions, but he wasn't cured. When he left the hospital, he began to think that a stronger preparation of salt (sodium chloride), might be more successful, so he got some "spirit of salt," which was hydrochloric acid, and painted it on the skin. This cured the sciatica, and when he returned to the hospital for another reason, he told the doctors. They were interested, and this resulted in a trial of a dozen patients. Brushing three to five applications of hydrochloric acid on the skin cured most of them.

A study was done of the hydrochloric acid treatment in England. It was painted over the tender areas, but if it resulted in redness and irritation, the treatment was stopped. The treatment was done every night for one to three weeks. Of the sixteen sciatics (who had received other forms of treatment without relief), two were completely cured, eleven were relieved of most pain and three had no results. In ten cases where the pain was present in the heels and plantar region of the feet, four were cured, one was relieved, and five had no results.

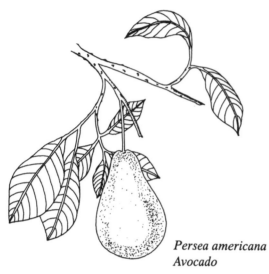

Persea americana
Avocado

A Mexican doctor accidentally discovered another sciatic treatment. He collected avocado seeds *Persea americana* for marking cloth. When the juice is exposed to light, it turns dark brown, and this makes good ink, which can be used in laundries. In order to preserve the seeds, he had to make a fluid extract. At the time he got malaria and suffered severely from intercostal neuralgia [pain between the ribs], and none of the traditional remedies, including morphine, gave him relief. He knew that the local Indians used avocado seeds steeped in rum to treat arthritis, so he had a servant rub his back with the tincture. The relief from pain was rapid. After two treatments he was completely free from the troublesome disorder. He tried the avocado seed extract on a number of people with neuralgia and intercostal neuralgia, and the treatment worked.

The natives of southern Mexico used avocado seeds to treat tapeworm, then took castor oil to expel the parasite. No harmful effects were noted in administering the extract to a dog. When the extract was administered by injection the pulse increased and in fifteen minutes there was complete relief from pain. Doctor Froehling wrote, "I

have not failed to procure relief after the first application, and have generally effected a cure after three or four."

In the Ayurvedic literature of India, sciatica was described under the name "gridhrasi." The legendary doctor Charaka divided it into the 'vatika' type in which the symptoms were pain, rigidity, tingling and restrictive movements and the 'vatashleshmik' type in which lassitude and anorexia were present. The marking nut *Semecarpus anacardium* was one of the chief remedies.

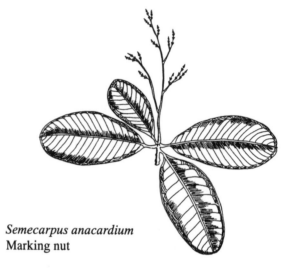

Semecarpus anacardium
Marking nut

In one study, eight sciatic patients were put on a placebo, but none of them had any relief after a week. The next week they were started on a quarter of a marker nut, which was gradually increased, until they were taking two nuts a day after a week. This was continued for a week, and then withdrawn. All of the people in the trial had unilateral pain, numbness, tingling, and a feeling of electric shock-like pains with nerve tenderness. Six of the eight people were free from pain at the end of two weeks. Nerve tenderness disappeared and they could easily stretch their legs. A year later, the patients verified that the condition had not returned. The remaining two people found no relief

The kidney herb *Orthosiphon stamineus* has some effect on sciatica. It is used in cases of painful urination with elevated uric acid levels. It quickly produces marked improvement when a patient drinks a tea made with five to ten grams of the herb. It also relieves nausea, headaches and facial edema. Could the ultimate cause of some nerve pain be due to poor elimination by the kidneys?

Glucurone is an oxidation product of grape sugar and is widely distributed in the body. It is the raw material for forming the jelly-like matrix called hyaluronic acid. The body uses this to make the cartilage between the joints, and the disks between the vertebrae of the back. It forms the sheath of the nerves. There was an attempt to treat arthritis with it in 1951, which wasn't very successful. It was noted, however, that several cases of sciatica were improved. This led to a trial in 25 sciatics. A gram of the sugar-like substance was taken three times a day by mouth. In 80% of the cases, the sciatica went away. The doctor theorized that in the remaining 20% of the cases, a physical cause existed, and the protrusion was pinching the nerve.

A 40 year-old woman with a history of lower back pain radiating into the right leg, failed to respond to all other treatments. She took glucurone four times a day and in two weeks the lower back pain had disappeared. Seventeen months later she was still normal. A 37 year-old man had shooting pains with tenderness down his left leg. After taking glucurone for three weeks, there was no more pain or tenderness.

Linnaeus, the father of modern botany, had a severe case of neuralgia and suffered from the pain. He was told that strawberries would relieve his pain, and he immediately said "Tenebo" [I will make the test.] He ate large amounts of strawberries and his pain went away. Every spring thereafter, Linnaeus practically lived on strawberries, and this is how he controlled his neuralgia.

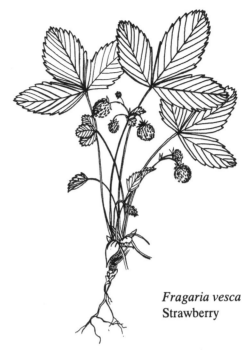

Fragaria vesca
Strawberry

Strawberries contain no alkaloids, or anything that even seems to remotely resemble medicinal chemistry. They are basically a delightful mixture of sugars, red coloring and water. I believe that it was the large amounts of grape sugar in the strawberries, which are oxidized in the body to glucurone. This acted as the healing agent for the cartilage and the nerve sheaths. Before the advent of refrigeration, it was rare to have fruit during the winter, and the neuralgias might have been much more common. Grape sugar occurs in many fruits, and it has been completely ignored as a dietary factor. It is just one of those strange substances that could make the difference between a bad back, irritating nerves and a healthy life.

✿ ✿ ✿

LOCAL ANESTHESIA

*"For let our finger ache, and it endures our other healthful members even to that sense
Of pains: nay, we must think men are not gods, nor of them look for such observances."*

William Shakespeare

"I say that the highest pain, and I say "highest," even if there is another ten atoms worse; is not consequently worse. I can name a number of worthy men, which according to their own account, have suffered tortures of pain from gout for several years."

Cicero -50

The Greek poet Homer is the first to mention the use of a local anesthetic. The subject of his story was the Greek army siege of the city of Troy in -1200. Homer wrote, "Having cut an arrow out of the thigh of Eunypylos, Petroclus put a bitter root on the wound, that took the pain away and ended all the anguish." Opium and mandrakes are not 'bitter roots,' and they are not local anesthetics, so Homer's anesthetic is unknown.

Pliny and Dioscorides mention that a stone from Memphis, Egypt was used as a local pain-killer. It was powdered, mixed with vinegar and applied to the place where pain was. The Memphis stone was the size of a pebble, and in soft black and hard white varieties. The identity has long been lost, but magnesium has some pain relieving properties, so the famous stone could be a form of magnesium. When mixed in vinegar it would form magnesium acetate, which would be more soluble.

At the time of Christ, Dioscorides mentions the anesthetic ability of rose oil for use in the eye. The oil contains beta-phenethylol, which has a high degree of efficiency, and a low degree of toxicity. It is less active in producing local anesthesia than cocaine, which is relatively inactive, except by injection. Perhaps the main reason why it did not become used more, was the loss of the secret of how to distill the oil from roses.

Each species protects itself through camouflage, speed, numbers or through some toxic material. Salamanders have a strong local anesthetic in their skins, which protect them from being eaten.

One of the best ways of curing a toothache was to make a tincture of ladybugs. Druggists in England sold this tincture as late as 1840. Wasps use anesthetics to paralyze prey, on which they lay their eggs. A study of nature's anesthetics could lead to better medical products.

Anesthesia officially came into being when ether was used to produce unconsciousness during operations in 1842. The word anesthesis first occurs in the *Dictionary Britannicum* in 1721. The idea of pain killing has been present for thousands of years.

The first people to have discovered the use of a local anesthetic were the Chinese. This was noted in 1891 when a Western doctor was doing an eye operation using the newly discovered cocaine. A Chinese doctor, who was present, said that they had used a similar substance prepared from the eye of a frog. The real material comes from glands on the back of toads. This is the brown waxy substance, which is sold in Chinese herb shops under the name of senso. It contains three alkaloids, which are considerably stronger than cocaine when purified.

The venom of the Chinese toad is sold in traditional Chinese pharmacies. When cocaine was discovered, doctors began to study other anesthetics, and experiments were done with toad venom in Russia. The alcoholic extract was named 'frynin.' A Russian article in 1904 described its use for cataracts, iridectomies, and blockage of the tear ducts.

One of the oldest popular toothache remedies is clove oil. It is a mixture of eugenol, caryophillin, and vanillin. An initial application of the oil produces a stinging sensation, with mild inflammation and then anesthesia. A case came to medical attention in 1983, in which a woman had accidentally applied some oil near her eye. A year later, the area still had no feeling and wouldn't sweat!

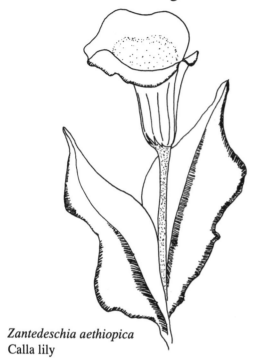

Zantedeschia aethiopica
Calla lily

The beautiful calla lily *Zantedeschia aethiopica*, which is known as the Easter lily, contains an active anesthetic. When it rains, the flower fills with water. Observers noted that birds stopped to take a convenient drink. They become temporarily paralyzed, and stand motionless with their wings outstretched for several minutes. As the anesthetic wears off, they recover and fly away. The alkaloid has been isolated, and it could be used in medicine.

Dental science became possible because of the discovery of local anesthetics. In 1874 the *Cincinnati Medical News* carried the story of a dentist who applied aconite roots to an aching tooth. This produced numbness and made it possible for him to fill the tooth without pain.

John Reed noted that during the dry years in Australia, cattle are forced to eat *Euphorbia drummondii*. The plant paralyzes them and causes death. When Reed applied the juice to his tongue, he could not taste quinine, indicating that his taste buds were paralyzed. He used the anesthetic for sprains and eye problems. When a preparation was sent to Europe, doctors found that it wasn't active,

and it was forgotten.

The Spanish explorers found that most of the inhabitants of the high mountains areas of Peru were addicted to chewing the leaves of *Erythroxylum coca*. Chewing the leaves by themselves does not release the cocaine, but the inhabitants mixed a little ash with the coca leaves to release the cocaine. In 1860 the German chemist Fredrich Wohler noted: "The alkaloid has a bitter taste and a peculiar effect upon the nerves of the tongue making the point essentially numb, and almost devoid of sensation."

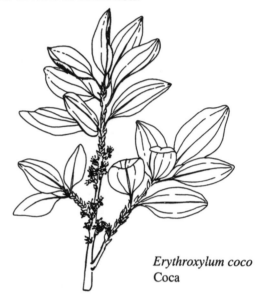

Erythroxylum coco
Coca

There are some 250 species of *Erythroxylum*. Cocaine comes primarily from *E. coca*, which contains up to 0.86% in the leaves. Another economic species is *E. novogranatense*, which contains up to 0.76%. The other species have no cocaine. The second council of Lima condemned coca in 1569 as a useless and pernicious leaf.

Cocaine had side effects, and it couldn't be used in dentistry. The first local anesthesia to gain recognition by dentists in the United States was a mixture of quinine and urea hydrochloride. The injection of a 1% mixture gave local anesthesia that lasted for four to five hours.

Plants related to quinine were tested by applying a solution to the eyes, and attempting to find the lowest dilution that would cause local anesthesia lasting more than 30 minutes. Quinine produces anesthesia in a 3% solution, cocaine in a 2 1/2% solution and hydroquinine in a 2% solution. The alkaloid isoamylhydrocupreine is active at 0.08% making it about 30 times stronger than cocaine.

This alkaloid comes from the false cinchona tree *Remijia pedunculata*.

Sigmund Freud believed that he had discovered a wonderful elixir, and at parties he had his friends take cocaine. After serious side effects and a death from the drug, he wisely turned to his famous couch, and made his place in history by talking, rather than taking drugs. But he got the cocaine anesthesia idea going at a party that he gave to taste cocaine. One doctor remarked: "How that numbs the tongue." The ophthalmologist Carl Koller remarked: 'Yes, that has been noticed by everyone that has eaten it." His statement resulted in a flash of inspiration, and the next day he put cocaine in the eye of a guinea pig. Then he tried cocaine in his own eye. After touching it with a pinhead and not feeling anything, the era of local anesthesia was born.

The problem with cocaine is that it is quite toxic and habit forming. In 1905 the German chemist Alfred Einhorn made a chemical derivative known in Europe as "Procaine," and in America as "Novocain." This was not habit forming, and had a seventh of the toxicity of cocaine. It does not penetrate the skin, so it must be injected.

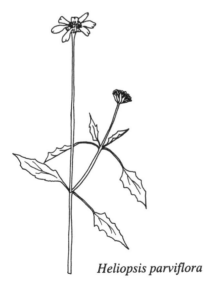

Heliopsis parviflora

Many of the plants known to kill insects are good local anesthetics. A central Mexican mountain plant *Heliopsis longipes* is a well-known toothache remedy. When a fresh root is pressed against an aching tooth, there is an intense numbing activity, which lasts up to an hour. The roots are added to food to make it extra 'hot.' The midwestern US plant *H. longipes* is also a good anesthetic. There

are chemical relatives of this anesthetic in the leaves and roots of *Chrysanthemum anethifolium*, *C. gracilis, C. frutescens* and *Matricaria pubescens*, which comes from North Africa. A local anesthetic with a similar structure is found in the roots of *Spilanthes acmella = S. oleracea*. These plants could be used by dentists, who would not have to inject a narcotic. A pad with the active substance would be pressed against the base of the tooth.

Ethnobotanical literature discloses a number of interesting local anesthetics. Russian researchers found that the roots of the *Fritillaria sewerzowii* lily contain alginine, which has about the same anesthetic activity as cocaine. In western North America the Indians found that the roots of *Wyethia amplexicaulis* numb the skin when applied to it. In central California the Indians mashed the roots of *Tauschia parishii* for toothache and local pains. They drank a tea of it for internal pain. Mexican doctors once used *Bocconia cordata = Macleaya cordata* as a local anesthetic.

In New Zealand the native Maori people chewed the leaves of *Macropiper excelsum* and *Pseudowinteria axillaris* as brush painkillers. The bushmen of the Kalahari Desert used *Sceletium tortuosum*, which has cocaine-like alkaloids. Others with anesthetics are the roots of *Echinacea angustifolia, Ludwigia prostrata, and Luffa echinata* in India. The Central American fish poison *Salmea scandens* is chewed to relieve toothache. In the Amazon *Triolena pustulata* is used for local pain killing. *Sedum acre* is another local anesthetic. The Chinese have a saying: "When knocked down, find *Daphne giraldii* quickly." Applied locally it produces reddening of the skin. When carefully diluted and taken internally, it markedly reduces pain.

Tomato leaves contain an anesthetic and a poisonous alkaloid. The leaves can be dried and powdered, and then extracted with a mixture of alcohol and acetone to remove the anesthetic and eliminate the toxic material. When tested on rats, a 2% solution proved to be as active as Novocain. Te fruits have no activity, and this is fortunate for tomato lovers. If the anesthetic substance was present in the fruit, you might feel like you were leaving a dentist's chair, after eating a tomato.

The Kurnool Medical College in India experimented with a 1-2% extract of the roots of **Anacyclus pyrethrum**. It provided anesthesia more than an hour longer than a 2% solution of xylocaine. In the third world, where hard currency is not always available to buy medical supplies, it may be better to raise an anesthetic, than to buy it.

There are few local anesthetics which penetrate the skin, but a fruit tree growing in India and parts of Africa has one. The leaves of **Ziziphus zizyphus** are chewed and applied to remove the pain of scorpion and insect strings. Both the duration and strength of the mixture of alkaloids is stronger and longer lasting than Novocain. The toxicity is low and the alkaloids have potent surface activity on the skin.

One of the oldest forms of anesthesia is the use of ice packs. Ice by itself is slow, but a mixture of two parts of crushed ice to one part of salt depresses the temperature and results in rapid anesthesia. It initially produces a burning sensation, then a numbness, and if it is not continued long enough to produce frostbite, there is no danger. It took about two minutes of ice anesthesia to operate for ingrown toenail, and six to ten minutes to

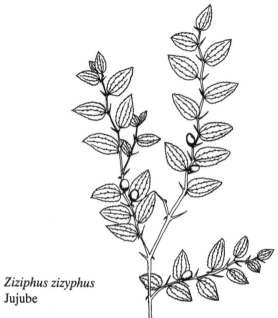

Ziziphus zizyphus
Jujube

remove an abscess from the breast. Minor operations can be done with virtually no pain or bleeding. It is useful for opening boils, removing splinters and small growths. Avicenna wrote a thousand years ago: "The most powerful of narcotics is opium, and among the less powerful are snow and ice water."

✵ ✵ ✵

GENERAL ANESTHESIA

Good News From America
"Hail, happy hour! That brings to glad tidings of another glorious victory. Oh what delight for every feeling heart to find the new year ushered in with the announcement of this noble discovery of the power to still the sense of pain, and veil the eye and memory from all the horrors of an operation. We have conquered pain. This is indeed a glorious victory of pure intellect. And from America comes the happy news from one's brothers in another land. It is the victory of knowledge over ignorance, of good over evil; there is no alloy. All our finer sympathies are enlisted in one universal prayer of grateful rejoicing. Benevolence has its triumph."
$\qquad$ Peoples London Journal January 9, 1847 (The article is talking about ether anesthesia.)

Five centuries before the time of Christ, Herodotus recorded that a Greek army operating in the area now known as Turkey was put to sleep. At that time, armies had little transportation, and they had to live off of the land or starve. They found beehives and eagerly ate the honey. The entire army fell into a deep sleep, which lasted an entire day. Finally they woke up feeling refreshed, but a little strange from losing a day. Bees gathered the honey from an abundance of **Rhododendron ponticum** flowers, which contain a narcotic.

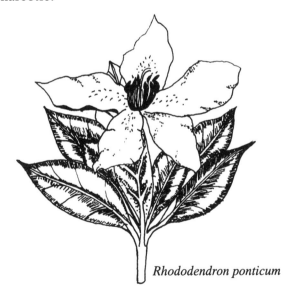

Rhododendron ponticum

During the Roman occupation of the Middle East at the time of Christ, life was harsh and punishment was severe for those breaking Roman laws. A society of women prepared a painkilling potion called "lebonadh," which was given to condemned criminals. This was generally a mixture of frankincense and wine, which was believed to enable the soul to escape from the pain-racked body. This drink was offered to Jesus dying on the cross.

The most powerful of all anesthetics is made by microscopic sea plants. Certain fish and shellfish concentrate the toxins. One of the most popular Japanese fish delicacies is sliced raw globefish eaten with horseradish, vinegar, and soy sauce. Japanese cooks must be licensed by the government to prepare it, because the poisonous liver and ovaries must be removed.

Pure tetrodoxin is 160,000 times stronger than cocaine. It was the source of U.S. patent #1,058,643, but it seems to have had little use, perhaps because it is so powerful. The results of its use are described in this old Japanese poem.

> *Last night, he and I ate globefish,*
> *Today,*
> *I help carry his coffin.*

Before modern times, pain was a part of sickness, and few doctors had any effective remedies. Pressing the carotid artery on the side of the neck temporarily blocks the blood supply to the brain and makes people unconscious for five to fifteen minutes. Aristotle wrote: "Again, those who press the veins of the neck become unconscious." A German doctor tried the method on 25 patients, and was able to put 17 of them to sleep.

The carotid artery runs from the heart, through the front of the neck to the brain. The word 'carotid' comes from the Greek word for 'sleep.' The native doctors on Java placed their hands on the neck and pressed the carotid artery with the thumbs. In a few seconds the head falls back, and the subject appears to be in a state of sleep.

The great French surgeon Ambroise Pare wrote of making patients unconscious for operations, by hitting them on the head with a mallet. He said that this should be done with great care, not too powerful a blow, on a nonvital spot.

On the march to Moscow, Napoleon's chief surgeon, Jean Larrey, found that wounded soldiers needing serious operations suffered little pain, because of the cold. Refrigeration anesthesia eased the pain of the suffering, after the battle of Eylau on the way to Moscow. There have been some experiments with cold anesthesia. Dentists have tried placing a cold probe against the jaw of the teeth needing work. Dental work can usually be done without pain, using cold to numb the teeth.

In an earlier era, alcohol was used for anesthesia. Concentrated alcohol was used in surgical operations, after distillation become widespread around +1500. The conclusion of experimenters is that alcohol does not reduce the pain; the person simply doesn't care about the pain.

The one great general anesthetic of the ancient world was the roots of the mandrake *Mandragora officinarum*. Hippocrates recommended mandrake roots soaked in wine for those "saddened in spirit and ready to destroy themselves." The Jewish historian Josephus said that it was useful for curing sick people dying from demons. Pliny mentions that taken properly, it brought sleep, but an overdose killed those taking it.

The mandrake became embodied with human qualities and digging it up meant death, unless an unlucky dog was used to pull it up. The root diggers who were glad to protect their monopoly and keep the price of the root high probably spread the legend. Doctors didn't understand that a 50-pound child wouldn't receive the same dosage as a 200-pound man. The lack of standardization was probably the reason why the plant fell into disuse. Too little and the patient was in pain, too much and the patient never woke up.

Pirates once captured Julius Caesar. He was ransomed with a large sum of money and mandrake wine. Polyaenus wrote: "The pirates rejoicing at the great amount of money, hastened to indulge in a sumptuous banquet and drank the drugged wine and were thrown into a stupor." Then Caesar put his sleeping captors to death. Roman troops used the same trick once in North Africa. They fled their camps on the approach of the enemy, leaving large containers of mandrake wine. The enemy then proceeded to drink themselves to sleep, and the Romans returned and captured them.

History has many references to mandrake wine. The Greek orator Demosthenes likened some of his hearers to those who had drunk mandrake wine, and were impossible to arouse. Xenophon said: "Wine, moistening the soul, lulls cares to sleep, just as the mandrake does man's body." The Roman army doctor Dioscorides wrote: "Physicians also employ this remedy when a necessity arises of amputation, or of applying the actual cautery." Avicenna wrote: "If anyone wishes any of his members cut, let him drink three obols of it in wine, and it will produce a stupor."

The use of mandrake wine gave way to the 'sleeping sponge' of the Middle Ages, which was a mixture of narcotic herbs. The sleeping sponge was an invention of Hugo de Lucca in +1220. The formulas for the sponge do not seem to have the anesthetic activity that was claimed for them. Without effective anesthetics doctors took to performing operations in minutes. On the other hand, patients preferred death to the operation, particularly if they were old.

Perhaps the Chinese were the first to discover general anesthesia, although it wasn't widely used. A tincture of *Jasminum sambac* was made with wine. It was claimed that one inch of an average root would produce unconsciousness for one day, two inches for two days, and three inches for three days. It is very poisonous, and if it was used, an overdose would often have meant death

In 1823 a Mississippi planter suffered from a fever. He requested that his servant bring him a tea from a certain root for his illness. The servant gave him the wrong tea, and the planter found that all power to move his muscles was gone. He couldn't move an eyelid, yet he could hear and understand the conversations around him. When he recovered from the paralysis, his fever left.

The planter tried yellow jessamine *Gelsemium sempervirens* on other persons. A patent medicine maker heard the story and produced "Electric Febrifuge," a tincture of yellow jessamine disguised with wintergreen oil. Doctors used it for anesthesia, but after losing too many people to overdoses, it was forgotten.

At about the same time William Hamilton was vacationing in Jamaica. He noted that the native fishermen used the bark of Jamaica dogwood *Piscidia piscipula* to paralyze fish. It was put into ponds and still water. The tree was believed to be the strongest during the full moon of April, and inert at other times.

He mixed an ounce of the powdered bark to 12 ounces of brandy and strained this 24 hours later. He added a drachm (3.7 grams) to a glass of cold water for a severe toothache. There was a burning sensation in the stomach, then sweating and then profound sleep for 12 hours. When he woke the next day, he was still holding the tincture bottle in one hand and the empty glass in the other. The plant was of considerable medical interest, but it fell into disuse with the discovery of anesthetic gases.

The Jamaica dogwood relieves mild to moderate pain and acts both as a local and general anesthetic. The active ingredient is rotenone, which was once a popular insecticide, used by farmers to control bugs. In large amounts it is potentially toxic, and could cause convulsions and death.

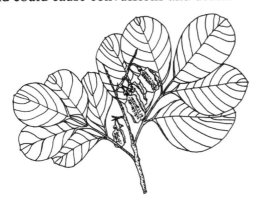

Piscidia piscipula
Jamaican Dogwood

During the early era of anesthesia, opium was conspicuously absent. Even though the opium poppy was widely grown in the Middle East, it was rarely used in killing pain. Plutarch wrote that those who gathered the juice of the poppy fell asleep. In +45 the Roman doctor Scribonius Largus described the process of making cuts in the unripe seedpod, to increase the amount of opium. Only in recent times, when we separated morphine from the opium alkaloids, has the opium poppy been a prominent painkiller.

A common garden plant which is a member of the same botanical family as the opium poppy, has strong narcotic properties. *Chelidonium majus* has a morphine-like chemical. It is less toxic, and gives marked relief of pain in cancer without a tendency to sleep, and without the troubling constipation which opium and morphine cause. Chelidonium sulfate has been given by mouth in amounts of 100-200 mgs. for cancer.

Embelia ribes is a common bush in India, and the black pepper-like berries are used in Ayurvedic medicine. When embelin is made into potassium embelate it can be taken by mouth, and it compares well with morphine. The anesthesia of morphine wears off in two hours, but embelin wears off in about four hours. In a week, morphine becomes less than half as active as the body adjusts to it, but potassium embelate does not. The anesthetic doesn't work on the opiate receptor sites, so it doesn't have the side effects of morphine.

One of the interesting chapters in the history of anesthesia was the attempt to make a useful anesthesia from puffball mushroom smoke. Beekeepers have long used the smoke to sedate the bees while gathering honey. In 1853 Benjamin Richardson began by experimenting on a kitten in a bell jar. The smoke from the dried mushroom anesthetized the kitten in half an hour. When it was removed, it was insensitive to pain and continued to sleep for the next two hours.

Richardson tried dogs and produced complete anesthesia in six minutes. The smoke was irritating to the throat and eyes, so he filtered it through potassium hydroxide to remove the carbon dioxide and particulate matter. He anesthetized a dog with a tumor, and the operation was without pain for ten minutes until the last stitches were put in.

He tried anesthetizing himself with burning puffball mushroom. In about four minutes he was in a stupor. The smoke irritated his throat and made his voice hoarser. With the availability of the new gas anesthetics his results were forgotten.

The modern era of anesthesia began with nitrous oxide in 1844, ether in 1846 and chloroform in 1847. James Simpson and his two assistants tested dozens of chemicals by sniffing them. On

November 4th, 1847 they found that a breath of chloroform put them to sleep so quickly, that they fell on the floor with a deep whiff. The editor of the *Lancet* wrote in an editorial in 1847 that anesthesia has "An unparalleled influence on the practice in this country." Only a year before the editor of the *Philadelphia Medical Examiner* had written: "We are persuaded that the surgeons of Philadelphia will not be seduced from the high professional path of duty into the quagmire of quackery by this will-o-the-wisp." But those who wanted pain-free surgery and dental work quickly put an end to his opinion.

☆☆☆

SLEEPING HERBS

"Now, blessings light on him that first invented this same sleep! It covers a man all over, thoughts and all like a cloak. It is meat for the hungry, drink for the thirsty, heat for the cold, and cold for the hot. It is the current coin that purchases all the pleasures of the world cheaply. It is the balance that sets the king and the shepherd, the fool and the wise man even. There is only one thing, which somebody once put into my head that I dislike in sleep. It is that it resembles death. There is very little difference between a man in his first sleep, and a man in his last sleep."

Don Quixote Michael Cervantes

Nobody really knows why we sleep, although there is no shortage of theories. It is theorized that the body builds up chemicals that are broken down during the process of sleep. Those who have forced themselves to stay awake for up to ten days develop a psychosis akin to mental illness, which disappears after sleep.

A small handful of people appear to need little or no sleep. Spanish scientists tested a man who hadn't slept for 30 or more years. He was a simple illiterate shepherd, but comfortable beds, hypnosis and powerful sleeping pills would not put him to sleep. He wasn't tired; he wanted to sleep, simply because he didn't have anything else to do at night. In England, a farmer who hadn't slept for 46 years was hospitalized. During his stay in the hospital, he was given sleeping pills, but they didn't help him sleep.

Most of us require about eight hours a night. Thomas Edison operated on two or three hours a night, but he took frequent short naps throughout the day.

Sleepwalking is rare, but individuals find their way in the dark and go through normal motions during sleep. It was reported in 1930, that an Italian family of four all walked in their sleep. One night they happened to come together during sleep at the kitchen table. They might have returned to bed without being aware of the night meeting, but one of the children happened to loudly scrape the leg of a chair on the floor and that woke everyone up.

The Greeks had a famous temple at Epidaurus, where pilgrims came to be healed in their sleep. They brought a sacrifice to the temple, then they were bathed and purified, and a gift was laid on the altar. One of the evening prayers said by the priests has been preserved: "O ye children of Apollo, who for many in past time have stilled the wave of sorrow, and shown a light of safety for those who travel, be pleased to receive our prayer which ye inspire in sleep and vision. Order it rightly we pray you, according to your loving-kindness. Preserve from sickness, give the body such measure of health and strength as may enable it to obey the spirit within, that our days may be passed in vigor and in peace." The lamps were put out and the pilgrims were encouraged to believe that the Greek God Asclepius would give them guidance and healing in their dreams. When the ruins of the temple were excavated, a stone stele was found on which grateful pilgrims listed 44 different cures.

In 1909 Doctor Lemesle set up a 'castle of sleep' in Touraine, France. Patients fixed their eyes on bright objects and heard the monotonous ticking of a clock to dull them before sleep. The windows were made of blue glass, because it appears to make people sleepy. The aim of the treatment was to get patients to spend as much time in sleep as possible, waking only to eat.

In the late 1950s a Chicago woman elected to take her two-week vacation under sleep-induced hypnosis. She was awakened several times a day for food and elimination. At the end of two weeks of sleep, old health problems disappeared, and she looked years younger.

There is no sharp line between sleep and waking, and army soldiers on long marches may fall asleep while marching. Insomnia may have physical causes, such as parasites and anemia. Sleep is more likely to be disturbed in dry air and deeper in humid air. Sleep is deeper when the air contains more negative ions.

Some smells may contribute to sleep, and hop pillows are a traditional aid. This use might have come from observations of hop-pickers that their children quickly fell asleep in the hop fields. King George III could not sleep without his hop pillow. One doctor spent many sleepless nights rather than take narcotics to go to sleep. He found that bunches of blooming heliotropes *Heliotropium arborescens* in the bedroom, put him into a deep restful sleep.

In Denmark it was common knowledge that black mussels *Cyprina islanica* made people sleepy. People ate them because they could easily be gathered along the shore, and when other foods were scarce, they were available. Parents noted that when children ate them, they became sleepy and weak in the knees. When sailors ate them, they became so sleepy that often the whole crew fell asleep together. The mussels were particularly active in September, which indicates that the sleepy substance was absorbed from the seasonal diatoms they feed on. Doctors in Iceland and Denmark recommended them to patients who had trouble sleeping.

Adenosine, which is present in some herbs, and nicotinamide, which is Vitamin B3, protect laboratory animals against audiogenic seizures. Adenosine has an opposite effect to caffeine. The combination of these chemicals elevates the amount of the energy-rich muscle driving compound known as ATP, and reduces the rate of breakdown.

In mice, which are subject to seizures, nicotinamide provides 20% protection, and adenosine provides 55% protection. A combination of the two substances protects all animals. When the mixture was given to mice, they could not stand on their feet, and rested their heads on the ground with their eyes half closed.

Italian researchers found that the blood of those suffering from insomnia had low levels of magnesium. By increasing the magnesium, sleep increased. A mixture of Vitamin B6 and magnesium was said to be especially effective in aiding sleep.

Perhaps the most interesting herbal sedative is the sleepy grass *Stipa robusta*, growing in the Sacramento Mountains of New Mexico. In the spring, the young grass puts grazing animals to sleep, without toxic effects. As the grass dries out in the sum-

mer, it loses its sedative power. The Mongolian species *Stipa inebrians* does the same thing.

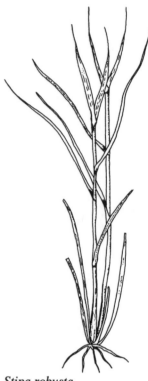

Stipa robusta

Horses are said to sleep up to ten days after eating the grass, although three days is much more likely. Usually the animal awakens and is hungry, so it eats a few mouthfuls of the grass, and then it falls asleep again, until, maddened by thirst, it rushes to the nearest stream. If your horse falls asleep after eating the grass, a thunk on his head will make him roll his eyes, but he will remain useless, until the effect of the grass wears off. Horses don't learn to avoid the grass, but cattle eat it only once.

Before the coming of white settlers, Indians used sleepy grass to tame wild horses. When horses wandered into the area and ate their fill, they awoke with a rope around their necks. While they were still groggy, it was a simple matter to break them. When cattle are transported long distances, they often become ill, and may not eat for days. If they could be fed sleepy grass just before shipment, they would be calm and unaffected.

The ranchers of Otero and Lincoln counties of New Mexico have another reason for disliking the grass. They face the problem that coyotes enjoy eating sleeping sheep, and they would love to have the grass eradicated. The chemical in sleepy grass has been isolated, but neither herbalists nor pharmacists have used it.

A medical experiment used German chamomile *Matricaria recutita*, to see if a strong tea was useful for heart patients. The doctors had twelve patients drink the tea before cardiac catheterization. Anxiety is common before the procedure, because there is pain. In this case ten of the twelve people fell asleep, some only ten minutes after drinking the tea.

There are 53 species of the water fern *Marsilea*

distributed over the world. This plant grows on the surface of ponds, where it forms a scum. It is listed in the Ayurvedic books of India, as a treatment for insomnia. Clinics in India used it for the mentally ill, because of the strong sedative properties.

In Bengal both ***Marsilea vestita*** and ***M. rajathensis*** are used in sleeping preparation. ***M. vestita*** contains up to 0.1% marsiline in the leaves, and laboratory tests show strong sleep-producing activity in rabbits. The roots of ***Zornia gibbosa*** are used by some tribes in India for sleep.

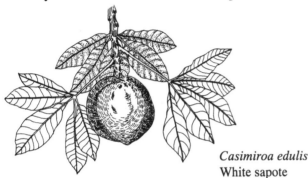

Casimiroa edulis
White sapote

The white sapote tree ***Casimiroa edulis*** produces an edible fruit, which is slightly bitter. Cultivated varieties of this tree are grown in California and Mexico. The old Nahuatl name for the fruit is 'cochiztzapotl' meaning 'sleepy sapote.' Extracts of the leaves, seeds and bark are used in Mexican folk medicine for sleep. Eating the fruit produces drowsiness, but it is not commonly available. The active chemical is disodium dimethylhistamine.

In Mexico there was an old magic sleeping drink known as 'sinicuichi.' Three separate plants were used in different areas to make the drink known by that name. The plant that had the most powerful effect was a tea of ***Piscidia piscipula***, which is the bark of the Jamaica dogwood. A small amount produces a deep sleep. The other two sleep plants were a fermented drink of ***Heimia salicifolia*** and the seeds of ***Rhynchosia precatoria***.

A study was done of a water extract of valerian roots by giving people either placebo tablets or valerian extracts. The sleepers had to evaluate the quality of their sleep. Poor sleepers found that they had a 30% increase with a placebo, but a 50% increase in good sleep with valerian. This was surprising, because the chemicals in valerian are relatively insoluble in water, and it was believed that they were not absorbed.

The Roman emperor Marcus Aurelius took the compound herbal tonic known as theriac. It made him sleepy, so he had the poppy juice removed. Then he had insomnia and couldn't sleep, so his doctor put it back in. Around +165, there was a rumor around Rome that Aurelius was addicted to the mandrake in his theriac.

Belladonna has narcotic action, and it was once used to promote sleep. Chaucer described it in *The Reeve's Tales* under the name of dwale: "To bed wente the daughter right anon; to bedde goth Aleyn, and also Jon, ther nas no more, hem neede no dwale."

There is an ancient Chinese remedy for insomnia, which was first described 2,000 years ago. It contains five herbs, but the only one by itself that is a sedative, is the seed of the jujube ***Ziziphus spinosus*** or *Z. ziziphus*. It has recently been the study of pharmacologists in Taiwan. It improves all of the measures of sleep; when you awake you feel rested. Peasants often used from 15-25 seeds of *Zizyphus*.

In China the young shoots and leaves of the common peanut plant ***Arachis hypogaea*** are reported to be a strong sedative. An ounce of the peanut shoots are put in boiling water, and the tea is drunk before bedtime. It has been tested on mice. None of the control mice went to sleep, but those receiving a tea of peanut leaves slept for 30 minutes.

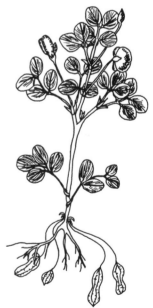

Arachis hypogaea
Peanut

A 54-year-old woman could only sleep one to two hours a night. Tranquilizers failed her, but after three days of fresh peanut plant tea, she was able to sleep four to five hours. Ten days later she was sleeping almost normally and didn't need the tea.

Among other things reputed to induce sleep are almonds, catnip, fennel, hops, lettuce, passion flowers and rosemary. Tinctures of mullein, oats and orange flower are reported to be actively sedative. The Menominee Indians made a tea of the partridge berry **Mitchella repens** for insomnia. The early American pioneers were reported to have found that the powdered root of **Cypripedium pubescens** was an effective sleep herb. No studies have been done on these folk remedies. A tea of orange tree leaves is said to be a strong sedative, which brings sleep.

Along the northwest Pacific coast, the sea milkwort **Glaux maritima** grew along the tideflats and sea beaches. Some of the coastal tribes dug and ate the roots. They only ate them in the evening, because they made the eaters very sleepy.

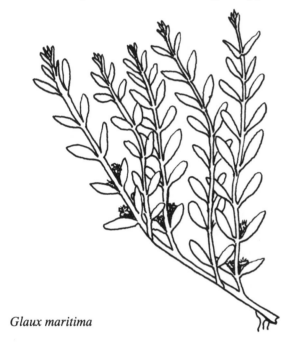

Glaux maritima

In the Amazon a tea of **Souroubea crassipetala** or **S. guianensis** is said to bring sleep. In the Caribbean the leaves of the soursop **Annona muricata** are used. In Central America **Passiflora ciliata** is the preferred sleep herb. Scientists have not found any sedative compounds in this plant. In Cambodia the fruits of **Diospyros decandra** are used for insomnia. In the Kalahari Desert of South Africa, Bushman mothers give a drop of the juice of **Sceletium anatomicum** to fussy infants. It puts them to sleep for up to five hours.

A sleep problem which many people suffer from, is sleep apnea, in which breathing stops momentarily. This is often due to nasal obstruction or high blood pressure. When the blood pressure is reduced, the problem goes away. Japanese doctors found that a thiamin supplement often corrects it.

One man suffered through ten years of sleep disturbance problems. He had great difficulty falling asleep and then awoke frequently. The army was hell for him, because it meant bedtime at 9 PM and rising at 4:30 AM. As a student he couldn't take early classes, for he simply couldn't stay awake. He tried all the sleeping pills and therapies. He even went to Europe for electrosleep therapy, but this didn't work well.

His thyroid was found to be underactive and he was able to function better with thyroxin. He ran across an article describing a relation between the hypothyroid condition and Vitamin B12. He began to take 0.2 mgs. of B12 and his sleep began to improve. In three weeks he was able to maintain a normal sleep schedule with relief from nocturnal body jerks. When he discontinued the B12 his sleep cycle began to deteriorate.

His experiences stimulated some research into B12 and sleep. It is not uncommon for the blind to follow a lunar cycle of 25 hours, which means that their 'sleep day' will drift one hour a day from the 24-hour day. A 14-year-old blind girl followed the lunar cycle since the age of one. When she was given B12 supplements she returned to a normal 24-hour cycle.

Three young people with delayed sleep syndrome weren't able to get up in the morning or get to sleep at night. They were given 3 mgs. of B12 a day, and in a few days the sleep cycle returned to normal. Other people with diffi-culty in falling asleep at night, or waking in the morning had the same result.

It is believed that Vitamin B12 sensitizes the body's clock to natural sunlight. The levels of the light hormone melantonin in the body are lower at night and higher in the daytime. This means that the vitamin increases the body's response to sunlight. This makes it of great interest in treating depression caused by lack of sunlight in the winter months.

☆ ☆ ☆

SENILITY

"He that has once the "Flower of the Sun", the perfect Ruby which we call elixir,
By its virtue.
Can confer honor, love, respect, long life, give safety, valor, yea and victory.
To whom he will. In eight and twenty days, he'll make an old man of fourscore a child. "

The Alchemist Ben Jonson 1619

"As in a dream I look on the shrubbery, aglow in the full moon on the sloping rock,
And my entire life passes before me like a vision.
The islands far below in the dim light of dusk, surrounded by the pale autumnal reeds,
This then is autumn, oh my soul. "

From the Chinese poet Tu Fu c. +750

When we picture ourselves as aged, we imagine being stooped and hobbling about. The real burden of age is not physical, but when the mind ceases to work normally. Consideration of this phenomenon has only taken place in the past 150 years. In the Middle Ages people did not generally live beyond the age of 40, although a few lived to an old age.

In the days of the Inquisition, *The Hammer of Witches* was used to eliminate all of those possessed by evil. The records show that a number of women who were victims of senile dementia were put to death. The inquisitors were punishing people who were merely suffering from the problems of old age.

In 1907, Alois Alzheimer published an account in a German psychiatry journal, of diffuse cortical atrophy with changes in the intracellular neurofibrils of the brain. This condition was thought to be present in about 5% of the aged. For the next 60 years, it was accepted that Alzheimer's disease was a rare condition, affecting only a small portion of those that we would call senile. In 1966, doctors reported that a full 50% of those suffering from 'senility' showed degeneration of the brain, as described by Alzheimer. The word 'senility' was dropped, and 'Alzheimer's disease' became the new buzzword of the doctors. However the other 50% did not show degeneration of the brain. So we are replacing a word with another medical term to give it more respectability. We still don't under-stand it, and most of those with 'Alzheimer's disease show only mild brain degeneration.

The chief signs of senility are the impairment of memory and intellect. Talk may become disjointed and ungrammatical, the dress may become untidy, and the person may be indifferent to his or her surroundings. With a CAT scan and magnetic resonance scanning, it is possible to tell which areas of the brain are working properly, and which are not. After spending thousands of dollars on testing, it doesn't help to be able to say "senile psychosis," when we have no cure, and we are simply using bigger medical words, to say what everyone knew all along.

There is a theory that Alzheimer's disease is actually a viral infection of the brain. When senile plaques were injected into the brains of monkeys, they produced a neurological illness equivalent to Alzheimer's. The viral disease known as 'kuru' of New Guinea mimics the signs of old age. People had hand tremors, slurred speech, jerky movements and their thinking capacity faded. The disease became notorious, because it only affected tribes of cannibals, and women were usually the victims. The women traditionally ate the brain, which was infected with the virus, and the men ate the body. With the extinction of cannibalism, the disease disappeared.

People with high intakes of soluble aluminum are known to show signs of senility. There is conclusive evidence that high levels of aluminum are correlated with the disease. Aluminum reduces the circulation in the brain, and this impairment of circulation, apparently fails to give brain cells the nourishment that is needed. Aluminum is not a factor in other cases.

Some who show signs of senility are often vitamin deficient. The chief deficiencies appear to be Vitamin B12, folic acid and iron. All of these are necessary to the red blood cells, which carry oxygen to the body. In England, these cases were chiefly elderly women, who lived on bread and tea. A change in diet did not cure them, but the addition of 20 mgs. a day of folic acid and an iron supplement produced a dramatic change in two months. Their minds went from confused to normal and their homes went from chaotic to tidy.

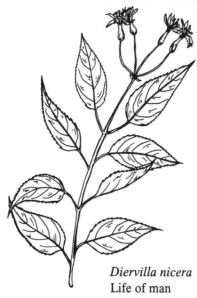

Diervilla nicera
Life of man

Herbal literature contains little help for the aged, but there are several notes that remain untested. The roots of 'life-of-man' *Diervilla lonicera* are said to provide a tea that cures senility. Gentian root was once prescribed for the 'softening of the brain.' In Colombia, South America, *Ranunculus peruvianus* is used as a stimulant tea for the weak and aged. In the Amazon, a bitter tea of *Pagaea recurva = Irlbachia recurva* is used to treat forgetfulness in the elderly, and the powdered leaves of *Cassia lucens* are said to help people remember. *Epimedium koreanum* is said to cure forgetfulness in Korea. In China *Ligusticum wallichii* is used to treat angina, because it improves blood circulation. It has shown promising results in treating senility.

The herbalist John Gerard wrote: "Sage helpeth a weak brain or memory, and restoreth them being decayed in a short time." In England, sage was widely believed to prolong life. It turns out that this may have validity. A screening of plants showed that sage oil inhibits acetylcholinesterase. This enzyme breaks down the chemicals that transmit nerve impulses. It may augment memory in the aged.

Richard Brook's herbal lists *Teucrium scordonia* as a brain stimulant for the elderly. Gerard's herbal mentions the "sickness called the forgetful evil." He recommended using the oil of cow parsnip *Heracleum maximum*. During the Middle Ages in Europe, rosemary in wine was used to treat failing memory. This may be why Shakespeare spoke of rosemary for memory.

In the South Pacific there is a slightly narcotic drink known as 'kava' which is prepared from *Piper methysticum*. German researchers found that it reduces some senile effects.

Many species of yams have crude steroids, and these serve as raw materials, for the production of commercial steroids. At a Moscow clinic Dr. Yurikov treated 26 patients suffering from cerebral arteriosclerosis with extracts of *Dioscorea polystachya*. Initially 50 mgs. were taken and this was increased to 800 mgs. It took from 12 to 75 days to restore the vitality and mental functions of the patients in the test.

Can senility be due to a clogged circulatory system? Dicoumarol is a product of spoiled sweet clover, and it is used to prevent blood from clotting. When it was tried on 13 people confined to a mental hospital with 'senile dementia,' ten improved. One patient could be discharged, and three were now able to feed and care for themselves.

In one case a successful 56-year-old lawyer began to forget the names of his coworkers. He became unmanageable at home, and had to be sent to an institution. By taking dicoumarol, he could take care of his work, but when he stopped, he became confused and uncooperative.

There are numerous herbs and therapies which decrease the amounts of cholesterol and increase the circulation. Trials should be done on combinations of these herbs known to increase circulation. These are dealt with in other sections of this book.

The ginkgo is one of the world's oldest surviving trees. It is related to the ferns, not to the other trees. It was found in the forests of China, and reintroduced to the US, where it had been the source of the petrified forests 70 million years earlier. The tree is either male or female, and only the female trees have the delicious ginkgo nuts. The nuts are surrounded by pulp, which contains butyric acid. This is one of the odorous components of human sweat. This is why nearly all city ginkgo trees are male.

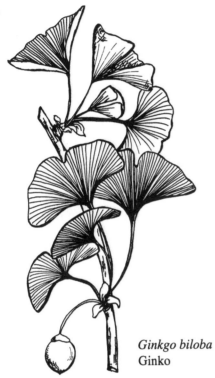

Ginkgo biloba
Ginko

A ginkgo leaf preparation has been the subject of many medical reports in Europe. In some cases, people who had been completely senile for 20 years took the preparation for six to eight weeks, and their minds began to clear. For the first time in years, they were able to recognize relatives and talk about things and events, which had long been forgotten. It was as if 20 years of their life had never existed, and now they were able to return to the world of the mentally active.

A test of the ginkgo extract, known as Tebonin in Germany, was done on 81 people with degenerative arterial and cerebral vascular disease. Fifty-one people reacted positively. The first changes happened in three to four weeks. There was better memory, hobbies were taken up again, and headaches and noises in the ears disappeared. It became easier to fall asleep and concentration improved. This extract has been used for years in Germany.

Ginkgo leaf extract is now available in health food stores. A friend gave this to her grandmother, who steadily improved in mental function over a period of months. When relatives came over who hadn't seen her for some time, they were surprised, and remarked about how much clearer her memory had become.

Chinese pharmacologists have isolated a chemical from *Huperzia serrata*. It shows a marked effect in increasing the efficiency of learning and memory in animals. When rats were given 100 micrograms of huperzine A, twenty minutes before training, there was a significant decrease in the number of trials needed to escape danger. The alkaloid showed strong anticholinesterase activity, and acted like physostigmine. Clinical trials of huperzine show good results in senile dementia, and it may soon be available for those suffering from the problems of age.

The American club moss *Lycopodium clavatum* is thought to have similar properties. The common European club moss *L. selago* was once used for medicine, and it has been found to contain the same chemical. This moss was said to be one of the secrets of the Druids of England, although they probably didn't use it for this purpose.

The fungus known as ergot *Claviceps purpurea* constricts blood vessels so that it would be expected to decrease brain function. A chemically processed ergot alkaloid known as hydergine apparently does just the opposite. It is a popular prescription drug in Europe, and it is often given before operations to reduce the effects of a lack of oxygen. In the US the maximum permitted dose is 3 mgs. per day, while in Europe it is 9 mgs. a day. At the higher levels it seems to act as a nerve growth factor, and it increases the level of neurotransmitters. This often results in a marked increase in mental function.

When rats become about two years old, they begin to show memory and learning loss similar to us. Japanese scientists tested an extract of an herbal mixture known as 'shosaikoto' in rats that were 110 weeks old. The old treated rats returned to the same abilities as six-week-old rats. The average learning time in rat tests was 63 seconds at six weeks, and this increased to 102 seconds after 110 weeks. The herbal extract enabled the old rats to learn at the same rate as the youngsters.

Shosaikoto is a water extract of 2 grams *Glycyrrhiza glabra*, 3 grams *Panax ginseng* roots, 7 grams *Bupleurum falcatum* roots, 5 grams *Pinellia ternata* tubers and 3 grams *Zizphus zizyphus*. The herbs were boiled and filtered and 120 mgs. of dried extract was given per kilogram.

Rats are tested for learning efficiency in mazes, and old rats show scores nearly double those made by young rats. In normal conditions young rats ran mazes in 23 minutes while making 27 errors. When allowed to remain in negatively ionized air they made 28 errors in 24 minutes. This is slightly worse for young rats, but within the limits of error in the experiment.

Old rats made 79 errors in 49 minutes in another trial. When they were exposed to negative ions, the score changed to 39 errors in 23 minutes. They were able to run the maze in the same time as the younger rats and their ability to remember the correct turns was much better. The experiment suggests that if your memory is fading, it would be of help to get a high capacity air ionizer for the bedroom. It will help you to sleep better and it may make a considerable improvement in your ability to function.

In Switzerland, tablets of an herbal preparation based on 500 mg. tablets of cinnamon, licorice, plantain, lettuce, marigolds, Iceland moss and other ingredients were taken for circulatory disorders. The tablets were taken twice daily, by a group of elderly people. In the area of sleep, energy and memory, 60% of the persons showed considerable improvement, and 30% reported some improvement.

Three centuries ago Bishop Hough said: "Whatever may be said in favor of it, old age is a losing game." It is not how many years we live, but how we make those years productive. Those who have many interests, and who get regular exercise, good foods and herbs, are more likely to remain healthy and active, until the time comes for us to leave the physical plane of existence.

✿ ✿ ✿

MEMORY HERBS

"My mind lets go of a thousand things, like dates of wars and deaths of kings,
And yet recalls the very hour – twas noon by yonder village tower,
And on the last blue noon in May – the wind came briskly up this way,
Crisping the brook beside the road; then pausing here, set down its load,
Of pine scents, and shook listlessly, two petals from that wild-rose tree."

"Memory" by *Thomas Aldrich, 1880*

Socrates explained memory this way: "There exists in the mind of man a block of wax. When we wish to remember anything we hold the wax to it, and receive its impressions as from a seal of a ring. We remember and know what is imprinted, for as long as the image lasts, but when it is effaced or cannot be taken, we forget and do not know."

Two thousand years have passed, and we still don't know what memory is. There is evidence that memory is the linking of proteins. When an antibiotic that breaks down proteins was given to fish, recently learned memories were lost. If we found something that enhanced the formation of memory proteins, perhaps we could have a super memory.

Several tribes have herbs that were supposed to make people forget. An Indian tribe along the San Juan River in Brazil used a preparation to make prisoners forget their homeland, and their loyalty to its rules. Boys in West Africa who witness secret initiation rites are given a potion to make them forget. In East Africa the Tonga tribes use *Annona senegalensis* to make babies forget the experience of nursing, when they are to be weaned.

There is a curious Mexican plant drink, which has a reputation as both a memory herb, and an aid to forgetting! Depending on the area of Mexico, 'sinicuichi' is either *Heimia salicifolia, Rhynchosia precatoria* or *Piscidia piscipula*. The bark of *Piscidia* roots kills fish and tastes somewhat like cinnamon. A tincture of this is known for putting people to sleep.

Heimia must be gathered wild, for in cultivation it loses its properties. The leaves are soaked in water and left to ferment. Farmers like to forget their troubles by drinking it, and it is often mixed with alcohol. It is a sedative, and the hearing decreases, and voices sound far away. On dark days it gives the vision a yellowish cast. People who drink it regularly forget things that have happened a few minutes ago. There seems to be a tremendous ability to remember things that have happened in the first years of life and even before this life!

There is a Mexican legend that before soul entered the underworld it drank a magic potion to forget its earthly existence. This potion is sinicuichi. The seeds of *Rhynchosia* cause memory loss, and they are taken as a narcotic rather than a mind stimulant.

The early explorers of the Amazon basin encountered a legend of a tribe of Indians who had perfect memory using a magic plant. If they wanted to recall any incident through their life, they ate a plant and then lay in their hammocks. They would swallow the fruit, concentrate on the event, and then everything would come back to them in exact detail. Nobody was able to track down the tribe or the plant.

It is known that the seeds of *Virola bicuhyba* are used by the tribes of southeastern Brazil as a memory reviver. The resin is used to treat sores and fungal infections. The seeds possess narcotic qualities. Could this be the source of the legend?

The first historic person to work with the art of cultivating the memory was the Greek poet Simonides. He was reciting poetry at a banquet, when he left the room. While absent the ceiling collapsed, crushing the guests. Simonides was able to identify the bodies, because he remembered exactly where everyone was sitting. He used pictorial association to impose ordered images on the mind. Nearly every book on memory follows this technique.

At the Greek town of Paros, archaeologists dug up a pillar inscribed with the great events of Greek culture and their dates. These were the invention of the flute, introduction of wheat, publication of Orpheus' poetry, and then dated at -477 was the memory system of Simonides!

St. Augustine considered this faculty as one of the three powers of soul, which were memory, understanding and will. Generations of Christian clergy used the association technique, to help their illiterate parishioners associate the various types of sins, with the proper regions of hell.

The art of associative memory became identified with the Roman lawyer Cicero, at the time of Christ. His name comes from 'cicer,' the wild pea, because of the peculiar dent in the tip of his nose. In early life he had asked the Greek oracle at Delphi how he could have the greatest honor in life. The pythoness replied that he was to make his own genius, and not the opinion of the people, the guide of his life. During the turbulent political times, he played a powerful role in shaping Roman justice. He remembered the names of thousands of Roman citizens, and although he probably didn't write any memory books, manuscripts on the Ciceronian art of memory circulated during the Middle Ages.

Galen, the great Roman doctor, was baffled when a patient came to him after losing his memory. He searched the book collections until he found a book by Archigenes on memory restoration. He didn't agree with the author that the seat of memory was in the heart, but the treatment was successful. The man was bled and mustard packs were applied to his head. He was told to eat mustard, artemisia and watercress. The tradition that watercress stimulated the memory survived in the proverb: "Eat cress and learn thereby."

There are many other suggestions in old herbals. Parsley roots finely chopped and added to wine were supposed to clean the brain, and help the memory. *Melissa officinalis* is known as the heart plant, but it is supposed to influence the memory. Another memory mixture was composed of marjoram, balm mint, nutmegs and cardamoms. The Cherokee Indians used a root tea of *Cynoglossum virginianum* for bad memory.

In *Gulliver's Travels* Jonathan Swift expressed the idea of eating a 'cephalic tincture' on a wafer in order to impart knowledge to schoolboys. The idea of 'smart pills' might have come from the famous insanity treatment center on the Turkish coast town of Anticyra. The Roman philosopher Careades visited it and took the treatments before entering into a long series of debates with other philosophical schools. He won his debates. He reasoned that if the taking of hellebore made the insane sane, it would make normal people brilliant.

The minerals in our bodies influence learning. Hair analysis shows that the best students have more zinc and copper, but the poorest students have elevated levels of toxic lead and cadmium in the hair. When cats were injected with a small amount of potassium salt before a training session, they learned as fast as the smartest cats of a group, and all 'potassium cats' were bright. All of the cats injected with calcium were 'dumb.' Would we learn faster by switching to diabetic salt, which is potassium chloride?

The classic memory herb was the nuts of *Semecarpus anacardium*. This is the marker nut of India, because the black ink in the husk is used to mark clothing. It was spoken of as 'the golden acorn that re-establishes memory and facilitates the perception of ideas.' Paulus Aegina, Rhazes, Serapion and Avicenna all recommended it for loss of memory. It was used to treat palsy and facial paralysis; and recent studies have focused on it as a cancer treatment. Nobody has tried to determine if the memory legends had any truth.

Another suggestive herb is found in *Medicine of the Prophet*. Iman Al-Jawziyya wrote, "Someone complained to Anas, God be pleased with him about a weak memory. Anas replied: 'Soak frankincense overnight in water and drink the solution in the morning on an empty stomach, for it benefits the memory.'" Paracelsus also recommended this bit of folklore.

Acorus calamus has a great reputation as a brain tonic in India. 'Vacha' was given to schoolchildren to help them with their studies. One study showed that it increased the percentage of alpha waves in the brain by 13%. These waves are believed to be associated with creativity and imagination. *Celastrus paniculata* has a great reputation in India and Ceylon as a brain stimulant. The seeds and oil are sold under a native name meaning 'brain polisher.' A double blind test indicated that the herb really didn't work, but many of the people taking it seemed happier, so it may have mood affecting properties.

Rats were either given an extract of the seed

oil, or a *Celastrus* seed extract by injection. In 15 days the rats showed an increase in the size of the nuclei in the granular layer, and the Purkinje cells of the brain. There was an increase in the lipids, phospholipids and protein content of the brain.

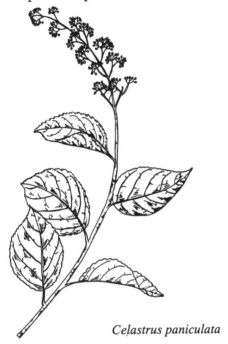

Celastrus paniculata

At Benares Hindu University in India, studies are in progress on an herb known as 'shankapashpi.' *Convolvulus pluricaulis* is known to reduce anxiety. The children receiving the herb increased their IQ by 7% over those receiving a placebo.

The witch doctors of South Africa are supposed to remember hundreds of facts, rituals and plants. When they are given their initiation into their profession, they take the African 'forget-me-not' *Myosotis afropalustris* to develop the memory. Many of these people have good memories, but this may be due to their system of mental training. Let's not forget the 'forget-me-not,' as a possible brain stimulant. But, let's remember that it does contain toxic chemicals among its possible beneficial ones.

Russian and Polish scientists have produced reports on *Schisandra chinensis* seeds as a treatment for fatigue. Experiments indicate that small amounts shorten reflex time and speed up learning, but larger amounts cause restlessness, aggression and insomnia. It is said to normalize brain waves after exhausting mental work. According to Russian reports, taking 100 mgs. of the seeds en-

ables people to double their mental work without experiencing fatigue.

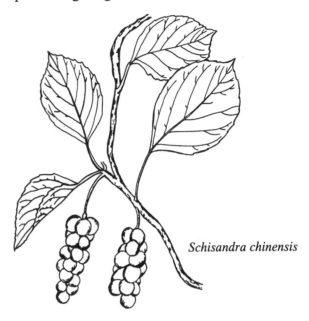

Schisandra chinensis

An extract of *Ginkgo biloba* is used to treat memory lack in the aged. Eight women took the herb in a double blind crossover trial. Six hundred milligrams of the extract significantly improved short-term memory. The reaction time to recall the memorization of six digits was cut in half.

Another study was done by giving people 40 mgs. three times a day of *Ginkgo biloba*. This produced an improvement in short-term memory and elevated the mood. It reduced headaches, vertigo and tinnitus. The results kept improving through the year of the test.

The general factor that we call intelligence may be due to the interconnections between the brain cells. Certain alcohols play a crucial role in encouraging increased neurite growth. A screening test was made for plant factors that influenced the growth of neurites. A southeastern Asian plant *Hygrophila erecta* increased neurite growth by four to six times and nearly doubled both the protein content, and the activity of two neuron-specific enzymes. The plant was used in folk medicine to heal wounds. It is not known if it would increase intelligence, but the prospect is interesting.

Wheat germ oil contains another nerve growth factor known as octacosanol. It was first identified in 1933 as a natural component of plants. The seedlings of rice are one of the richest sources at 481 micrograms per gram. Wheat germ oil has four alcohols, which stimulate nerve growth. They are the 24-carbon tetracosanol, the 26-carbon hexacosanol, the 28-carbon octacosanol, and the 30-carbon triacontanol.

A friend of mine developed memory problems. Years before, he had been treated with the antifungal agent Griesofulvin. His memory became so bad that he had to stop the treatment. Now he was approaching 60, and his once excellent memory was poor. One day he heard two women talking in a health food store about cod-liver oil. "I'll try some," he thought, so he bought a bottle. This brought about a remarkable improvement in memory. In a few days he was able to remember names and dreams. The effect seemed to wear off after about a month, although the memory remained better than before.

This goes along with the discoveries of Aryeh Routtenberg about the nature of memory. He found that a chemical inside cells called PKC forms both short and long-term memory. When the cell is alerted that it needs to form a memory, a chemical notifies PKC, which starts a chain of brain cell connections. Routtenberg found that corn oil was a good stimulant of PKC production. Mice given supplements learned up to 20% faster than control mice.

Scientists have not done much work into investigating natural substances for altering the memory, but there are a few hints. Volunteers, who could remember an average of six nonsense words with a placebo, could remember an extra word with choline. If they took the narcotic scopolamine, they could remember about one less word. A Japanese report indicates that the brain becomes more electrically active after taking plant growth hormones. Vitamin B6 acts as a plant-rooting hormone, and there is some indication that it stimulates the memory.

Scientists have found that memory gets better with constant work in remembering. When volunteers worked every day memorizing long lists, their ability to remember increased, because they made the effort to remember. It may take a while before we have herbal smart pills, but the possibility of memory improvements through herbs and nutrition seems good.

DEAFNESS

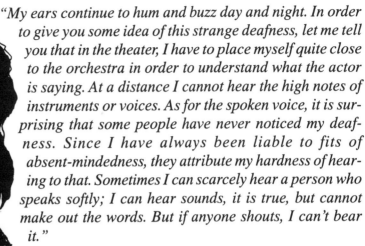

"My ears continue to hum and buzz day and night. In order to give you some idea of this strange deafness, let me tell you that in the theater, I have to place myself quite close to the orchestra in order to understand what the actor is saying. At a distance I cannot hear the high notes of instruments or voices. As for the spoken voice, it is surprising that some people have never noticed my deafness. Since I have always been liable to fits of absent-mindedness, they attribute my hardness of hearing to that. Sometimes I can scarcely hear a person who speaks softly; I can hear sounds, it is true, but cannot make out the words. But if anyone shouts, I can't bear it."

A letter from Ludwig van Beethoven to Dr. Franz Wegeler on June 19, 1801.

Perhaps the first person to understand the nature of sound was the early English poet Geoffrey Chaucer (+1340-1400). In *The Hous of Fame*, he is taken to a place between the sea, earth and heaven where everything spoken and done on earth was stored. The eagle that took him explained that sound is merely broken air, and that words and music break air into sound. The eagle explains that this can be demonstrated by throwing a stone into water and watching the waves.

The nature of sound as vibrations was a subject of the earliest physics studies. On August 8, 1666 Samuel Pepys wrote in his diary: "I discoursed with Mr. Robert Hooke about the nature of sounds, and he did make me understand the nature of musical sounds made by strings, mighty pretty; and told me that having come to a certain number of vibrations proper to make any tone, he is able to tell how many strokes a fly makes with her wings by the note that it happens to in music."

Around 1875 a small surveying party were working near what was to become Yellowstone National Park. Doctor Charles Turnbull and a teamster in charge of the horses and mules, were the only people in camp. The teamster was deaf, so sign language and writing had to be used. Nearby was a large gathering of Crow and Nez Perce Indians on the Yellowstone River.

A medicine man rode into camp, and kept asking about the deaf man. Then he walked down to the stream, and returned with a flat rock the size of a man's head. This was to be heated, placed in a hole in the ground and covered with a wet blanket. The patient was to pour rattlesnake liver oil into his ears for 'six sleeps,' and then the ear was to be steamed, and this would restore his hearing. The Indian doctor was given a fee of coffee and sugar, and he rode away to join his gathering. His remedy was sold for deafness, because the AMA announced in 1926 that they had put "K-17" (rattlesnake oil for deafness), out of business.

Before the modern era of sign language, little was known about the world of the deaf. The Law of Moses said that no one should curse the deaf — after all, it was the will of God that they were deaf! The Christian church looked down on their intellectual capabilities, but it permitted marriage using sign language.

The deaf were often ignored, because they had no way of communication. Sir Walter Scott painted an interesting picture of Zara in *Peveril of the Peak*. Charles Dickens wrote about Sophy in *Dr. Marigold*. She was a deaf child who was bought for a song and renamed for a lost daughter. Dr. Marigold taught her the alphabet and she responded by learning quickly.

In an earlier era, hearing disorders were marked by superstition. The dominant figure of learning of the 13th century, Albertus Magnus, wrote, "Lion's brain if eaten causes madness; but remedies deafness, if inserted in the ear with some strong oil." The saintly German monastic leader, St. Hildegard of Birgen wrote, "Deafness may be remedied by cutting off a lion's right ear, and holding it over the patient's ear just long enough to say, 'Hear, Adimacus, by the living God and the keen virtue of a lion's hearing.'"

A 14th century manuscript at the Bibliotheque Nationale of Paris is perhaps more rational: "Take a houseleek *Sempervivum tectorum* and rub it up carefully. Then roast four fresh fat eels of equal length on a spit. Collect the fat as it melts, and mix it with the fat of foxes and the juice of the houseleek. Drop the mixture in the sound ear at bedtime, and it will run through into the diseased organ. The following day drop it into the diseased ear, and on the third day as hot as possible, into the sound ear, and thou wilt be cured."

The minute amounts of energy that vibrate the air are funneled into a drumlike structure, and then transferred to three tiny bones that shake special nerve cells. As the ear be-

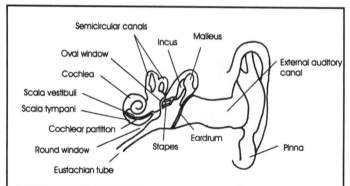

Sempervivum tectorum
House leek

comes less sensitive, we lose the ability to hear the fricative consonants- ch, f, s, sh, and th. As hearing decreases further, we lose the hearing of the explosive consonants, which are b, d, k, p, and t. Normally we hear the sentence: "The sounds of the deaf." With moderate loss others hear "e ound o e dea." With severe hearing loss people hear "e oun o e ea." A child who is deaf to high tones, will say 'f' for 'th' and 'th' for 's' and 'y' for 'l'. If the speech isn't right, perhaps the hearing isn't right, and a test is in order.

Hearing loss may be selective. If we are exposed to a constant industrial pitch, the cells responding to that pitch will cease to respond. Loud noise decreases the hearing sensitivity, and eventually permanently damages the hearing. A father walked his daughter to a rock concert, and asked: "Can you hear the sound of your footsteps?" When he picked her up after the concert, he asked the same question, but this time she couldn't hear her footsteps on the sidewalk.

About 12% of the adult population suffer some hearing loss. The problem of deafness is directly correlated with blood circulation in the ear. The thicker the blood viscosity, the poorer the circulation, and the greater the hearing impairment. When blood cells clump together, the surfaces are smothered, and oxygen availability is reduced. Heat and fevers reduce the fluidity of the blood and cause hearing loss. Chlorophyll is known to reduce blood sludging and often it reduces deafness and tinnitus.

In one case a 61 year old man became increasingly deaf over a 15-year period, and he was totally deaf in his left ear. Before being given the blood thinning agent dicumarol, he couldn't hear his own voice. When he took chlorophyll supplements, ear noise (tinnitus) ceased to be a problem and he could hear better.

Another indication that hearing loss is a circulatory problem comes from the fact that briefly breathing high levels of carbon dioxide can markedly improve hearing. This gas makes us pant when we run, and it dilates the circulatory system, in an automatic effort to release it through the lungs when we work hard. It produced a significant improvement in hearing in 55% of those treated.

One promising solution to the problem of treating the inner ear is by mixing vasodilative agents, with the skin penetrating solvent DMSO. This was tried on a group of 15 people, who sprayed a solution into the auditory canal every four days. Nine recovered completely from the buzzing in their ears, and half of those with dizziness were cured. The ear temperature rose from 36.8 C. to 37.9 C. indicating an improvement of blood flow to the inner ear.

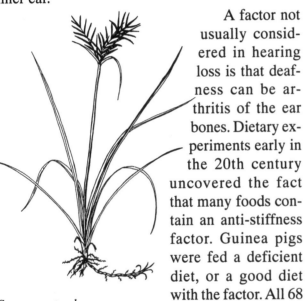

Cyperus rotundus

A factor not usually considered in hearing loss is that deafness can be arthritis of the ear bones. Dietary experiments early in the 20th century uncovered the fact that many foods contain an anti-stiffness factor. Guinea pigs were fed a deficient diet, or a good diet with the factor. All 68 guinea pigs on the good diet had no hearing problems; but those fed the deficient diet produced 19 deaf animals. A common anti-stiffness factor is sitosterol, and several closely related natural steroids. The roots of *Cyperus rotundus* are particularly rich in this factor. This could be the secret of earwort *Dysophylla auricularia = Pogostemon auricularia*, which was once used to treat deafness.

The one herb known to affect the buzzing and dizziness of Meniere's disease is black cohosh *Cimicifuga racemosa*. It was used by gradually increasing the drops until you become dizzy! This meant that it was affecting the inner ear, for this is the balance organ of the body. Often there was a remarkable increase in healing when Meniere's disease was treated. The herb is a good way of treating arthritis. If deafness is due to arthritis of the ear bones, the herb could be particularly valu-

able. Nobody has bothered to do a controlled test of it.

"Bee glue" also known as propolis comes from plants and is gathered by bees to seal spaces in the hive. It was made into a tincture with 40% alcohol and mixed with corn or olive oil in a 1:4 concentration. It was put into the ears of 382 people in Russia. It improved the hearing in 314 people, but there was no improvement in the rest. Ear noise troubled 106 people; but after treatment the noise disappeared in 62 and decreased in 16.

Several reports claim that high levels of Vitamin A could improve hearing, although this is disputed. Dr. Lobel injected 50,000 units of Vitamin A in olive oil twice weekly for six weeks. He found a measurable improvement in 15 of 30 deaf people. There was a reduction in ear noise as well.

Other doctors claimed that thiamin could improve hearing and Meniere's disease. Thiamin and nicotinamide are claimed to bring about a slow improvement in hearing. Hearing loss is linked to zinc deficiency and when older people take zinc supplements, they claim to hear better, and troublesome ear noises disappear.

In 1960, a large French study was done on the treatment of deafness with vitamins and amino acids. Twelve injections were given every other day for 24 days; then there was an interval of 15 days. This course of treatment was repeated four times over a five-month period. Within 30 minutes of each injection, there was often an immediate improvement in hearing. Children generally benefited the most, with a marked ability to hear high frequency sounds. About 60% had good results, and some 25% had no results.

One of the long forgotten remedies once used by 'aurists' for treating deafness is putting glycerin into the ears. In 1851 Thomas Wakley, the editor and founder of the Lancet, ''rescued' the remedy so it could be used by doctors. He found that in many cases in which the eardrum appeared to be dry and scaly, glycerin drops had a fair chance of success. In one case a 49 year old woman had been deaf for six years. After seven weeks of glycerin, the woman's hearing was restored, and the eardrum surface was now a healthy pink.

In another test of glycerin, a doctor claimed that four out of six cases had hearing improvement. In the two cases in which the patients said there was no improvement, the relatives noticed that they no longer had to shout to them. Some of these people might have suffered from impacted earwax, and not all cases had a true hearing improvement. Glycerin is available at any drugstore and earplugs can be used to hold it in place at night. It is worth trying for two months, for many people seem to have had remarkable benefit.

The Taiwanos of the Amazon treat deafness with the leaves of *Heteropterys olivacea* in oil. Culpeper wrote, "The juice [of *Glechoma hederacea]* dropped into the ear doth wonderfully help the noise and singing of them, and helpeth the hearing which is decayed." At the time of Christ, Celsius wrote:, "The dropping in of the juice of unripe grapes mixed with rose oil is fairly effective against deafness."

There are a number of short articles on the use of mullein *Verbascum thapsus*, as a tincture made with alcohol in the treatment of deafness. In one case two girls were rejected from school, because they couldn't hear. When two to three drops of mullein mixed with glycerin was put in their ears daily, the hearing improved enough in three weeks, so that they could return to school.

In 1912 an Eclectic doctor reported that a mother brought her boy to him saying: "He's becoming deaf like his father." The doctor gave the boy mullein drops to put in his ears. Weeks later, the father dropped into the doctor's office to thank him for restoring his hearing. He used the extra drops in his son's formula.

There are a number of old reports that pilocarpine injections can cure some cases of deafness. The alkaloid in this herb causes sweating. This substance comes from the Brazilian herb known as jaborandi *Pilocarpus microphyllus* or *P. trachylophorus*.

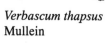

Verbascum thapsus
Mullein

After experiencing profuse sweating a few times, the hearing would often markedly improve. Other cases had no improvement with jaborandi.

In the inner ear, there are special hair cells, which transmit the vibrations of sound to the nerves. When these cells die or are damaged by loud noise, we lose our hearing. Hearing aids cannot regenerate the cells. Scientists have found that that chemical forskolin which is present in *Coleus barbatus* actives the cAMP protein activator. This activation leads to the regeneration of the hair cells of the inner ear. This finding has aroused hope for hearing regeneration.

In 1932 two German doctors presented evidence that the bone marrow of young animals contains some sort of growth factor. When they gave raw bone marrow to two older people, their senile deafness disappeared.

In areas of China with low levels of iodine in the soil, there are many deaf young children. When iodine supplements are added, their hearing gradually returns to normal in one to three years.

Another curious way of treating hearing loss is adding Epsom salt to hot bathwater, and immersing the ears in it for ten to fifteen minutes. The salt baths are used every other night, for the first weeks, and then are progressively reduced. A 42-year-old man could hear a test sound five feet away in the right ear and two feet away in the left ear. After a week of soaking the ears in a pound of Epsom salts, the hearing was 15 feet in the right ear and nine feet in the left ear. When he continued the baths for some time, he could hear a whisper in each ear at thirty feet. In another case a 64-year-old business manager was about to lose his position. He could only hear a sound four feet away on the right side and four inches on the left side. After two months of soaking in the baths he could hear sounds at ten feet on the right and two feet on the left.

In the era of hearing aids, we no longer attempt to restore lost hearing. These old accounts taken from medical journals indicate that many people could lead a life without hearing aids, through the use of simple remedies.

MENIERE'S DISEASE

"This morning, sitting in a bed, I had a fit of giddiness; the room turned round for about a minute, then it went off, leaving me sickish, but not very. I saw Dr. Cockburn today, and he promises to send me the pills that did me good last year; and likewise has promised to send me an oil for my ears, that he has been making for that ailment, for somebody else."

Jonathan Swift 1710

"Feverfew Tanacetum vulgare *dried and made into powder, and two drams [seven grams] of it taken with honey or sweet wine, purgeth by siege melancholy and phlegm; wherefore it is very good for them that are giddy in the head, or which have the turning called vertigo, that is, a swimming and turning in the head."*

Herball, or General Historie of Plantes *John Gerard*

If you can hear a slight bit of buzzing or tingling noise in quiet circumstances, you're normal. The faint noise in our ears may be due to the circulation of the blood, past the sensitive hearing nerves. We don't normally notice it, unless we plug our ears. If we listen to the 'roar of the sea' in a seashell, we are really amplifying the faint sounds of the inner ears. If the noise is disturbing, then it is known as tinnitus.

It is a common belief that when your ear tingles or buzzes, somebody is talking about you. Variations of this belief are that tingling of the right ear means somebody is speaking well of you. If the left ear tingles, somebody is speaking badly of you. Noise in the right ear is also supposed to mean that a woman is talking about you, and noise in the left ear means that a man is talking about you.

I once knew a woman who would extend her arms when her ears buzzed. She would slowly rotate until the noise stopped, and then stop to think of who lived in that direction. Then she would say that so-and-so must be talking about her. She was doing what Pliny had written about 2,000 years before: "And then besides, it is a notion universally received, that absent persons have warning that others are speaking of them, by the tingling of the ears."

Hearing voices in your head can be a sign of insanity, but it can have some mundane causes. Several cases are known where individuals living near powerful radio stations could hear the broadcast. What seems to have happened is that metal fillings in the teeth picked up the signal and transformed it into pulses sufficient to be heard. There are cases of farmers who claimed to hear radio stations while out in their fields. What apparently happened is that the zinc coating on the fence wire crystallized and formed a detector. When a powerful radio transmitter was nearby, the cows got a free concert.

The same nutritional and physical factors which act against deafness also act in tinnitis and Meniere's disease. The therapies used in deafness are of interest here. Anemia and high blood pressure may also cause tinnitus. Ear noises usually occur on one side, and 'buzzing' is a common description. The first treatment for the disorder is attributed to the famous medical school of Salerno, Italy. They recommended mixing wormwood *Artemisia absinthium* with ox-gall and putting it into the ears.

Ear noise is much more common when the blood clumps or sludges. The fluidity of the blood is increased by heat, and having a fever may decrease noise in the ears. However, high fevers can cause the blood cells to clump and increase the ear noise. The fluidity of the blood is in relation to the charges on the surface of the blood cells. In theory, a supplement of potassium citrate ought to decrease the noise in the ears. Tablets can be obtained in health food stores.

Chlorophyll, the green pigment in plants, reduces sludging of the blood and generally decreases deafness and noise in the ears. In one case a 71 year old man took chlorophyll supplements for four months and the deafness and tinnitis decreased in both ears to bearable levels. Chlorophyll supplements stopped attacks of Meniere's disease in a 33 year-old man.

A 61 year-old man became increasingly deaf for 15 years until his left ear became totally deaf, and he could no longer hear his voice. Using supplements of dicumarol and chlorophyll, he slowly recovered the ability to hear his own voice. The tinnitus ceased to bother him until he had a car accident, and then the stress brought back the ear noise.

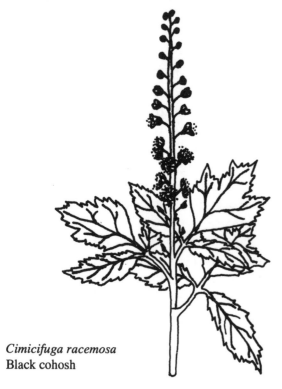

Cimicifuga racemosa
Black cohosh

Black cohosh was first collected in New England in 1680. Linnaeus named it *Actea racemosa*, and later the botanical name was changed to **Cimicifuga racemosa**. It was widely used by the Indians for snakebite and for helping women at the time of birth. In 1823 it was introduced into American medicine as a cure for tuberculosis. The pulverized roots are mixed with alcohol to make up the tincture.

If too much of the tincture is taken, it produces a spinning sensation in the head. The theory that like cures like, may have been the impetus for trying it in ear disorders. By 1898 reports began to

appear in the medical literature that it was very valuable in curing ear noise. The average amount taken is about 30 drops of the tincture, although the dosage varies from 10 to 60 drops in the reports. The amounts probably reflect the different strengths of the solution. The number of drops is increased daily, until the head begins to spin. This is done several times and Meniere's disease is then said to disappear.

There is a peculiar phenomenon, that when hot or cold water is put into the ear we get giddy. The discovery of 'caloric vestibular stimulation' of the ears won a Nobel Prize. The heat stimulates the balance center and produces vertigo. There is an old German treatment of steaming the middle ear to cure tinnitus. German doctors claimed that most cases could be cured or improved in 30 days with the treatment.

We hear with our ears, and we balance our bodies with them as well. There is a constant flow of nerve impulses from our ears to our nervous systems as we walk, telling us to make slight shifts in position. This is all done automatically, so that we do not realize that our balance is only partially controlled by the eyes. The realization that the inner ear controls balance came from finding that deaf persons did not get seasick.

Prosper Meniere was born in southwestern France in 1799. He became an associate professor at the University of Paris where he took up the study of the ear. He died of pneumonia in 1862, in the same year he described the new disease he found. In his papers he describes a sudden onset of deafness, and ear noises with vertigo, nausea, and vomiting. He correctly placed the problem in the semicircular canals of the ears.

Martin Luther was probably a victim of the disease. He attributed the whistling and roaring in his ears to the devil. He had attacks of dizziness and nausea that made him so giddy that he would fall off of his stool while at work.

The use of glycerin for treating deafness has long been forgotten, but taking glycerin internally is a test to distinguish Meniere's disease from other conditions. In testing, the patient fasts, and then takes 1.2 grams of glycerin per kilogram of weight. Many people will get headaches after taking 60-90 grams of glycerin orally, but it brings a tremendous improvement in hearing ability and some tones may improve by up to 40 decibels. The hearing improvement is only temporary.

Manganese has an effect on the formation of the otoliths of the inner ears, which control the balance. In families where deafness is hereditary, it may be prevented by extra manganese during pregnancy.

Mink farmers found an unusual pastel color in mink, which was registered under the trademark of 'Autumn Haze.' Along with the color came a high rate of head tilting, and the inability to swim normally. The mink farmers were able to reduce the defect by careful breeding. Eventually, they found that supplements of manganese during pregnancy eliminated the disorder.

French doctors found that Meniere's syndrome could be treated with injections of magnesium salts. A 5 cc. solution of 50% magnesium sulfate was injected two or three times a week. It is given at an extremely slow rate, so there is no sensation of heat.

Eighteen patients, who had no success with other treatments, were treated with injections. The giddiness disappeared and the hearing improved. It takes from ten to fifteen injections to cure the disorder. In seven cases there were no attacks during the following year, seven people were greatly improved and four had no change.

A 50 year-old woman suffered from severe vertigo, nausea and vomiting for fourteen years. She had daily spells, and was treated with normal methods without effect. After 15 injections of magnesium sulfate she was able to live a normal life. She lasted for 14 months without spells, and then another set of injections gave her a troublefree life.

The first attempt to treat Meniere's syndrome with vitamins was published in 1940. Injections of 10 mgs. of thiamin and 250 mgs. of nicotinic acid were done to 20 people. This resulted in 17 people becoming free from vertigo, and others showing improvement. Tinnitus was cured in ten cases and relieved in another ten. A high protein and vitamin diet was recommended along with the treatment. Vitamin deficiency was quite common among many people, and it may be that many cases of Meniere's syndrome were due to deficiency at this time.

A Chicago doctor was treating a patient who was becoming progressively deaf and complaining of hearing a slapping noise in one ear. Niacin

didn't help his hearing. When he was given 100 mgs. of Vitamin B6 his hearing improved. Further study showed that half of those with Meniere's disease had a significant improvement with this vitamin.

A 70 year-old woman wasn't able to walk without holding onto something. Vitamin B6 relieved her of instability to the point where she could walk alone, but she wasn't completely cured. A 56 year-old man suffered from dizziness, vomiting and diarrhea. Three doctors failed to help his dizziness. By taking 100 mgs. of B6 he was able to return to work in three weeks.

Vitamin B12 has been shown to be in short supply in 47% of the persons suffering from noise induced hearing loss and ear noises. A survey of 'normal' people shows that 27% are slightly deficient. A preliminary study has shown that B12 lessens ear noise. Since these conditions are linked, supplements may improve Meniere's disease.

One of the early explorers of the Hudson's Bay area of Canada was James Isham. He wrote, "The English in these parts make a drink of it [Labrador tea], going by the name of wishakapucka tea, being of a fine flavor, and reckoned very wholesome – I was troubled very much with a nervous disorder, and by constant drinking one pint made strong for three months, it entirely cured me."

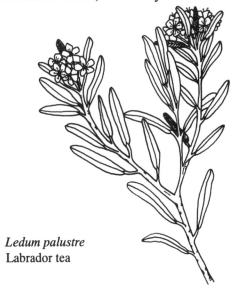

Ledum palustre
Labrador tea

Later in his account he gives us clues that his problem may have been Meniere's disease. "I can observe that the plant wishakapucka [*Ledum palustre*] entirely cured me, being very much affected with a nervous disorder, when I went into that country last, and have known a person since my arrival in England, which troubled with a giddiness in his head, and subject to fainting fits by using this plant made strong, twice a day."

Pueraria tuberosa

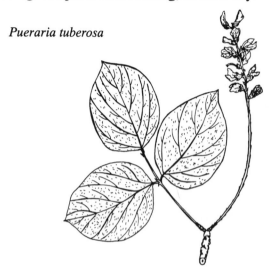

Sudden deafness, tinnitus and Meniere's disease may be due to tiny blood clots in the hearing mechanism. Sudden deafness may be a sort of 'coronary ear attack.' A study on the use of the roots of *Pueraria tuberosa* on sudden deafness was published in China in 1975. A tincture of 1.5 grams of the herb was taken three times a day. If it was begun the first week after the deafness, it was 55% effective in restoring hearing. If it was taken one to three months later, it was only 5% effective.

One of the old treatments that was said to work very well, was the use of jaborandi tea *Pilocarpus jaborandi* to produce sweating. This was drunk for several days, and produces severe sweating. The patient was put to bed and wrapped up, so that they could continue to sweat. In one instance a woman was so dizzy that she couldn't get out of bed. The sweating treatment cured her.

The same treatments that work in deafness may give some relief in Meniere's disease. In old herbal literature the blessed thistle *Cnicus benedictus* is mentioned as a certain cure for giddiness. Culpeper, the English herbalist, mentions *Tanacetum vulgare* and *Bellis perennis,* which is the English daisy, as a cure. Chinese doctors used *Nauclea sinensis* to cure vertigo and scintillations of the eyes. In Russia *Passiflora incarnata* was claimed to help most people with deafness and Meniere's disease. In Nepal the herbs used to correct dizziness are a combination of *Lecanthus peduncularis* and *Dichroa febrifuga.*

✯ ✯ ✯

ANEMIA

"This being done, I work to fortify the blood and consequently the spirits which have their source there, and for this I order the patient to take, for thirty days some remedy drawn from Mars. Nothing else succeeds better on such occasions. The Mars communicates to the mass of weakened blood a certain fire and volatility which raises and reanimates the broken down spirits. An evident proof of this, is that when one gives Mars in the pale color, the pulse becomes at once fuller and slower, the pallor disappears and once again the face is rosy and ruddy."

Thomas Sydenham is using iron (Mars) as a tonic for anemia. +1661

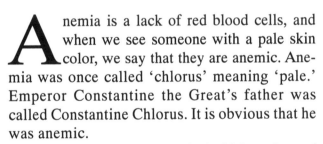

Anemia is a lack of red blood cells, and when we see someone with a pale skin color, we say that they are anemic. Anemia was once called 'chlorus' meaning 'pale.' Emperor Constantine the Great's father was called Constantine Chlorus. It is obvious that he was anemic.

Iron was the ancient symbol of Mars, the god of war. A shield and the spear symbolized it. The soldiers adopted it as their symbol, and gradually the combined symbol became the symbol for man. In astrology, Mars controlled the blood, and iron was its specific element. In India the famous Nagarjuna wrote the *Lauha Sastra* meaning "The Science of Iron."

The first person known to have used iron specifically to treat anemia was Thomas Sydenham. In 1681 he wrote: "Next to steel in substance, I prefer a syrup. Steeping iron or steel filings in cold wine makes this. When it is sufficiently impregnated, strain the liquor and add sugar and boil to the consistency of syrup."

The molecule known as hemoglobin serves as the oxygen carrying part of the red blood cell. At the center of this wheel-like molecule is an atom of iron in the ferrous (+2) state. Iron exists in the +2 or the +3 ferric oxidation state, but the body can only use iron in the +2 state. We need one milligram of iron daily, and we get 10 to 15 milligrams in our diets, although most of it is +3 iron and can't be absorbed. Most of the iron in our bodies comes from recycling the iron from old red blood cells, but the rest must come from ferrous iron.

The green pigment known as chlorophyll in plants is chemically identical to the pigment of red blood cells. The difference in pigment comes from an atom of iron in the red cells where an atom of magnesium would appear in plants. Chlorophyll is known to stimulate the regeneration of the blood and increase the metabolic rate. When chlorophyll is added to embryonic cells, there is an immediate growth response, suggesting that it is a powerful healing agent in accidents.

During WWI soldiers who bled a great deal were given a mixture of one part spinach juice to 50 parts of wine. It may have been the chlorophyll that restored the red blood cells.

Several studies have attempted to identify the hemoglobin forming properties of spinach *Spinacia oleracea*. Small amounts of copper are needed for the synthesis of blood. Spinach contains an ideal ratio of 37 parts of iron to one part of copper. Spinach regenerated blood twice as fast as an iron-copper mixture. The level of red blood cells was 25% above the mineral combination.

Rabbits were made severely anemic by injecting them with saponine-collargol. Then they were given 2-3 injections of a water extract of powdered spinach. This increased the number of red blood by an average of 1.5 million red blood cells. The effects were more lasting than those observed after injections of liver extracts.

Both copper and manganese are necessary for the formation of red blood cells. When mice are fed only on milk, they developed anemia, which was remedied by the addition of copper. The role of manganese in the formation of blood is unclear. At the turn of the century, many doctors mixed it with iron tonics, because they discovered that it cured anemias that were untreatable with iron supplements.

In 1922 rats were injected with 1-2 mgs. of germanium dioxide per kilogram of body weight. This resulted in a marked increase of red blood cells. Smaller doses were just as marked and significant.

Further tests showed that germanium dioxide was ineffective taken by mouth. Mixing it with sodium hydroxide produced sodium germanate. A small amount of this produced a 10-20% increase in the number of red blood cells over a short period of time. The use of germanium has been revived by Japanese experimenters in a different chemical combination, although I believe that sodium germanate is probably a more effective compound.

The activity of germanium dioxide was tested in a hospital. Sodium hydroxide was added until the solution became neutral, then it was brought to a pH of 7.6 with hydrochloric acid. Only freshly prepared solutions were active. Most cases of secondary anemia responded to the injections.

In a typical case a 25 year-old man had nausea and loss of appetite. He steadily grew weaker until his blood cell count dropped to 1,760,000. Three injections of germanium raised this to 2,200,000 and enabled him to leave the hospital. This is less than half the normal number. In other cases germanium doubled the number of red blood cells, but this was uncommon. It usually improved patients, but it wasn't a complete solution.

In 1852 Karl Vierordt became the first person to do an accurate count of the number of red blood cells. He used a fine capillary tube and spread a minute amount of blood over a slide and counted the red blood cells with a microscope for the next three hours. Adaptations of this method are used today.

In 1906 Paul Carnot injected normal rabbits with serum from anemic rabbits. This stimulated the production of red blood cells, and he theorized that there was a substance he called 'hemopoietine,' which was a signal for producing more red blood cells. It took almost 50 years to discover a signaling hormone known as 'erythropoietin'. It is controlled by an oxygen feedback system. Low levels of body oxygen increase the hormone, which generates more oxygen carrying blood cells.

The first understanding of how our bodies construct the oxygen carrying hemoglobin molecular came in 1945, when the American chemist David Shemin swallowed 66 grams of the amino acid glycine over a three day period. The glycine was made with a nitrogen isotope, so it was traceable with mass spectometry. The level rose quickly in the blood as the glycine was converted into hemoglobin. The level remained constant, and then dropped quickly four months later, when the body destroyed the old red blood cells. The mystery here is how the body recognizes and destroys cells that are 120 days old.

Since anemia does not come suddenly, we don't usually know that we have it. We feel chronically tired and fatigued when we work. Friends notice our pale appearance with pearly eyes, and slightly waxy skin. Our problem can be described as 'tired blood,' but it is due to a lack of oxygen, because of the lack of cells to transport it.

Many types of anemia have no connection with iron. A new anemia was discovered in 1821, which was eventually named 'pernicious anemia' in 1876. In 1926 doctors discovered that liver cured this type of anemia, but the patients had to eat a half-pound of liver daily in order to be cured. The Nobel Prize for medicine in 1934 was shared by three men for their discovery of the treatment of anemia with liver. In 1948 the anemia factor was isolated and named Vitamin B12. It was so active that a few hundred micrograms cured the worst cases of pernicious anemia. About one out of 200 Scandinavians suffer from pernicious anemia, because they lack a protein that enables them to absorb Vitamin B12. Large doses overcome the body's inability to absorb it.

Another mysterious anemia generally occurred in pregnancy. It responded to liver and brewer's yeast, but Vitamin B12 was not the cure. In 1943 scientists isolated a vitamin which they called pteroylglutamic acid, which they later renamed folic acid. Supplements of the new vitamin cleared up difficult cases of diarrhea and sore mouths with cracked tongues and the associated anemia.

A rare form of anemia responds to the amino acid methionine. If rats are fed a diet low in methionine, red blood cells counts drop. This produces anorexia and the rats don't want to eat. A 70 year-old Frenchman had only a quarter of the normal number of red blood cells and a low number of white blood cells. When he was given three grams of methionine daily, the red blood cells doubled in a month and were almost normal in two months. The white blood cells tripled in the same period of time. Methionine can be obtained in many health food stores, for it is used to treat the enlarged livers of alcoholics.

Medical scientists fed onions to dogs to see if it would protect them against black tongue. At a level of 50-200 grams of onions per kilogram there was a marked decrease in red blood cells. They reached a minimum in seven to twelve days. The animals remained in good condition, and with continued onion feeding, the blood count slowly began to return to normal.

In the years of 1926-1930 physiologists ran a long series of experiments on dogs, trying to find foods which regenerated the blood. Liver had the greatest regenerative ability, followed by blood, and all meats and fish had some ability. Most vegetables were inert, and only fresh spinach had some regenerating ability. The real surprise was that both fresh and dried peaches, apricots and prunes had blood-regenerating abilities, not much inferior to liver.These findings surprised the researchers, because these fruits contained very little B12 or folic acid. Raisins, grapes and apples were less active, and berries were inert, although they had high iron content.

In many parts of the world the major cause of anemia is hookworms. These parasites suck blood from the intestinal walls and create severe anemia. The hookworm problem was once common in the southeastern US due to the habit of going barefooted. A study financed by the Rockefeller Institute found that hookworms were the reason why so many people felt tired and run down. Mass treatment programs were started. At first it was considered shameful to admit that you might have worms, but a massive public campaign with prominent figures testifying that they felt better after treatment worked wonders.

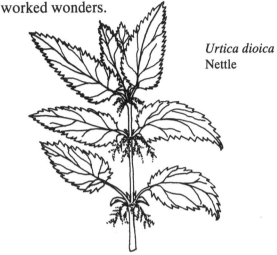

Urtica dioica
Nettle

In Sweden the traditional spring tonic generally included fresh nettles. Tests in 1898 showed that anemias not responding to iron, were quickly cured with nettles. Nettles have a red blood cell proliferating compound. They were used in heart conditions, because the heart enlarges when the blood is anemic.

There are several herbs which are red blood cell stimulants. In Russia, rats were made anemic by bleeding, and various herbs were given to them. *Sedum telephium* was found to rapidly regenerate the blood. French scientists used extracts of *Sophora japonica* in laboratory animals. Thirty minutes after administration the blood count stood at 3,260,000. An hour

Sedum telephium

later it rose to 3,440,000 and in another hour it rose to 4,000,000. ***Codonopsis tangshen*** from western China was also found to be a powerful blood cell proliferant.

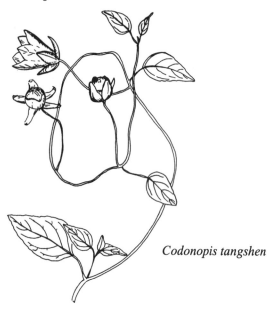

Codonopis tangshen

The first descriptions of sickle cells were made in 1840 on deer. Epidemics have been reported from Michigan in which deer died due to sickle cell anemia. It may be a virus, but the cause remains a mystery. Sickle cell anemia was first described in humans in 1910. The red blood cells became shaped like oats, and they are now short and thin.

In 1948 Linus Pauling investigated sickle cell anemia. He found that as a negative ion normal hemoglobin moved to the left, but as a positive ion, sickle cell anemia hemoglobin moved to the right in an electric field. Pauling felt that this was a true molecular disease. Eventually it was found to be a genetic defect, in which one amino acid was altered in the hemoglobin.

Vitamin B6 relieves painful body cramps caused by sickle cell anemia. When 50 mg. tablets of the vitamin were taken by five people, the cramps decreased in frequency and severity. All the patients reported that their general well being improved. One person was hospitalized by sickle cell anemia about once every two months. After taking B6 supplements, he no longer needed hospital care.

During painful episodes of sickle cell anemia, the body suffers from acidosis. In order to overcome this, sodium citrate was given with codeine. This reduced the average duration of the painful periods from six days to two days. This might have been due to the increased electrical surface charges on the blood.

One herbal help for sickle cell diseases was discovered by a child. When she drank a little juice of an unripe papaya ***Carica papaya*** the severe bone pain and sickle cell problems were gone. The doctor took her blood cells and added a solution of sodium metabisulphite. Under a microscope, all the cells sickled within 30 minutes. Then he added a drop of unripe papaya to another vial of blood, and now none of the cells sickled in two days. If the blood cells started to sickle, it reversed them. Unripe papaya juice is used in some meat tenderizers.

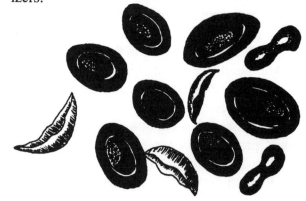

Normal blood cells and sickle cells

Common ordinary food flavoring vanilla has moderate antisickling activity. Rats taking vanilla show no ill effects. No clinical trials have been made of this simple substance.

In most parts of the world, toothsticks are used in place of toothbrushes. Nigeria has a high rate of sickle cell anemia, because the gene that causes it confers some protection against malaria, which is very common. The most common toothstick is ***Zanthoxylum zanthoxyloides***. This tree contains an antisickling agent, and it is under active investigation as a treatment for the disease. The seeds of the Nigerian plant ***Cajanus cajan*** have a significant antisickling action.

✧ ✧ ✧

SALTS AND THE BLOOD

"The leperous distilment, whose effect
holds such enmity with blood of man
That, swift as quicksilver it courses through
the natural gates and alleys of the body;
And, with a sudden vigor, it doth posset
and curd, like eager droppings, into milk,
The thin and wholesome blood."

Hamlet William *Shakespeare*

Sydney Ringer was born at Norwich, England, and went to University College in London, where he became a doctor in 1863. He became a professor of materia medica, pharmacology and therapeutics. He spent his days attending patients in the wards, but after work he spent hours studying physiology. In 1869 he prepared a *Handbook of Therapeutics*, which became the standard textbook of his time, and went through 13 revisions.

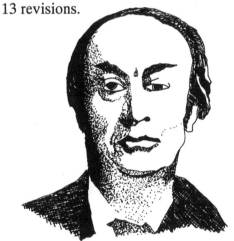

Sydney Ringer

In 1880 Ringer began to experiment on mixtures of salts for keeping the hearts of laboratory animals beating outside the body for prolonged periods of time. He was able to demonstrate that the duration of cardiac contraction depend on the minerals in the body. This work led to a solution of sodium, potassium and calcium salts for keeping the heart beating, which is known as "Ringer's solution." The solution is composed of 0.85% sodium chloride, 0.03% potassium chloride and 0.48% calcium chloride.

Ringer discovered the role of calcium in the contraction of the heart, when a solution kept isolated hearts beating much longer, than he had been able to do previously. His laboratory assistant ran out of distilled water for preparing the solutions and substituted tap water. After studying the components of the tap water, Ringer realized that it contained a significant amount of calcium. He then started studying the effects of mineral mixtures on the heart.

If more potassium was added to the mixture, heart contractions decreased and eventually stopped. The addition of more calcium strengthened the contractions and lengthened the intervals, until the heart stopped in a state of tonic contractions known as 'calcium rigor'. Calcium aided the action of digitalis, strophanthus and squill. It was particularly important in congestive heart failure.

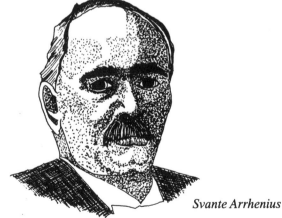

Svante Arrhenius

At the same time Ringer was studying mixtures, the Swedish chemist Svante Arrhenius was developing a theory of electrolyte dissolution. Normally we would write CaCl2 for calcium chloride; but Arrhenius showed that a liquid solution of minerals was composed of ions, which could be written Ca++ and 2 Cl-. It is these ions which travel across cell membranes and alternatively allow the muscle tissue to relax and contract. Arrhenius was originally thought to be a crank, but eventually it was realized that his theory provided the basis of understanding cellular phenomenon.

Experiments done with sea urchin eggs disclosed the fact that a single salt has toxic effects, but a mixture of mineral salts protects the eggs from harm. This is true of the heart; calcium is necessary, but potassium and magnesium protect it against toxic agents. Experiments with these eggs led to the concept of physiologically balanced salt solutions. Most table salt is pure sodium chloride, but sea salt is a balance of minerals. Experiments suggest that our table salt would be healthier if it was a mixture.

The largest amount of calcium in the body is bound up in the form of calcium phosphate, which makes up the bones and teeth. By using low concentrations of various calcium salts in the laboratory to stop the heart in either diastolic (filling) or systolic (emptying), we can understand the need for each

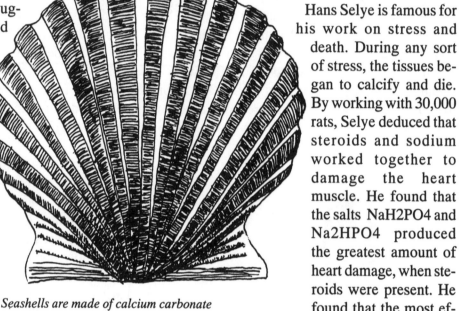
Seashells are made of calcium carbonate

salt. Without phosphate the heart stopped in diastole at 1/30th of the normal calcium concentration. If phosphate was added, the amount of calcium could be reduced to 1/300th the normal amount.

Most people are not fond of hard water, because it leaves a ring around the bathtub, and a milky film on dishes rinsed with it. Water softeners prevent it from clogging our pipes with scale, but the reverse seems to be true for our heart and circulatory system. Hard water contains extra calcium and magnesium and we soften the water by replacing the ions with sodium.

There have been many studies of the death rates from heart and circulatory disease, compared to the elements present in the water. In general, the harder the water, the lower the death rate from cardiovascular disease; the softer the water, the higher the death rate from cardiovascular disease. People living along the Ohio and Columbia rivers where the water is soft have higher rates of heart attacks, than people do along the Missouri and Colorado rivers where it is hard. A study in England where the water was changed from hard to soft showed a 10% increase in cardiovascular related deaths.

Death rates show significant variations in water with magnesium, calcium bicarbonates and sulfates. Silica, iron, potassium and nitrates in the water do not affect heart rates. As a general rule, water with large amounts of calcium and magnesium had a lower death rate, and an autopsy will show less heart damage resulting from the water.

Hans Selye is famous for his work on stress and death. During any sort of stress, the tissues began to calcify and die. By working with 30,000 rats, Selye deduced that steroids and sodium worked together to damage the heart muscle. He found that the salts NaH_2PO_4 and Na_2HPO_4 produced the greatest amount of heart damage, when steroids were present. He found that the most effective agents for preventing heart damage when damaging salts were present, were $MgCl_2$ and KCl. Selye found that a deficiency of thiamin produced heart cell damage, but no other vitamins affected the heart in this way. This was used by the breeders of silver foxes, who had a disease known as "Chastek paralysis," which damaged the heart and liver cells. It was curable by adding thiamin to the diet.

Canadian doctors found that the addition of calcium chloride to the diet lowered the high blood pressure in 58% of patients. It lowered the systolic pressure by 30 mm. and the diastolic pressure by 12mm. The treatment had to be continued for three to four weeks in order to get results. The doctors found that 13% of those taking potassium chloride had a significant lowering of blood pressure. These salts improved cardiac symptoms and reduced water retention.

In 1907 Lauder Brunton announced that he was able to treat pneumonia accompanied with heart failure, with calcium chloride. He observed that it was often useful in cardiac disease when the heart was failing, but it did not always produce good results. About one person in three with heart conditions, benefited measurably with calcium supplements.

The combination of calcium and digitalis is especially significant. If calcium is given along with digitalis, the heart slows down for four to five hours. In 1921 G. Singer recommended that people taking digitalis alternate the use of digitalis and calcium. This was less toxic, and controlled dropsy. It counteracted the bad effects of the prolonged use of digitalis.

Russian researchers found that Epsom salts taken by mouth were successful in the treatment of angina pectoris and relieved pain from other heart conditions. South African doctors found that the salt produced dramatic clinical improvement in many cases of coronary heart disease. The action of magnesium sulfate is unclear, but it dilates the arteries and clears up lipids. Magnesium acts as a stimulant to the ATP, which powers the heart, muscles and normalizes the electrocardiogram.

When blood flow to the heart was constricted in laboratory animals, it caused the death of some of the heart cells. A mixture of potassium and magnesium asparaginates was highly effective in regenerating the damaged cells. Magnesium asparaginate causes a prolonged increase in blood flow, and decreases the peripheral blood resistance. It is much more active than magnesium chloride.

The action of the salts is complicated, but the evidence indicates that a proper mixture of these salts in the drinking water could produce significant benefits in cardiac conditions. When we eat foods we are eating solutions of minerals, so we are affecting our bodies, in ways that we normally have no realization of.

✦ ✦ ✦

THE ELECTRIC CHARGE MYSTERY

"Flat outstretched upon a mound of earth I lie; I press my ear, against its surface and I hear,
Far off and deep, the measured sound, of heart that beats within the ground.
And with it pounds in harmony, the swift, familiar heart in me.
They pulse as one, together swell, together fall;
I cannot tell my sound from earth's, for I am part of rhythmic, universal heart."

Elizabeth Odell +1884

When the early users of microscopes studied the capillary flow of blood they noted that red blood cells tended to repel each other. They found a higher incidence of agglomerated blood cells during disease. This fact became a standard medical test of how fast a patient was improving from a serious illness. If the red blood cells increased their repellency, it reduced the blood sedimentation rate.

Studies of 600 patients showed that the common feature of burns, diphtheria, eclampsia, leukemia, malaria, whooping cough, measles, multiple sclerosis, scarlet fever, and the common cold was clumping of the blood. The researchers didn't have a way of liquefying it, so they put down their observations as a major feature of medicine. It stands to reason that patients could heal much faster if we could keep the blood more liquid.

When the circulation is poor, little plugs of blood temporarily block the capillaries in the back of the eye. They can be viewed with a special microscope. It is also known that psychiatric patients have disturbances following infectious disease, for the disease increases the sedimentation rate of the blood, decreasing the efficiency of the blood in carrying oxygen to the brain. The sludging of blood and a slowing of the rate of blood flow is particularly noticeable in rheumatoid arthritis. While these facts have long been noted, few doctors have used them in treating the disorder.

Suspended particles, such as silt in water, or red blood cells within blood, have an electrical mechanism for staying in solution. Each particle or blood cell forms an electrical surface known as a 'zeta potential.' The layers of absorbed ions on the surface charge the particle. Each blood cell is repelled from its neighbors by a negative charge.

If you have played with magnets, you know that two negative poles repel each other. The principal is similar with two red blood cells and negative surface charges.

Before doctors could give blood transfusions, they had to keep the blood from clotting. In 1774 William Heuson found that Glauber's salt ($Na_2 SO_4$) would keep the blood from clotting. In 1866 Braxton Hicks added sodium phosphate to blood to keep it from clotting. The blood didn't clot, but his first three patients died in shock, because he didn't know anything about matching blood types. In 1914 citric salts were successfully used in blood transfusions and they have been used thereafter.

The person who nearly discovered the secret of coronary thrombosis was Doctor Ernest Klein. Each day he checked the blood of some 200 people at the University Hospital of New York City. He used blood coagulation units known as sahli. In normal healthy individuals the blood was about 85 sahli, but in those with coronary thrombosis it nearly doubled. In these individuals blood would often begin to clot as quickly as it was drawn.

After three years of research work, Klein formulated three rules for people who were prone to heart attacks. He asked that they eliminate "dry" foods like bread and potato chips. Secondly, they were to eliminate red meats like steak. Thirdly, they were to drink six to eight glasses of a mixture of water and citrus juices each day.

In 1949 he published his findings in a New York journal for doctors. The next day both he and his daughter were fired from their jobs at the hospital. He did not realize the function of the surface electrical charge, but he did come close enough to the truth to disturb the medical profession.

The mystery of electrical charges is explained

somewhat in this manner. A salt can be balanced in charges like NaCl (sodium chloride) which has a +1 and a −1 electrical charge on its ions. A salt like K_2SO_4 (potassium sulfate) has two −1 charges balancing a +2 SO_4 ion. Potassium citrate $K_3C_2H_3O_2$ is a compound, which balances three +1 charges against a single −3 charge. If the salts are added to the blood, we find that the ions form an electrical double layer; the negative or electrical repulsive action increasing rapidly with ions of multiple negative charge, balancing ions of a single plus charge. When ions of this type are mixed with blood, it becomes very resistant to coagulation and is suited for transfusions.

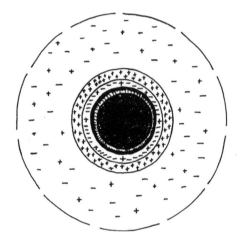

Red blood cell surrounded
by electrically charged layers

The most powerful blood coagulation agents are metals with a +3 electrical charge. In the case of calcium chloride $CaCl_2$, a single +2 charge balances two −1 charges. In aluminum chloride a single +3 charge balances three −1 charges. Aluminum adds a positive charge to suspended particles and coagulates them. This is why cities purify water with alum (aluminum sulfate and other aluminum salts). When added to muddy river water, the suspended particles quickly coagulate and fall to the bottom. Particles in a muddy river are kept in suspension by negative charges, and when the charge is neutralized with multiple positive ions, the particles are no longer suspended.

Thomas Riddick was the inventor of a special device to measure the charges of particles in solution. The zeta meter is a microscope focused on a fluid-filled tube marked with fine lines. When electrical current is applied to the fluid, the particles

move at a speed proportionate to their charge. The time it takes for the particles to move a short distance, is a measure of electrical charge. This meter is used in water treatment plants and paper mills, where it is important to coagulate particles in the water.

Riddick had a heart condition in which his heart skipped every fifth beat. He also had frequent heart attacks, with profuse urination. He analyzed his urine during heart attacks, and found that it contained 13 times more aluminum than his normal urine. The body was purging the excess aluminum from the body during the attacks

Riddick began to study the electrical charge on his blood, and that of people with heart conditions. He found that young healthy people had high negative charges on the red blood cells. People with heart problems nearly always had lower changes on their red blood cells. The severity of heart conditions was in direct relationship to the electrical charge on the blood cells.

A young healthy person has an electrical charge of −17 millivolts on each cell, and the red blood cells are equally spaced. When the charge drops, two or three blood cells group together into 'comets.' As the charge drops more, progressively larger groupings form. A drop in charge to −12 millivolts means that the blood becomes extremely clottable. This means that the blood clots are much more likely to form that damage the heart. It also means that the arteries are more likely to become clogged with debris.

The doctors told Riddick that nothing could be done for his heart condition, and they were doing the best they could. He began to wonder if the real problem was a low electrical charge on his blood. To test the idea, each day he drank a quart of water, with a gram of dissolved potassium citrate. In six weeks, his heart stopped skipping beats and his electrocardiogram returned to normal. A number of his friends had heart conditions, so he began asking them to try

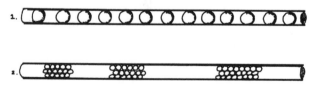

Normal red blood cells found in capillaries (top) and
clumped blood cells from low electrical charge (bottom)

doing the same thing. Many of them found that their heart conditions began to improve.

One of his friends was a bachelor who had been eating canned foods for years. Canned foods usually have larger amounts of metals with high positive charges on them. When he measured his friend, he found the lowest blood electrical charge he had ever seen, and he asked him to see a cooperating doctor at once. His friend never made it; an hour after the meeting, he was found behind the wheel of his car, dead from a stroke.

The electrical charge mystery is part of the explanation of high blood pressure. Pressure depends on the friction of the blood, and the resistance to flow in the tissues. When the viscosity (thickness) is reduced, blood pressure falls. There have been several studies on the use of potassium and sodium citrates to reduce blood pressure.

While Riddick was studying the electrical charges of the blood, his pet parrot stopped talking and the feathers began to fall out. The veterinarian recommended B vitamins for the bird. When he took his pet home, he noticed the peck marks on the cast aluminum bird dish. He replaced it with a ceramic dish, and added potassium citrate to the water. Two days later the parrot was asking for crackers and growing feathers again.

Riddick noted that his parrot's cold feet turned warm in a few days after drinking the citrate solution. This could be attributed to an improvement in the blood circulation of the capillaries of the feet. A letter to the bird supplies company, brought about a switch to porcelain bird dishes. Science is protecting the health of parrots, but it ignores the health of humans, especially when we use aluminum cooking pans. Heart attack rates also may be higher in towns where the water is treated with aluminum salts. Riddick tried to determine this, but the government wouldn't release the data.

In 1931 Lettinte Cooper published a short book *The Danger of Food Contamination by Aluminum.* The book kicked off some discussion in the medical literature. Doctors cited a 1914 study by the Department of Agriculture on feeding alum (aluminum sulfate) to young healthy college students. They found no problem and concluded that aluminum was nontoxic.

But a number of letters written to the medical journals expressed the opposite. One man wrote to say that he suffered from abdominal pain for years. After reading about aluminum, he stopped using the cookware, and he was free from pain, except when eating a certain prepared food. When he wrote to the makers, they told him it was prepared in aluminum pans. He mentioned that he knew of six other people, who had suffered from pain caused by cooking in aluminum pans.

One family had constant trouble with nausea and diarrhea. This stopped when they switched to nonaluminum pans. Another woman drank hot milk warmed in aluminum pans and suffered from stomach trouble. It should be added that today's aluminum pans are hardened, and are better than they were in 1930. The lesson remains the same for susceptible persons.

Arthur Coco discovered that the pan you cook from affects the pulse. Copper pans caused the greatest increase in heart rate, and aluminum was next. Enamelware had a slight increase, but Pyrex glass cookware didn't affect the heart at all. He wasn't aware of the electrical charges produced by heavy metals on the blood.

Chelation therapy is done by adding a substance, which strongly unites to heavy metals in the body. The first use of chelates was published in 1941 when sodium citrate was used to remove lead from the body. Six people were treated at the Philadelphia General Hospital with two to four grams of sodium citrate three times a day. In three weeks, the high levels of lead fell into normal range, as the citrate united with the lead, and the kidneys removed it from the body.

This form of chelation therapy has a major advantage over the therapy practiced by many doctors. Sodium and potassium citrates are readily available and can be taken by mouth. One vitamin company sells potassium mineral supplements in the form of potassium citrate.

Citrus fruits contain citric acid, and both potassium and sodium citrates. In areas where they are commonly eaten, the death rate from heart conditions is probably lower. With the rise of a negative charge on the blood it doesn't sludge, and the higher charge aids in the dissolution of cholesterol and cellular deposits along the blood vessel walls. These salts are not thought of as health supplements, but they should help to overcome the conditions which bring on heart attacks.

PREVENTING BLOOD CLOTTING

"When I returned unto my mill, I met my servant John,
He asked me why I looked so pale, An' yet so very warm."
An' what occasion so much blood, upon my hands an' clothes?
The sad an' only answer was, a bleeding from the nose.
An English ballad known as The Noel Girl

"Of course, day say, Brer Rabbit ain't a reg'lar doctor wid a sachel of powders and pills, but he do have some herbs an' erntments dat he got from de witch-rabbit down in de swamp."
Doctor Rabbit Cures de King *Joel Chandler Harris*

The use of leeches was extremely popular during the sixteenth and seventeenth centuries, when these annelid worms were used as a standard treatment for taking the 'bad blood' out of people. After the leeches had been removed the punctures continued to bleed. The blood in the body of the leeches remains fluid, because of an anticoagulant. This anticoagulant factor was isolated and named hirudin. It is used by laboratory workers to keep blood fluid, and it is being investigated as a medicine now that gene splicing can produce it in quantity.

When a mosquito bites us, it leaves a raised area. The mosquito injects a tiny amount of an anticoagulant, which causes an allergic reaction. The eel-like creatures known as lampreys also use an anticoagulant when they suck the blood of fish.

In 1938 a young man was admitted to a New York hospital with blood clots in his legs. He was given an intravenous infusion of heparin for the next sixteen days. Then the supply of heparin ran out, and the patient relapsed. Heparin is a natural anti-clotting enzyme in the body. Until recently it could not be made; it had to be isolated from the blood, so the supplies were low. Something better was needed, because many circulatory conditions need something to prevent blood clotting.

Back in 1933, Ed Carlson, a frustrated Wisconsin farmer drove 190 miles through a blizzard to the Agriculture Experimental Station in Madison marched into the building with a dead calf and a bundle of spoiled sweet clover hay ***Melilotus officinalis,*** and shared his bafflement with Dr. Karl Link. In wet years, farmers couldn't wait for the hay to completely dry in the field. Stored in the barn, the damp sweet clover hay spoiled, producing some abnormal chemical, and killing the cattle. Many farmers had experienced the same problems, and whole herds of cattle had been decimated.

The chemists began a research program to isolate the bleeding agent, and by 1938 they succeeded. One of the coumarin chemicals caused rats to bleed to death in low amounts. Since the <u>Wis</u>consin <u>A</u>lumni <u>R</u>esearch <u>F</u>oundation was backing the project, they named the rat killer "warf" and added an "arin" from the word coum<u>arin</u>. The new anticoagulant proved to be an extraordinary potent rat killer. After eating small amounts of it, they bled to death. It took 30 years for rats to develop resistance to it.

An army veteran decided to commit suicide with the new rat poison. After taking warfarin for five days, he changed his mind and checked into the naval hospital with 'hemorrhagic sweet clover disease.' He was given blood transfusions, and large doses of Vitamin K. He recovered without complications.

When the doctors speak of 'coronary thrombosis,' they mean that small blood clots have blocked portions of the heart. Blood clots in the head can result in paralysis and brain damage. What began as a dead calf, and later as a case of suicide, had important medical implications for treating blood clotting, and anticoagulants have been used in medicine ever since.

Onions have a chemical which prevents blood from clotting. German scientists found that a water extract of onions had little direct effect on the heart, but an alcoholic extract increased the volume of the pulse, and improved the blood flow.

The active agent in onions and garlic has been found to be a chemical known as 2-ajoene. At a level of 20 mg/kg. it completely prevents all platelet aggregation for the next 24 hours in rats. The regular eating of onions and garlic could significantly help those affected by blood clotting.

Blood contains fibrin, which clots protein in the blood. When we are cut, the fibrin forms a clot, so we do not continue to bleed. Enzymes in the blood keep the fibrin in check, and decrease the possibility of spontaneous clotting. Volunteers ate 60 grams of fried or boiled onions for breakfast and then had their blood tested. The onions increased the fibrin dissolving enzyme by 50% in the next few hours. The blood was significantly less able to clot.

In 1980, a laboratory worker was testing a sample of blood for coagulation. He had been doing an experiment on blood coagulation over a period of time, to study the changes in coagulation. On this day, his blood completely failed to coagulate and ruined his experiment. He tried to find out why his blood had suddenly ceased to clot, and he eliminated all of the normal reasons.

On the previous day he had eaten "Ma po dou fu" soup at a Chinese restaurant. One of the ingredients in the soup was "mo er," a black tree fungus commonly used in Chinese cooking. *Auricularia polytricha* is a shell mushroom growing on tree trunks, which had a reputation in Hong Kong of 'thinning the blood.' The potency of the fungus varies widely, so it rarely poses a danger to people. People have experienced nosebleeds or severe bruising after eating the fungus, but this was uncommon.

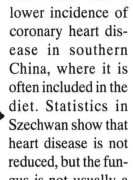

It was suggested that there was a lower incidence of coronary heart disease in southern China, where it is often included in the diet. Statistics in Szechwan show that heart disease is not reduced, but the fungus is not usually a regular part of the diet either.

Auricularia polytrichais
Mo er (the two sides of the fungus)

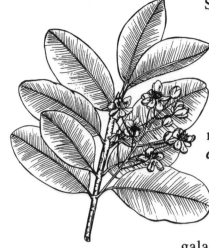

Calophyllum inophyllum

Seaweeds have weak anticoagulant activity, and they have been of interest in treating clotting disorders. Irish moss *Chondrus crispus* is about 1/25th as active as heparin. The carrageens are sulphated galactans present in seaweeds that prolong the time of blood clotting. They have been suggested as a treatment for peptic ulcer because they stimulate the formation of fibrous tissue.

Plants with enzymes in them often have some ability to inhibit coagulation, because they dissolve the proteins that make the blood clot. The sap of *Ficus glabra* inhibits coagulation, but *F. doliaria* and *F. retusa* don't.

An herb in India known as *Calophyllum inophyllum* contains a highly effective anticoagulant agent. It also has significant antiarrhythmic activity on the heart. It is not quite as active as dicumarol, but it does the same thing, and can be easily grown.

Cinnamon *Cinnamomum aromaticum* is a tree bark, and was a common ingredient of Chinese and eastern medicine. An alcoholic extract of cinnamon is useful in treating headaches and inflammation. It is effective in treating blood coagulation disorders. The active part has been identified as cinnamic aldehyde.

It seems that nature has an interesting variety of clot preventing substances in common herbs.

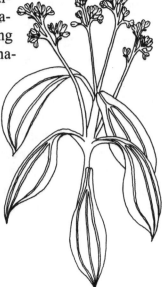

Cinnamomum aromaticum

AIDING BLOOD CLOTTING

"There come three lovely maidens to earth down from the sun. The first is called blood-leter [the lancet], the second is blood-geter [the basin], Blood-go-away! Blood-have-done!"
Medieval blood charm
*"Go to the place where shepherd's purse [*Capsella bursa-pastoris*] grows and say there three Marias and three Paters on your knees. Repeat this verse: 'I pray you, O Lord, that you may relieve this bleeding, which is on your servant, whom you redeemed through your own blood', then pluck the herb and apply it to the bleeding."*
The Rose *An Irish poem written around +1466 by Donnchadh O'Bolgaudi*

In 1890 the British Prime Minister William Gladstone addressed a group of herbalists. He told them the story of how he was cutting down a tree with an ax, when he received a severe cut on his finger. He had no handkerchief with him, so he bound the injured finger with the leaf of a nearby tree. The bleeding stopped at once, and the wound healed faster than his previous injuries had done before. He wondered if the tree leaf contained some special medicine.

In ancient Greece cheese was made by breaking off a twig from a fig tree and stirring milk with it. The white sap coagulates the milk, which is the first step in making cheese. Doctors believed that blood clotting was similar to making cheese. In 1666, Marcello Malpighi repeatedly washed a blood clot, and then examined the remainder under a microscope. He found little bundles of white strands, which were named fibrin.

In 1954 John Hageman went to Cleveland for peptic ulcer surgery. The doctors found that his blood couldn't clot, and they named the missing ingredient, the Hageman factor. The Hageman factor is activated by ellagic acid. This acid is part of the tannins in tree barks, and many fruits contain it. It is active in a single part per 100 million. When dry it is a dark purple powder, which makes a faint yellow solution.

The self-sealing mechanism of the blood, is like the 'stop leak' solutions that are added to seal leaks in car radiators. The mechanism is very delicate, because blood must flow through the narrowest of openings. If the clotting mechanism is too active, it will plug the capillaries and damage vital parts of the body. Blood clotting is a complex process requiring enzymes, Vitamin K and calcium. Alfalfa is high in Vitamin K, and the addition of 1% alfalfa to the diet of chickens with bleeding problems quickly stops this.

As more blood leaks from the body, the remaining blood clots quicker. Adrenaline increases the rate of blood clotting. If the blood coagulates too quickly, there is danger from clots and heart attacks.

The raw material of the fibrin fibers are the same amino acids that make up the skin. Gelatin is made by chemically dissolving the skin, and other by-products of meat packing plants. If a gelatin solution is put on a bleeding wound, the blood immediately begins to coagulate. French surgeons once did operations by using gelatin solutions to control bleeding. A measured amount of gelatin was fed to a dog and a blood sample was taken. The gelatin cut the blood clotting time in half.

In 1755 the *Philosophical Transactions of London* published two letters on controlling bleeding. A British surgeon found that when agaric of oak *Polyporus igniarius* was applied to amputated limbs, it had a remarkable effect in stopping bleeding. When the dressing was removed two days later, the stumps didn't bleed.

Philippe Lafosse was the farrier (horse doctor) for the king of France and a writer of veterinary books. He noted that peasants used the puffball mushroom *Lycoperdon* species to control bleeding. He cut off the tail of a horse and applied lycoperdon powder. In 24 hours a skin formed over the arteries and behind it was a plug of congealed blood. Members of the French Academy of Sciences came to see this. He cut off the tail of another horse and applied puffball mushroom powder. When the dressings were removed 15 minutes later, three of the four arteries remained stopped.

Fine powders can act as sites for fibrinogen to clot in wounds. The doctor who called attention to this experiment wrote, "I think this strongly deserves the notice of the world. If the same effects are produced on human bodies, the painful tying up of the arteries and the uncertainty of the agaric will be fully compensated in this noble powder." In one instance, a man was literally bleeding to death after a tooth extraction. The gap was packed with puffball spores and the bleeding stopped. A surgeon once performed operations with puffball spores. This apparently caused little irritation, and controlled emergency situations.

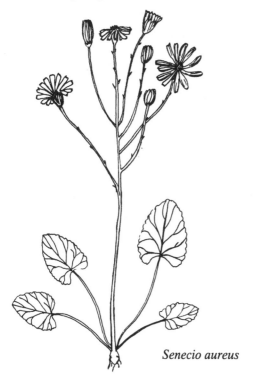

Senecio aureus

The common nettle *Urtica dioica* has a reputation of stopping bleeding. In the nineteenth century French doctors reported that nettles were better than ergot, iron or tannins in controlling bleeding problems. In 1885, a dentist used a tincture of nettles to stop bleeding, three days after a tooth had been extracted. Another account involves a priest who was said to have tried all remedies, but only nettles would stop his frequent nosebleeds. Nettles were once used as a woman's herb, to reduce menstrual bleeding.

A man had problems with blood in the urine,

and he had been treated by two doctors for six months and steadily grew weaker. The new doctor didn't do any better, and he asked the advice of an old country doctor. "Put your patient on a teaspoonful of the fluid extract of *Senecio aureus* three times a day and you will soon clear up his urine." In two days the urine was as clear as spring water, and the doctor continued to use the herb on other cases.

Another herb used in bleeding was fleabane *Conyza canadensis*. In 1865 Dr. John Moorman used 15 drops of the oil to cure a man suffering from profuse bleeding from his lungs. In half an hour the bleeding ceased entirely.

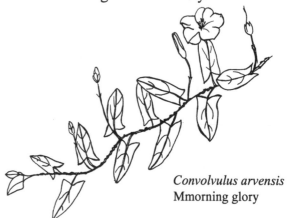

Convolvulus arvensis
Mmorning glory

Researchers were chopping up morning glory roots *Convolvulus arvensis* for a chemical study. Whenever they cut their fingers, the bleeding seemed to stop almost immediately. They made up a 5% solution of the roots in water, and tested it on eight people with a 'standard cut.' The length of time blotter paper would continue to show bleed spotting was a measure of the effectiveness of the root. A controlled cut stopped bleeding in 19 seconds, extracts of the leaves reduced this to 14 seconds, and root extracts reduced the bleeding time to 12 seconds.

The cowboys of the American West split the pads of the prickly pear cactus *Opuntia* and used them for wounds. The cactus contains high levels of pectin, which is the material in jams and jellies. It is soluble in the blood, and calcium clots it at the site of an injury.

There are several highly effective blood coagulant herbs. In Nigeria *Aspilia latifolia* is known as 'bleeding weed.' It is said to be a powerful vasoconstrictor, and bruised leaves and flowers are applied to wounds. Africans say it stops the bleeding even from a severed artery. In the Amazon jungle severe wounds are treated with the sap of **Croton salutaris**. A man who slashed his arm with a machete would have bled to death, if the juice of the plant hadn't been put on the wound. The juice stopped the bleeding quickly.

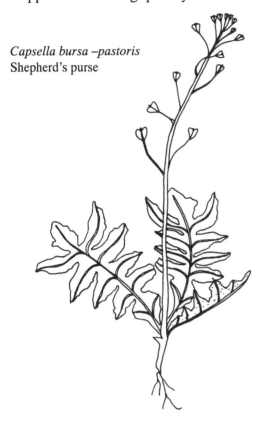

Capsella bursa –pastoris
Shepherd's purse

Shepherd's purse **Capsella bursa-pastoris** is an old traditional homeostatic agent. It was used at a New York hospital for doing prostate surgery. During a nine-year period beginning in 1930, 503 patients were operated on, and only three cases involved postoperative bleeding. There were no controls, but the doctors considered this a remarkably low rate. The active hemostatic chemical in it is bursinic acid.

A trial was made of shepherd's purse extracts injected into hemophilia patients to see if the uncontrolled bleeding could be stopped. In one case coagulation time returned to normal. In other cases it increased the clotting potential of the blood, but it really didn't help that much.

The old horse farriers (horse shoers) used **Alnus incana** to stop bleeding. A man received a severe blow with a sickle, and some of the external arteries were severed. The bleeding was persistent, and all domestic remedies were exhausted. A farrier advised cloth soaked in alder bark, placed over the cut. In a short time, the clot was firm and the bleeding stopped.

In another instance a laborer cut his leg with an ax. Bleeding was so severe that his friends feared for his life. The doctor ordered a cloth soaked in alder bark tea. This quickly checked the bleeding.

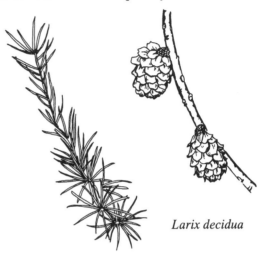

Larix decidua

In Mexico and the Caribbean, many people use the blood flower **Asclepias curassavica**, which is applied to the cut or drunk as a tea. Around 1860, Irish hospitals used a tincture of larch bark **Larix decidua**, which was taken by mouth to control bleeding. It was said to be successful, where all the usual remedies failed.

The Indians of California used **Commelina oelitus = C. tuberosa** to stop bleeding. This herb is used in Mexico and other countries to stop bleeding. **Tradescantia erecta** was used in South America as a homeostatic in cockfights. Sharp spurs worn by the fighting cocks would kill their opponents, unless the bleeding stopped. Other herbs used in folklore are mullein, horsetails, sassafras leaves, alum root, sunflower leaves and the smartweed **Polygonum bistorta**.

The bite of the carpet snake **Echis carnata** prevents coagulation, and the wound keeps on bleeding. A clerk of the tax collection office in India was bitten in 1873. He was treated by an Ayurvedic doctor who used a root, which quickly stopped the bleeding. After a good deal of persuasion, he found that it was from **Pogostemon purpuricaulis = P. parviflorus**.

Rabbi Judas first mentions the condition of hemophilia in a discussion in the Babylon Talmud. A woman had three sons who bled to death after circumcision. Even though circumcision was part of religious law, the next son was excused from it. The idea that a few people did not have blood that clotted normally was first discussed by John Otto in 1803. The word hemophilia was coined in 1828 when Willy Helmholtz studied a family of bleeders.

Hemophilia is a genetic disorder in which the blood loses the ability to clot. The disorder was common in the royal families of Europe, and any male child unlucky enough to inherit the gene, was likely to have a short life. The fall of the Czar of Russia is attributed partly to the fact that his son had hemophilia. The mad monk Grigori Rasputin, alone seemed to be able to stop the bleeding. The nobility became opposed to the Czar over this, and this led to the downfall of the old Russian monarchy. Rasputin could have known some herbal secrets, for he was a friend of Peter Badmaef, the famous Mongolian-Tibetan healer. There was speculation that it was a ginseng preparation, but the most popular Russian anti-bleeding herb was betony **Stachys officinalis**.

In southern Uzbekistan and Northern Tadzhikistan, the "intoxicating mint" **Lagochilus inebrians** or **L. setulosus** is used to treat hemophilia and bleeding conditions. A strong tea of this mint produces the sensation of drunkenness, which is why it was known as the intoxicating mint. The leaves were gathered in October, and boiled with honey for tea. It was a well-known woman's remedy for excess menstrual bleeding.

There is a simple cure for the bleeding of hemophilia that grows throughout much of the United States. Around 1857 a carriage driver had hemophilia. Every time he began to bleed from a cut, he chewed a piece of ragweed **Ambrosia artemisiifolia** to stop the bleeding. John Hill got the remedy from him, and used it to treat a number of cases of uncontrollable bleeding. A young woman from Goldsborough, North Carolina had her ears pierced and almost died from the bleeding. When she chewed a little ragweed, the bleeding stopped in 15 minutes.

In 1882, Doctor Hill was called to treat a boy bleeding from the nose, gums and bladder. His family had a history of dying of bleeding, and cuts were almost uncontrollable. Hill found some ragweed in the corner of a fence, brewed up some tea, and gave him tablespoonfuls of it. In 15 minutes the oozing of blood from the gums and the nose stopped. Within a day, his urine ceased to contain blood.

In 1885 John Hill was called to the bedside of a woman in Goldsborough. The woman was dying from unstoppable bleeding. He pulled out a package of ragweed, and had the woman chew somewhere he brewed up a tea. In a few minutes the bleeding stopped, and the next day the woman was able to get up and have breakfast.

Ragweed is probably the most hated weed in America. Millions of people in the Midwest suffer from allergies to its pollen after the oats and wheat is harvested. The stubble is covered with these plants. Folk medicine hardly refers to it, but *Simmons' Liver regulator* was a mixture of it with licorice and cascara.

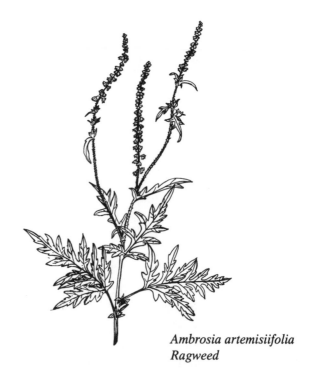

Ambrosia artemisiifolia
Ragweed

We have totally forgotten the old bleeding herbs and substituted whole blood clotting factors for hemophiliacs. This resulted in a high risk for AIDS and hepatitis. Thousands of hemophiliacs come down with these diseases. The problems of bleeding could be easily taken care of with simple remedies like nettles and ragweed. They are not just cost effective; they are safe as well.

✿ ✿ ✿

THE ACID-BASE BALANCE

For coffee it's 5; for tomatoes it's 4;
while domestic ammonia is 11 or more.
It's 7 for water, when in the pure state,
but rainwater is 6 and seawater is 8.
It's basic at 10, quite acid at 2,
and if above 7, it will turn litmus blue.
Some find it quite troublesome, doubtless their fog
has something to do with that terrible log.
An anonymous chemistry poem describing common pH readings

There is a hidden regulatory mechanism that rigidly controls the alkalinity of the body. The normal pH of our bodies is about 7.4, but it fluctuates a little. We normally have little conception of acid-base relationships. We do eat acid foods like sauerkraut, which forms by fermenting due to lactic acid bacteria. When the pH of the blood of a hundred people were checked, the average was about 7.43. Four people had a pH over 7.6 and seven people had a pH of 7.3 and under.

Those familiar with western American history remember the great cattle drives across the plains. The cowboys tried to keep the thirsty cattle from stampeding towards the alkaline water holes, which would surely kill the cattle. A major change outside the narrow acid base range means death for us, as well.

There is considerable literature about which foods are 'acid' or which are 'basic,' and how one should mix certain proportions of acid and base foods. These ideas date from an old Department of Agriculture report about the mineral contents of foods. Foods with high mineral content were supposed to be alkaline, and those with low mineral content were supposed to be acid. This has little to do with the acid-base balance of the body.

The pH of the blood varies with external factors. Blood samples were withdrawn from six dogs over the period of a year. During the time, the pH varied from 7.28 to 7.68. The pH tends to rise with the rise in the barometer, and it falls as the temperature falls. The pH of humans had exactly the same type of fluctuations. The lowest (most acid)

pH's were in the spring and fall, when epidemics of sickness are prevalent. There is evidence that a fall in pH is the trigger for colds and other illnesses.

The word 'acid' derives from the Arab word 'acaid' or 'sour' referring to vinegar. Most acids have an 'acid' taste, and what makes that taste is free hydrogen, written as H+. Sugar is not an acid, but when it is fermented with yeast, it forms an alcohol. With further fermentation in the presence of air, it forms vinegar, which is an acid.

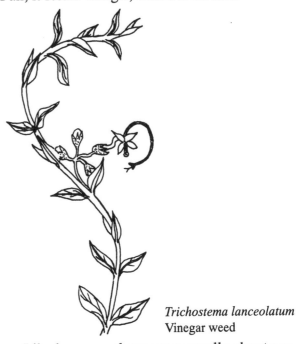

Trichostema lanceolatum
Vinegar weed

Like humans, plants are normally about neutral in pH. Vinegar weed ***Trichostema lanceolatum*** is an exception for it contains about 0.2% acetic acids in the leaves and stem, giving it the taste of vinegar. When deer and sheep eat the weed, it inhibits the digestive microbes in the rumen.

The French chemist Antoine Lavoisier named 'oxygen,' from the words 'generator of acids.' Soon it was learned that the oxidation of sulfur, phosphorus and carbon also made acids. In 1825, Sir Humphry Davy correctly proposed that the real acidifying property was hydrogen. In 1884 Svante Arrhenius explained acidity in terms of the ion H+ on his doctoral thesis, and that is the way we understand it today.

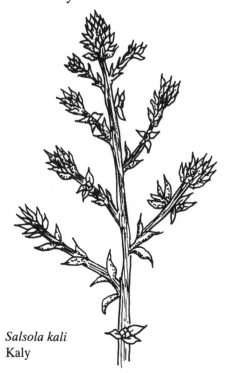

Salsola kali
Kaly

The word 'alkaline' comes from the herb 'kaly' ***Salsola kali***, which was once burned to concentrate the alkaline material known as 'sal kaly.' The words ran together over time and became alkali and then alkaline. When the alkaline material from ashes was heated with animal fats, soap was formed. This basic chemical process is still used to make soap.

Instead of writing <u>p</u>ouvoir <u>H</u>ydrogene, (literally hydrogen power), we have shortened this to pH. This is an abbreviation used by chemists to express how acid or how alkaline a solution is. Pure distilled water has a defined pH of 7.0. This means that an equal number of H+ ions, balance the same number of OH- ions. The pH scale is not linear, it is logarithmic. If we began by making water acid by adding vinegar in small quantities, a pH of 6 means that there are 10 times more H+ ions than a

pH of 7. A pH of 5 means that there are a hundred times more H+ ions that a pH of 7. A pH of 5 means that there are a hundred times more H+ ions that a neutral pH. As the scale goes up into the alkaline range a pH of 8 means that there are ten times more OH- ions than at a neutral pH. Chemists and physiologists use the pH scale, because it emphasizes the delicate balance in biological life, near the neutral zone.

If we put one drop of vinegar into a cup of water with a neutral pH of 7, the pH falls to 5.5, which is a level that, in our bodies, would instantly kill us. We know that we can easily drink several tablespoonfuls of vinegar and no harm will come to us, in spite of the fact that a lowering of the pH below 7 usually means death. The blood is carefully regulated with a 'buffer' which is a solution of a weak acid H_2CO_3 (carbonic acid) and $NaHCO_3$ (sodium bicarbonate, which is baking soda).

In 1797 the doctor of the Duke of Orleans of France invented a process for making soda from salt. Nicolas Leblanc mixed sulfuric acid with common salt to make sodium sulfate. This was burned with coal and limestone to form baking soda. Our bodies form it naturally in the blood.

The regulation of pH of the blood is kept constant by ordinary baking soda. The measure of how much baking soda you have in your blood, is known as the alkaline reserve, and the body tries to keep this constant. Drinking several teaspoonfuls of vinegar does not kill us, because the acid combines with sodium bicarbonate, and the pH remains the same. The body keeps the mixture of carbonic acid in the blood, and the bicarbonates at a ratio of 1:20. If the pH drops, we breathe out more CO_2, to regulate the pH.

Since the bicarbonate: carbonic acid ratio is about 20:1, this keeps the pH of the arterial blood regulated. If the pH drops below 7.35, the carbonic acid reacts with sodium or potassium to stop the pH drop. The kidneys regulate the pH, by adjusting the amounts of bicarbonates in the urine. If we have too much CO_2, the blood becomes acid, then the breathing increases, which releases it, and the blood goes back to the alkaline side.

Doctors rarely check blood pH because of a belief that nearly everyone is normal, so why bother. One man suffered from pruritis of the anus for eight years. He had an operation, took alcohol injections and had to wear a pad. His blood pH turned out to be a high 7.84. He was advised to eat an acid forming diet of meat, fish and eggs and take 40 drops of hydrochloric acid three times a day. The itching and discharge disappeared in a week, and didn't return.

A woman had severe pain after eating, and she was advised to eat an alkaline diet. Her blood pH was 7.84. She was given an acid diet and dilute hydrochloric acid. The symptoms cleared up within a week.

On the other hand, an examination of the urine and blood of 250 patients suffering from sinus problems, showed that all but three had acid or low pH blood. All cases of colds and sinus infections are marked with symptoms of acidosis. We become short of breath easily, and instead of being able to comfortably hold our breath for 40 seconds, we can last only 25 seconds. More acidity means breathing faster and shallower. Acidosis is marked by diets with white bread, meat, excess sugar, and potatoes. A diet with whole grains and vegetable juices produces a more normal pH.

When you have diabetes your body cannot burn sugar, so it is forced to burn acids without insulin. The cells take a fat such as steric acid, which is 18 carbon atoms long. The enzymes break it down two carbon units a time, degrading the chain to C16, then to C14 etc. The buffer capacity gets used up by acid generation, and the diabetic begins to breathe hard. When the pH falls into the range of 7.3 to 7.1, the diabetic goes into a coma, which will mean death, if it is not taken care of.

In 1877, the first experiments were done on the effects of acids. Rabbits were given large amounts of hydrochloric acid by stomach tube. As the acid combined with the sodium bicarbonate buffer, most of the carbon dioxide left the blood. The pulse and breathing became rapid, and the animals went into a coma, and then died. The animals could quickly be restored to life, in the coma, by giving them a half-gram of sodium bicarbonate per kilogram of body weight. By 1885 Ernst Stadelman realized that the diabetic coma is an acid condition, which could be treated by administering sodium bicarbonate.

The great physiologist J.B.S. Haldane did numerous experiments in shifting the pH of the blood to study the effects. He took large amounts of ammonium chloride, in order to depress the pH. Just walking down a level street with an acid pH was such an effort that he was panting, and had to stop repeatedly to catch his breath.

Some cases of asthma don't respond to asthma medications, because of respiratory acidosis. A 12 year-old girl whose blood fell to 6.66 in an acute asthma attack holds the record for a low pH. She was given injections of a sodium bicarbonate solution. When the pH rose to 7.27, the airway resistance began to clear, and she regained consciousness. She was then able to respond to epinephrine and recovered.

Vomiting and illness of pregnancy is often, but not always marked by a low blood pH. In many cases, there is a marked improvement by raising the pH of the blood, with baking soda. This rise in pH reduces water retention (edema), which is a marked feature of acidosis.

The immune system works in an alkaline pH, and generally speaking, the higher the pH, the poorer the survival of the virus. The herpes virus thrives in solution at a pH of 6.3. When the pH rises to 7.8, the virus is inactivated and can't reproduce. These experiments suggest that alkaline salts could control herpes attacks.

Calcium and other minerals are soluble in the presence of a high alkaline reserve, for it is the formation of bicarbonates, which hold them in solution. In some forms of arthritis, where the solution of minerals is involved, a slight shift in the pH of the blood might be a key in reducing the symptoms. Most cases of arthritis have no relationship to pH.

Increasing the alkaline reserve may be a key to controlling seasickness, vertigo and Meniere's disease. An excess of bicarbonates dissolves some of the calcium of the otoliths of the inner ear. It seems improbable that a simple kitchen chemical could control Meniere's disease, but it is true. In 1950 a Japanese researcher reported that he was able to relieve ten of eleven cases of vertigo, including four cases of Meniere's disease, with baking soda.

If the pH of the blood shifts towards the acid side, the stomach cannot secrete hydrochloric acid, and digestion is poor. After the pH is brought back with baking soda, digestion is restored. This is the real secret behind the use of baking soda in indigestion. Baking soda stimulates the intestinal movements and increases the amplitude of the heart.

In cancer, the blood usually becomes slightly more alkaline. In 1882 a short report was published on a woman who took ammonium chloride and a lump in her breast disappeared. Eighty years later researchers found that they could cure rat cancers by giving them the acid salt ammonium chloride, but this was not applied in a practical way to human cancer.

In 1968 a doctor noted that patients with advanced cancer have highly alkaline blood. Patients who didn't have a high pH in advanced cancer had little pain. When patients with severe pain took from 500 mgs. to one gram of ammonium chloride three times a day, there was a dramatic reduction in pain. The more alkalinity, the more dizziness and light headedness, which was relieved when the pH returned to around 7.4

It is normally assumed that painkillers block the pain receptors in the nerves. However, Doctor Evand found that painkillers sharply reduced the pH of the blood. Even aspirin compounds make the blood more acid.

If you are ever wandering in the Amazon jungle and get shot with a poison arrow, don't give up hope. Get out your box of baking soda, and take a few spoonfuls in water. When dogs were injected with curare, the pH fell steadily until they became paralyzed. When they were given 2.5 grams of baking soda by injection the paralysis reversed itself, and they were completely normal.

The kidneys control the acid-base balance by excreting excess acids or bases into the urine. When toxins are added to the body, the blood becomes acid. The toxins act in the liver, so the liver must play a part in regulation of pH. I suggest that many of the liver stimulating agents such as *Silybum marianum* and *Cynara cardunculus* leaves are alkaline shifting agents. This would account for part of their effects in pregnancy toxemia, seasickness and Meniere's disease.

The pH of the body is constantly shifting with the temperature and the barometric pressure. It is also slightly shifting with the food we eat. The old acid-base dietary conception has little to do with internal shifts of the body's pH. Vegetable foods are constantly making small shifts to it, although little has been done in the way of a study on the subtle shifts of diets.

Most people know that vitamins are essential cell nutrients. One of their most important jobs is the regulation of pH, so that normal cellular functions can go on. When French researchers tested the vitamins in relationship to the blood pH, the neutral vitamins were biotin, inositol, and folic acid. Acidgenic (acid shifting) vitamins include C, D and choline. Alkalgenic (alkaline shifting) vitamins are A, B group, E, F, K and the bioflavanoid rutin. Taking vitamins to shift the pH into a more healthful range, is a way of giving us better health.

ARTERIOSCLEROSIS

"The artery and vein, which in the old people extend between the spleen and liver acquire so thick a coat, that it constricts the passage of the blood, which comes from the mesenteric vessels. This blood passes through the liver to the heart and two great vessels, and consequently through the whole body. These vessels apart from the thickness of their coats grow in length and become twisted like a snake. The liver loses its sanguineous humor, which was carried to it by the vein. Consequently this liver becomes desiccated and like congealed bran, both in color and substance. When it is subjected to the slightest friction, its substance falls away in small flakes like sawdust, and leaves behind the veins and arteries."
Leonardo da Vinci

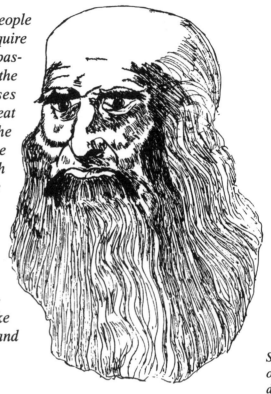

Self-Portrait of Leonardo da Vinci

Anatomy was a rare science in the ancient world, because of the prohibitions against cutting up dead people. Aristotle mentions a hardened coating, which he describes as 'a bone in the heart,' although he didn't observe it. In 1575, the Italian anatomist Gabriello Fallopio, wrote of a woman whose arteries had 'turned to bone.' At first this wasn't accepted by many doctors, but eventually "arteriosclerosis," meaning "artery-hardening," became the accepted word to describe the condition.

By 1506, Leonardo da Vinci did two dissections at the Hospital of Santa Maria Nurova in Florence, Italy. He found that a two-year-old child had no 'coat' on the capillary vessels, but an old man had a thick coat blocking the flow of blood. Leonardo wrote, "As a consequence of this, the old dread cold more than the young. Those that are very old have a skin the color of wood or dried chestnut, because the skin is almost completely deprived of nourishment. The coats of the vessels behave in man as in oranges. The peel thickens and the pulp diminishes the older they become. If you say that it is the thickened blood, which ceases to flow through the vessels, this isn't true. The blood in the vessels does not thicken, because it continually dies and is renewed."

Leonardo had the first theory of arteriosclerosis. He studied the flow of fluids, and noted how slow moving water forms S curves in a glass tube. He noted that the rivers of Italy formed S curves. As the rivers changed courses, they left silt on one side, and he applied this idea to the blood.

The problem of cholesterol has only been recognized in the twentieth century, but it has existed throughout time. When Marc Ruffer made a medical study of the mummies of Nubia, Egypt, he found that many of them had hardening of the arteries. These people didn't smoke, and they probably didn't drink that much. We assume that they didn't have the worries of civilization, although building pyramids might have been stressful. Their diet must have caused hardening of the arteries.

Cholesterol is a steroid wax that deposits on blood vessel walls. Cholesterol is just one of many sterols, of which digitalis, cortisone, Vitamin D, and the male and female hormones are members. People with circulation problems are often put on a low cholesterol diet. Cholesterol narrows the blood passages, and the surrounding tissues have less nourishment. Low cholesterol diets were very common a few years ago, but so many foods have cholesterol, and their value wasn't that great, so most doctors no longer prescribe them.

In 1908 a Russian scientist fed rabbits milk and egg yokes, and the rabbits developed arteriosclerosis. When rabbits were given corn oil, it lowered their cholesterol, but coconut oil raised it. High blood pressure caused more cholesterol to deposit on the cell walls.

Since egg yokes are high in cholesterol, they are normally excluded from special diets. When 31 Japanese volunteers were fed three egg yokes per meal for two weeks, nine of them had a marked rise in cholesterol. Avoiding dietary cholesterol does not necessarily decrease blood cholesterol, but it seems to help about 30% of people.

A comparison of European and Chinese people reveals much lower levels of gallstones (which are lumps of cholesterol), and coronary thrombosis in China. The Chinese diet includes lots of rice and soybeans with sesame, peanut and soybean oils. The difference in diets was graphically demonstrated during the Korean War, when it was found that 50% of the dead Western soldiers had visible atheromas on the aortic wall. An incredible 10% had at least one coronary artery reduced by 50% of its diameter by deposits. By contrast, there were no deposits found in autopsies of Chinese and North Korean soldiers.

Vegetable oils with high iodine numbers (i.e. unsaturated) are known to lower plasma cholesterol. It is the linolenic acid in the diet that lowers cholesterol. The amounts of this unsaturated fat vary by 55% in flax oil, 8% in soybean oil, 7% in millet seed oil and 0.5% in corn oil. With increased amounts of linoleate in the diet, cholesterol concentrations fell by 29% in two months and continued to fall. This means that we need to choose cooking oils or foods with high amounts of linolenic acid.

In 1877 Dr. William Ord had a patient with an enlarged nonfunctional thyroid gland. This uncommon disorder is known as myxedema. He studied nearly a hundred patients with the disorder, and published a booklet on his findings. He noted that in all cases, the arteries showed advanced arteriosclerosis. The iodine used by an active thyroid seems to prevent deposition of cholesterol in the body. This is why iodine supplements are active in removing angina pains. They gradually clear up the cholesterol from the arteries.

A number of common ordinary foods have significant cholesterol-lowering properties. Cabbages contain s-methyl-1-cysteine sulfoxide. When added to the diet of rats both compounds decreased the blood cholesterol from the control levels of 400 mgs. to 266 mg./100 ml. of blood. When rats were given supplements of the amino acid methionine, it lowered the cholesterol to 291 mg./ 100mg. The chick pea *Cicer arientinum* lowers cholesterol, and in areas in India where it is a staple food, people have low levels of serum cholesterol and a low incidence of heart disease.

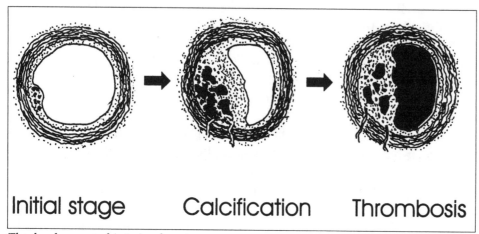

Initial stage   Calcification   Thrombosis

The development of Arteriosclerosis

Beets contain betaine, which resembles choline in molecular structure. Betaine was given to 21 people suffering from coronary arteriosclerosis. These people were on a low cholesterol diet and they had taken choline and inositol to reduce cholesterol. The addition of six grams of betaine daily resulted in easier breathing and a reduction in angina pains. In six months the serum cholesterol fell from an average of 275 to 214 mg. per 100 cc. of blood

Cholesterol is a curious substance, because the liver excretes it into the bile. Then it goes into the digestive tract, and most of it is reabsorbed. The leaves of the eggplant **Solanum melongena** have an active cholesterol-lowering substance. With radioactive tracers, scientists showed that eggplant leaves lowered the absorption of cholesterol by 77%. It prevents absorption in the digestive tract, but it isn't particularly helpful in the diet.

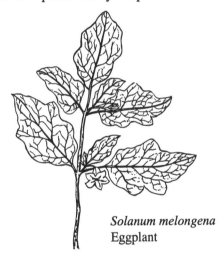

Solanum melongena
Eggplant

The yellow coloring principle of turmeric **Curcuma longa** is curcumin. When rats were fed levels of 0.1% in the diet, the serum and liver cholesterol levels fell to half of normal levels. Curcumin stimulates the liver to turn cholesterol into bile acids which are eliminated from the body.

Hindu catnip **Nepeta hindostani** is an active medical plant. Pigs were put on a high fat diet and half of them were given an extract of 20 mg./kg. of the plant. On this high fat diet, the heart muscle fibers under a microscope showed swelling and smudging. The pigs given a tincture of catnip showed no swelling or acid staining, and the fibers retained their original structure.

The story of silicon in medicine began in 1874 with a report that it was quite valuable for diabetics and cancer patients. Other doctors reported that silicon supplements could help gout, diarrhea and dyspepsia. Some of the mineral springs of France are high in silicon, and this aroused interest in drinking high silicon waters.

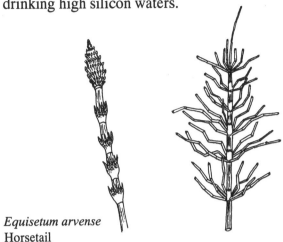

Equisetum arvense
Horsetail

In 1905 several experimenters began to work with sodium silicate, which is soluble in water. It is relatively nontoxic when taken by mouth, but quite toxic when injected. Three experimenters showed that sodium silicate removed the deposits in the arteries. High blood pressure, dizziness, angina, labored breathing and dyspepsia slowly disappeared.

Studies show that there is a relationship between the water supply and arteriosclerosis. The 'water protective factor' is silicon, and the more silicic acid in drinking water, the less coronary heart disease is found. Rich sources of natural silicon are rice straw at 2.7%, rice hulls at 2.3%, oat hulls and oat straw at 1.7%. Most health food stores carry a preparation of silicon extracted from horsetail **Equisetum arvense**.

When 31 rabbits were fed a diet high in cholesterol, 77% of them developed arteriosclerosis. In a similar group of rabbits with silicon supplements, only 21% showed artery damage. This finding extends to humans. Those people with damage show low silicon levels; those with clear arteries show higher levels of silicon.

By 1911 French doctors published their first results on silicon in arteriosclerosis. Patients who were bedridden saw their dizziness and backaches disappear after taking silica supplements. Many bedridden patients were able to walk and lead a normal life. Further studies confirmed that high levels of silicon lead to low artery clogging.

Rats were put on a high cholesterol diet and then divided into dietary groups. The rats eating rice had no change in cholesterol levels, but those on wheat, barley, whole wheat and milk powder had slightly reduced levels. The rats given oatmeal had much lower levels of cholesterol.

Then the doctors followed up the experiment by having 21 male volunteers eat two slices of bread a day, which was made by using 50% oatmeal. In three weeks the average cholesterol of the volunteers fell from 251 mgs. to 223 mgs. When the volunteers switched to wheat bread, their cholesterol levels rose to 246 mgs. in two weeks. We eat bread, because wheat has a quality of stickiness and rises well. The public is conditioned by advertising to accept bleached wheat bread, as the only real bread. My grandmother made oatmeal bread, and its slightly nutty flavor was always a special treat.

It is now recognized that oat bran selectively lowers the low-density lipoprotein cholesterol concentrations. Oat bran makes delicious bread, muffins and cereal. There is ample evidence that the use of oatmeal and oat bran could significantly improve the health of the nation.

Among the many plants mentioned in medical literature for reducing cholesterol are dandelions, turmeric, rosemary and *Orthosiphon staminaus*. In 1934 it was discovered that the leaves of the common artichoke *Cynara scolymus* are very active in lowering cholesterol. They were used in Italy for a wide variety of complaints. A kilogram of the leaves yields about 150 milligrams of cynarin. The agent becomes inactive when the leaves are dried, so it was not readily available until it was synthesized in 1960.

The active agent is a chemical called 1-4 dicaffeyl-quinic acid. When 1.5 grams a day were given to 23 people with arteriosclerosis, the average cholesterol level fell by 25% over a period of two months and was still falling. The people felt better, and there was less heart pain. The chemical sped up the conversion of cholesterol into bile, which was excreted from the body.

Around 1960 the US Army Quartermaster Corps asked nutritionists to test the C rations for nutrition. When they fed the jelly included in the rations to chickens, the birds had less cholesterol. The pectin in the jelly was then tested. Animals given pectin ate more, and gained less weight than

the controls. They excreted three times as much fat and twice as much cholesterol, as the other chickens. It takes around 5% pectin in the diet to produce a significant lowering of cholesterol.

Yogurt lowers cholesterol, and it is theorized that it blocks a regulatory enzyme. Regular use of yogurt can lower the cholesterol level by a third. When yogurt is discontinued, cholesterol levels quickly go back to their original values.

It has recently been recognized that fish oils reduce cholesterol. A woman did a trial for eight weeks under a skeptical doctor's supervision. The systolic blood pressure went from 175 to 138; the cholesterol fell from 253 to 195 and the triglycerides fell from 150 to 104.

In 1948 scientists put a group of rhesus monkeys *Macaca mulatta* on a synthetic diet. Vitamin B6 was removed from the diets of healthy monkeys. For the first six months, there was little change. Then they become hyperirritable and jumpy. Their hair was thinner and lighter. It was found that they developed severe arteriosclerosis.

A theory developed from this. When the protein methionine is broken down it forms homocysteine. When homocysteine is injected into baboons it produces arteriosclerosis. Homocysteine is a toxic amino acid that causes the cells lining the artery to degenerate and slough off. Where this happens, clumps of cholesterol and tirglycerides form what is called an atheroma. The clump of material is a roadblock, which restricts the flow of blood. Extra Vitamin B6 converts homocysteine to the nontoxic cystathionine, and prevents the process that forms arteriosclerosis.

Angina is a condition in which arteriosclerosis restricts the flow of blood, and reduces the oxygen to the cells. A study was done in South Africa on 17 patients. They were given a low meat, high vegetable diet. Along with a B vitamin supplement, they were given 100 mgs of B6. All of them had a complete or partial relief of angina, with more energy and a sense of well being.

The pain from angina pectoris is due to cholesterol blockage of oxygen around the heart. A supplement of Vitamin B6 alone could prevent many heart by-pass operations. Other studies prove that a diet high in unsaturated oils, silicon and herbs can reverse these unhealthy conditions.

☆☆☆

BLOOD PURIFIERS

"Dr. Croone told me, that at the meeting of Gresham College tonight, there was a pretty experiment of the blood of one dog (a little mastiff), let out, till he died into the body of another (a spaniel) on one side, while all his own ran out on the other side. The first died upon the place, and the other pretty well, and likely to do well. This did give occasion to many pretty wishes, as of the blood of a Quaker to be let into an Archbishop, and such like. As Dr. Croone says, it may if it takes, be of mighty use to man's health, for the mending of bad blood by borrowing from a better body."

Diary of Samuel Pepys *November 14, 1666*

When I was discussing a plant, a friend remarked: "Well, I suppose you consider that one a blood purifier?"

I remarked: "What do you mean by blood purifier?"

"I don't really know," he admitted. Although the meaning seems self evident, the words "blood purifier" are meaningless. In 1898 *Popular Science* published a humorous spoof on "Directions on becoming an 'Indian Doctor.'" "Buy up a job lot of senna, and make it into senna tea with a few other 'yarbs.' Bottle it and take it out on the road with a wagon. Name it 'yokotami, the great blood purifier of the Pugwash Indians.' Men will throng to the wagon to get it, and going to the edge of the crowd, will take a furtive swig to see how much better they feel. They usually think they do and after their bowels have moved the next morning, they know they do."

In 1682 Thomas Ash became one of the first to mention the blood herbs of the New World. "The China **Smilax tamnoides** grows plentifully there, whose root infused yields us that pleasant drink, which we know by the name of China ale in England; in medicinal uses, it's far more excellent. In all pestilential distempers, as plague, smallpox and malignant fevers, it is a noble specific. When stung, they eat the root, applying it to the venomous wound; or they boil the roots in water, which drunk fortifies and corroborates the heart exciting strong and generous sweat, by which the endangered nature is relieved and the poison is carried off and expelled. It modifies and sweetens the blood. It is good in fevers, scurvy, gonorrhea and the lues venerea."

The Pennsylvania Dutch used 'blood thinning remedies' in the spring, for presumably the thick winter blood was poorly adapted to the warm months. These "bluteinigungsmittel" remedies contained such items as dandelions, lettuce, watercress and plantain. The herbs that they spoke of as blood purifiers were sassafras, sarsaparilla, burdock and devil's bit.

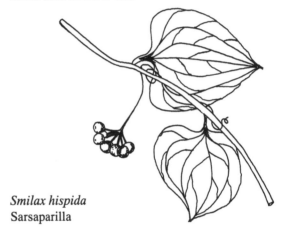

Smilax hispida
Sarsaparilla

In the nineteenth century, the regular doctors believed that they could draw off bad blood by bleeding. The Thomsonian doctors believed that the best way to remove bad blood was to sweat out the impurities. They used hot teas to open the pores of the skin, and heated rooms to sweat their patients.

Nearly a century ago, the British Medical Association put out a book called *Secret Remedies*. The sections are listed by category, and the contents of the remedies were listed. An example is Harvey's Blood Pills. They contained sarsaparilla, dandelions, burdock, quinine and potassium iodide.

Clarke's Blood Mixture was said to cure scrofula, scurvy, scrofulous sores, glandular swellings, cancerous ulcers, bad legs, syphilis, piles, rheumatism, gout, dropsy, sore eyes, and eruptions on the skin. The main ingredient was potassium iodide.

Hood's Compound Extract of Sarsaparilla was made from sarsaparilla, dandelion, mandrake, dock, pipsissewa, juniper berries and other vegetable remedies. The bottle read: "...designed to act upon the blood, and through that upon all the organs and tissues of the body."

Hughes' Blood Pills were made with aloes, japap resin, cinchona bark, ginger and oil of cloves. The bottle stated: "The blood being therefore the life of the living body, it stands to reason that if it is poisoned, you poison the whole system, and eventually destroy the life of the man. When the blood is chilled, or distempered through breathing impure air, unhealthy food etc., it at once gets disturbed, and breeds disease in some form or other."

The use of color is obvious in the choice of blood purifiers. The most popular blood purifier of the Appalachians was sassafras tea, which has a red color and a pleasant odor. Sassafras was the main taste of the original 'root beer.' Root beer was originally a beer, which was brewed with a mixture of six roots for the purpose of purifying the blood.

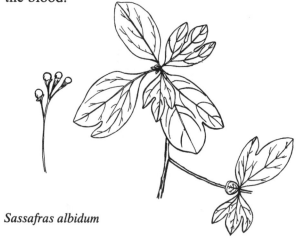

Sassafras albidum

A tea of sassafras roots *Sassafras albidum* was once known as a "spring tonic," and it was common knowledge that sassafras thins the blood. The truth behind this bit of lore was accidentally discovered in 1939. A woman came to Doctor Vander Bogart's office and said, "My head feels so funny; I cannot describe it, I feel so funny all over; trebly, nervous, and I cannot seem to control myself." The doctor found that the woman's high blood pres-

sure had dropped by 30 mm. in one week without any apparent cause. He gave her medication for her headache, and she left.

The next week she returned to the doctor, and he found that her blood pressure rose back to its usual level. She wondered if it was the sassafras tea that she had drank the previous week. The doctor asked her to try sassafras tea for a week, out of curiosity. Soon she had headaches and her blood pressure dropped by 30 mm. By ceasing to drink the tea, she had no further problems.

Doctor Bogart had a 42-year-old patient with a dangerous blood pressure level of 240. For nearly 12 years he wasn't able to find a cause or a suitable treatment for her. She began to take a sassafras tincture, and her blood pressure quickly dropped to the healthy range of 100/154. All of the doctor's hypertensive patients had major blood pressure reductions simply by using a tea or tincture of sassafras.

In popular herbal literature, the blood purifiers are generally either red or yellow. If you were sick with jaundice, your skin was yellow, but you treated it with either red or yellow herbs. You could take 'yellow dock,' dandelion tea, primrose flowers, yellow perilla, or Oregon grape which is a bitter yellow tea. The most popular red blood purifiers were beet roots, wild cherry bark, red clover flowers, red wheat, sassafras and red cedar. Red roots mentioned for blood purification were ***Salix alba tristis***, ***Lachnanthes caroliana***, and ***Ceanothus americanus***.

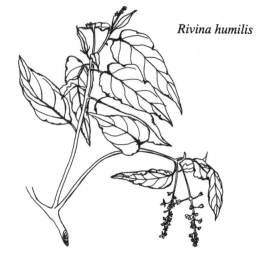

Rivina humilis

A survey of the flowers shows that about 50% are white, 20% are yellow, 20% are red, and 10% are the remaining colors. There are more than 60 species of flowers called 'blood flowers' from their blood red color. Among popular names are the 'bloodberry' *Rivina humilis*, the 'blood root' *Potentilla erecta*, and the 'fire weed' *Epilobium angustifolium*.

The germ theory of disease began with the work of Louis Pasteur around 1875. Before that time, bad humors, bad vapors and bad blood were popular explanations of disease. Because of the idea that disease was caused by poisons in the blood, it was popular to bleed, to treat almost anything, Bleeding removed the bad blood, and the body replaced it with good fresh blood.

The lore of bad blood is present in many societies. The Mackenzie River Eskimos have few plants to use in medicine, but the blood letter's knife is the cure-all. They do not associate snowblindness with the glare from sunlight, but with bad blood. In the spring the sun returns and thins the blood, so it flows into the forehead and the eyes. This influx of bad blood causes snowblindness, so it must be drained by making cuts above the eyebrows. Cutting in front of the ear cures earaches, and cutting treats headaches over the painful area.

In Chinese medicine the word 'oketsu' means 'accumulation of bad blood.' The herbs used to treat it are diuretics. What they are really treating is congestive edema, which they believe is an excess of bad blood. The popular diuretic herbs are *Akebia quinata*, *Platycodon grandiflorum* and *Polygala tenuifolia*.

The 'oketsu' syndrome of Chinese medicine can mean 'blood stagnation' and also indicates a fever. One herb that is used to treat it is *Angelica acutiloba*. It decreases blood viscosity, and increases peripheral blood circulation after oral administration. The active component is about a milligram of adenosine per gram of the root. Other herbs containing adenosine are *Ganoderma lucidum*, and *Verbena officinalis*.

There are a number of traditional definitions of blood purifiers. John Lust says in his herb book that blood purifiers are herbs that eliminate toxins and uric acid. It is obvious from the old herb books that anything reputed to cure snakebite is a blood purifier. The idea is that the snake injected a toxin, and the herbal cure removed the toxin. A third definition of blood purifier is anything that takes away skin problems.

The main idea behind the words 'blood purifier' in nineteenth century herbalism is that skin disease is a result of bad blood. Boils were not present on thin, anemic-looking people, but on ruddy person whose faces suggested too much drinking. The French have a saying: "Se faire de mauvais sang," which means, "to make some bad blood." When we get angry, emotions cause our face to break out. Syphilis was a disease of bad blood, and it caused terrible skin disorders.

The traditional meaning of 'blood purifiers' are herbs which clear up the skin. These were the herbs used to treat ringworm, eczema, psoriasis, and boils. The most active herbs for several of these disorders were the berberine-containing plants such as goldenseal or species of *Berberis*.

Potassium iodide is a very well known 'blood purifier.' This was once widely used for the skin disorders following syphilis. It was known as a blood purifier, alliterative or deobstruent. It was used to clear opacities in the eye.

The makers of iron tonics advertise their products for 'tired blood.' Of course they are speaking of anemia, which is generally curable with iron, B12, folic acid and methionine. The red blood cells have an average life span of 120 days, and then the body breaks them into bile, which provides the brown color of the feces. We do not know how the body determines which red blood cells are 'old,' and thus breaks them down. We do know from radioactive tracers that we get three complete changes of red blood cells each year of lives, so we never really have 'tired, old blood.'

If we are to use the words 'blood purifier' in a scientific way, then it should be divided into the categories that deal with the blood. Every fifteen minutes all the blood in the body passes through the liver, where enzymes convert waste products into forms that the kidneys remove from the blood. The average lifetime of a drug is often less than an hour, because the liver enzymes convert it into another form. The liver stimulants are thus true blood purifiers.

The adult function of the spleen is still largely unknown, but it plays a part in the regulation of the blood. The spleen is on the left side of the body under the diaphragm. In the prenatal embryo the spleen participates in the formation of blood. The spleen also regulates the number of white and red blood cells.

Emanuel Swedenborg was a Swedish scientist and mystic who founded a religion out of his experiences. In his work *Animal Kingdom*, he extensively discussed the activity of the organs and blood purification. Swedenborg wrote, "There are these three vicera- the liver, pancreas, and spleen, whose special province is to purify the blood. But the main duties depend on the liver. From their association in function, their succession of operations, their connection with each other and with the aorta; and from the nature of each, and the power it possesses of demanding its tribute, at will from the system."

The other categories of blood purifiers are red blood cells stimulants, bile stimulants, gout herbs, and kidney stimulants. The herbs which deal with these problems are discussed elsewhere. Combination of these herbs are real 'blood purifiers.' An understanding of this gives meaning to a generally meaningless term.

✲ ✲ ✲

LOW BLOOD PRESSURE

"I dreamed that the visible universe is the physical universe is the physical person of God; that the vast worlds that we see twinkling millions of miles apart in the fields of space are the blood corpuscles in His veins; and that we and the other creatures are the microbes that charge, with multitudinous life the corpuscles."

Following the Equator *Mark Twain*

"We also have our spring when the little arterioles dilate, the lymph flows in a brisker stream, the glands work harder, winnowing and straining. Each year nature readjusts the whole machine. I can feel the ferment in my blood at this very moment, and as the cool sunshine pours through my window I could dance about in it like a gnat."

Arthur Conan Doyle

The first person to attempt a measurement of the blood pressure was the remarkable English clergyman scientist, Steven Hales. He tied a horse down, and cut the artery of the neck. Since rubber tubing wasn't invented yet, he attached the artery with the windpipe of a goose to a long glass tube tired to a tree. The blood rose to a height of eight feet three inches and went up and down with the beat of the heart.

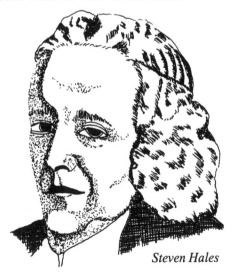
Steven Hales

To understand this experiment it is necessary to understand blood pressure. If you could isolate and weigh an air column an inch square, which extended to the limit of the earth's atmosphere, you would find that is weighed. 14.7 pounds. A column of water an inch square by 34 feet long is equal to the weight of that column of air. If air were the same density as water, we would be at the bottom of a 34-foot deep swimming pool.

If the heart of Steven Hales' horse had pumped the blood to a height of 34 feet, the blood pressure would have been 14.7 pounds per square inch. Instead of saying that the blood pressure is 3.7 pounds per square inch (it was pumped about a quarter of the way), we use mercury units based on a sea level reading of 760 millimeters of mercury. This was first worked out by the French scientist Jean Poiseuille with a mercury manometer. When we convert to millimeters, we find that Stephen Hales' horse had a blood pressure of 190 mm. of mercury.

When the doctor puts a cuff around your arm, he is approximating the height in mercury, that the blood would be pumped to. Greater pressure means greater restriction of the flow, so blood pressure is a measure of resistance. Higher pressure means that the heart must work harder to pump blood, and there is a greater chance of malfunction and heart attacks. Lower pressure may mean a feeble heart action, or excessively dilated capillaries.

After the cuff is put around your arm and inflated, the doctor listens to the sounds of the blood with a stethoscope. As the pressure restricts the flow to the cutoff point, the heart makes 'Korotkoff sounds.' We hear these sounds in home plumbing, when water is constricted and the pipes vibrate. When the 'water hammer' sounds disappear, it means that the blood flow is cut off, and at this point the reading of air pressure on the cuff establishes the blood pressure.

An English company did a survey of the blood pressure of all 3,400 employees. In men from 15-19 years of age, this ranged from 56/108 to a high of 95/143; while women in the same group ranged from 58/101 to 92/138. In men who were 60-64 years old, this ranged from 71/123 to a high of 92/184. A comparable age group of women had blood pressures, which ranged from 72/125 to a high of 108/180. In each five-year interval the blood pressure of the men increased by 3 mm. systolic and 1.4 mm. diastolic. In the same time period, women increased by 3.5 mm. systolic and 1.7 mm. diastolic.

In 1956 Jakob Boe published a study of the blood pressure of the people of Bergen, Norway. Blood pressure of men below the age of 40 is gaussian, i.e. it is a bell shaped curve, with approximately as many people on the low side as on the high side. After the age of 40, the blood pressure curves are separated into two groups. One group retained an average sytolic (emptying) pressure of 140 mm. of mercury. The second group had a mean (most frequent) pressure of around 200 mm. of mercury and a range of 170-240. Of course, blood pressures ran all the way from readings of 110 mm. to life-threatening readings.

Doctors don't agree on what constitutes low blood pressure. For adults the standard might be below 110 mm. diastolic or below 90 mm. systolic pressure. Low blood pressure may be a symptom of a real heart problem, i.e. the heart is too weak to pump the blood around the body. The person may feel weak and tired. If it is not heart weakness, he will probably live a lot longer than those of us who have high blood pressure. His body is adapted to it, so it isn't a medical problem.

Blood pressure is inherited; if your family has high blood pressure, you probably will too. For unknown reasons small families have lower pressure, and large families have higher pressure. People who do hard physical work, tend to have lower blood pressures, then people who sit at a desk and do light work all day.

Many tribes in East Africa tipped their arrowheads with a toxin from the seeds of **Strophanthus gratus**. Ouabain is a steroid hormone, which increases the force of the heartbeat, and slows its rate. Digitalis, ouabain, and many other substances of the same nature increase the blood pressure.

Scientists investigated a mysterious 'sodium pump' inhibitor in the blood. This inhibitor raised the blood pressure, and it appeared that people who had more, had higher blood pressure. To their surprise they found that mystery substance was ouabain. It is probably made by the adrenal glands, and more of it in the blood raises blood pressure.

Blood pressure is like obesity: there is no boundary separating out low and high groups. When either weight or blood pressure is increased, there are increased risks. Both low and high values indicate that something is likely to be wrong. What is normal for one person can be high for another.

I knew a long distance bicycle racer who wore a medallion around his neck giving his blood pressure and heart beat. Constant hours of racing dropped his resting heartbeat to 55, and greatly lowered his blood pressure. The medallion was a reminder to doctors, if he was involved in an accident; he was not in shock, it was his normal blood pressure and heart beat.

Blood pressure is not a constant; it depends on what time of day it is, or whether you have recently eaten, and what your emotional state is. As you go to sleep it drops by 20-30 mm. in the first two to three hours. Then it slowly rises as the waking hour approaches, and jumps 10-20 mm. in the first hour of waking. The blood pressure curve continues to rise and dips about 1 P.M, and then rises again to reach the highest value for the day around 6 P.M. New measuring techniques show that it varies greatly when you are involved in conversation.

One of the problems with low blood pressure is known as orthostatic hypotension. This is a sharp decrease in blood pressure, when a patient afflicted with it stands. The blood pressure is normal when we lie down, but the pulse does not increase in some people when they stand up, and then they are dizzy and barely able to function. Vasoconstricting drugs raise the general level of blood pressure, but they don't prevent a decrease in blood pressure when people stand. The disorder improves during the day, so it isn't bothersome later on.

People with orthostatic hypotension shouldn't sleep on a flat bed, but should lie in a semi-inclined or 'head-up' position. A 59 year-old man had a lying down blood pressure of 80/130. After he was standing for five minutes the pressure dropped to 45/55. He couldn't stand up very long, because his heart wasn't performing enough work. When the head of his bed was elevated by 18 inches, improvement occurred rapidly. He was able to stand erect for longer periods. After four days he could stand for an hour without problems. When he switched to a level bed, his problem returned. When he went back to the elevated bed, he was able to return to normal work in two weeks.

A doctor working at the Mayo Clinic complained of exhaustion and attacks of unconsciousness. It started when his father was ill, and he spent long nights with him. There was a pronounced weakness in walking and several times he lost consciousness. Hypoglycemia was suspected, but his blood sugar was apparently normal. When he switched to a bed which was elevated by about 18 inches the problem went away in a few days.

Blood pressure is regulated by a complex interaction between the nervous system, and the catecholamines secreted by the adrenal gland. The catecholamines are made largely from the amino acid tyrosine. It is interesting to find that when rats with high blood pressure are given tyrosine, the pressure is lowered. Glutamic acid is known to elevate the blood pressure.

When rats are made hypotensive by bleeding and then are given tyrosine, the blood pressure rises. An amount of 50 mg./kg. produces a significant increase in five minutes, and double this amount produces a faster response and higher blood pressure. The blood pressure may increase by up to 50% in fifteen minutes and then it drops off. Tyrosine has been considered for treating people with shock or excessive bleeding.

In 1940, an experiment was done at Rochester, Minnesota, to see what a deficiency of Vitamin B1 would do. In three to six months the volunteers became irritable, depressed and quarrelsome. People dropped things, and were unable to concentrate. Two persons threatened suicide and others developed anxiety neurosis. The blood pressure dropped sharply to levels of 50-60 diastolic and 85-100 systolic. When people stood up they became pale and giddy. The vitamin may be useful in low blood pressure.

A 70 year-old man had a horizontal resting blood pressure of 99/160. When he stood up, his blood pressure dropped to 70/110, which resulted in unsteadiness and giddiness. The only thing that the doctor's could find wrong was a low level of Vitamin B12. As a last resort he was given a daily injection of 100 micrograms of B12 for a week, then one injection of a milligram each week was given. The problem improved and was completely gone in two months.

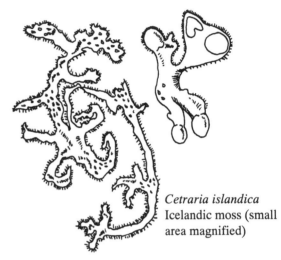

Cetraria islandica
Icelandic moss (small area magnified)

The first herb found that raises blood pressure was Icelandic moss *Cetraria islandica*. Anemic patients were given 100 mg. tablets of *Cetraria* twice a day. This resulted in a 30% increase in red blood cells and a 13% increase in white blood cells. The 3% of cetrarin in the herb raised the blood pressure.

Licorice *Glycyrrhiza glabra* is a strong stimulant of the adrenals. The adrenal hormones in turn raise the blood pressure. A doctor formed the habit of eating several licorice bars a day, when he passed a health shop in England. He didn't realize what was happening until he checked his blood pressure. It was normally 70/120, now it stood at an alarming 160/240.

Glycyrrhiza glabra
Licorice

There are many herbs known to treat high blood pressure, but few studies have been done for low blood pressure. A test in India showed that a water extract of **Convolvulus pluricaulis** lowers blood pressure. The paradox was that small amounts of a tincture of the same herb raised blood pressure! Both yohimbine and quebrachine produce a protracted elevation in blood pressure. This hypertensive effect is a result of direct action on the vasomotor center. Vitamin B12 raises the blood pressure, in cases of pernicious anemia.

The regular taking of ginseng is known to increase the blood pressure and elevate the mood. For this reason taking large amounts of ginseng should be viewed with caution. Poke weed **Phytolacca americana** was once a popular folk remedy for arthritis. It raises the blood pressure of nearly all people who take it. This is possibly due to kidney damage, so the plant should be used with great caution.

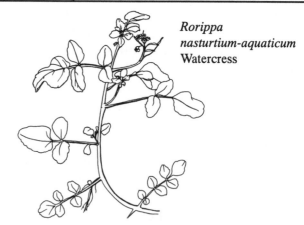

Rorippa nasturtium-aquaticum Watercress

A study was made of the herbs used by native herbalists in Brazil to lower the blood pressure. Two of the herbs used actually raised it. Watercress **Rorippa nasturtium-aquaticum** and **Mikania glomerata** had a pronounced effect on raising the blood pressure and the heart beat. While low blood pressure is comparatively rare in comparison with high blood pressure, nature does have remedies.

✧ ✧ ✧

HIGH BLOOD PRESSURE

"Keep thy heart at seventy throbs in a minute, all more than that wears away life too quickly. If thy respiration be too quick, think with thyself that thou hast has sinned against natural order and moderation.

Drink not wine nor strong drink; and observe that this rule is worthiest in its symbolic meaning. Bask daily in the sunshine, and let it rest on thy heart.

Eat no spiced meats. Young chickens, new fallen lambs, fruits, bread four days old, milk, freshest butter, will make thy fleshy tabernacle youthful."

Nathaniel Hawthorne

Until William Harvey discovered the circulation of the blood, there was little idea of either blood pressure or circulation. The English scientist Stephen Hales (1677-1761) began his scientific work by studying the flow of sap in trees, and then he applied his techniques to the study of blood pressure. He determined the volume of blood pumped by the heart by taking a freshly killed sheep's heart and pouring it full of hot wax from a gunbarrel. He then multiplied the volume of wax, by the number of beats per minute, to obtain the first real measure of the heart's output.

The modern era of blood pressure measurement began in 1897, when the cuff sphygmometer was invented. In 1905 it was linked to the stethoscope, and correlated with 'Korotkoff sounds.' When these hammering sounds disappear, the circulation is cut off, and the air pressure indicates the blood pressure.

Using a series of ingenious blood pressure measuring devices, scientists found that the average blood pressure remains constant throughout the body. They also found that higher than normal pressures were accompanied with headaches and mental confusion. The Italian physiologist Karl Vierdont put subjects on a delicately balanced board. When problems were given to them, so that they had to think hard, the head went down and the feet came up. He attributed this to a greater supply of blood to the head. He believed that the time of one complete blood circulation in all animals and man remained constant at 27 heartbeats. Another study places the complete circulation of blood at just about double this figure.

The study of high blood pressure (hypertension) began in 1836 when Richard Bright was struck with the frequency of large hearts without disease, along with small kidneys. Since he did not know that hypertension was the cause, he suggested that kidney problems were due to chemicals in the blood, which affected capillary circulation and forced the heart to work harder. When the heart had to work harder, it enlarged.

Many of the nineteenth century doctors made observations indicating that high blood pressure was not good. Since they had no easy way of measuring pressure, doctors checked the pulse. A 'hard pulse' was a sign of something wrong. But they had no specific remedies to 'soften the pulse,' so there was little they could do about it.

In modern times studies involving more than 400,000 people show conclusively that lower diastolic blood pressure reduces stroke and coronary heart disease. The lower the blood pressure, the lower the risk. A reduction of 10 mm. blood pressure resulted in 56% less stroke and 37% less coronary heart disease. Countries like the US and Russia have a high average blood pressure and a high risk of stroke. In areas like South America average blood pressure is low and heart disease is rare.

It has long been known that people who are overweight have higher blood pressure. Overweight is associated with heart palpitation, knee pain, neuritis and vertigo. Generally about two days after a good weight reduction diet is started, relief is felt in shortness of breath and palpitation. It is not unusual to have a drop of 20 mm. in systolic blood pressure in the first week.

A woman suffered from headaches, backaches, shortness of breath, and swelling of the ankles. Her weight was initially 190 pounds and the blood pressure was 110/204. In four weeks her blood pressure dropped to 92/170, and when she got to 158 pounds the blood pressure was 98/165.

Doctor Wesley Norwood of South Carolina discovered the first real remedy for hypertension around 1850. He found that a tincture of green hellebore could reduce the frequency of the pulse at will. He administered it to adults in quantities beginning at eight drops every three hours, increasing it by a drop at each dose, until the pulse was reduced or until vomiting was produced. In that case the dose had to be reduced by half.

In 1856 Ephrim Cutter dug a quantity of green hellebore **Veratrum viride** roots from a stream and dried them. After soaking them in 95% alcohol for a week, he distributed the tincture to the Massachusetts Medical Society. The doctors were enthusiastic about the new remedy; it was a wonderful 'arterial sedative,' and it quickly and drastically lowered the pulse. The use of the tincture lowered the pulse rate by 20-40 beats a minute.

The green hellebore remedy was forgotten until it was briefly revived in 1948. A patient had a blood pres-

Veratrum viride

sure of 170/270. The man was confused and disoriented, and the normal drugs weren't working. A few drops of the veratrum tincture lowered the pressure to 70/150 in eight hours. The drop in blood pressure lasts about 12 hours, so it has to be taken twice a day.

The second herb which was found to reduce blood pressure, was the Brazilian shrub jaborandi *Pilocarpus jaborandi.* It received tremendous attention around 1880 with a report that it grew hair on bald heads, but disappointed doctors found that this was uncommon. A few leaves of the plant caused heavy sweating; so it is used in small amounts. Pilocarpine is used to treat glaucoma, which is high eyeball pressure, so it is not surprising that the herb also reduces blood pressure. The leaves of jaborandi yield about 0.5% pilocarpine.

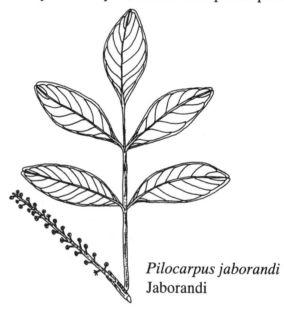

Pilocarpus jaborandi
Jaborandi

In 1914 Doctor William Robinson gave all of his cases of hypertension and enlarged hearts pilocarpine. The average dose was 2 mg. per day, although it occasionally had to be reduced. The alkaloid was taken after meals with water. This reduced the blood pressure from 30-40 mm. in 4-6 weeks. It reduced headaches and kidney disease caused by high blood pressure. Harsh dry skin became soft, possibly due to the sweating effect.

In a typical case, a 68-year-old woman suffered from stroke, impaired speech and headaches. Her systolic blood pressure was 214, and her pulse was 84. In four months the pressure fell to 182 and the pulse fell to 74. A 66 year-old man suffered from insomnia, vertigo and headache. In three weeks his blood pressure fell from 208 to 188, and the symptoms were going away. In eight months the blood pressure remained constant at 166, and the man enjoyed better health than he had in years.

The third herb found that reduced blood pressure was watermelon seeds *Citrullus lanatus*. Doctor Barksdale ground them, boiled them, and extracted them with various solvents. He was able to isolate a glucoside saponin, which he called "cucurbocitrin." He gave this to frogs and looked at their capillaries under a microscope. Their size nearly doubled after taking the extract.

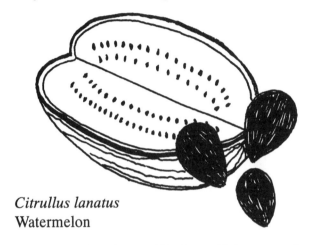

Citrullus lanatus
Watermelon

Constricting the capillaries will increase the blood pressure, but dilating them will reduce the pressure. Cucurbocitrin is active when taken by mouth and is completely safe. A study showed that it improved 56 of 68 patents with high blood pressure. People who were practically invalids became useful and started to enjoy life again.

These herbs were forgotten because most doctors did not measure blood pressure, nor did they see a link between it and illness. In 1929 Samuel Levine found from a study of 145 heart attack patients that 60% of them had high blood pressure. He had nothing to treat it, but the study was the first recognition that it was important to check blood pressure and reduce it. Further studies showed that one of seven adult whites had elevated blood pressure and about one in four adult blacks.

The leading cause of heart disease, strokes, and kidney failure is high blood pressure. About half of those with elevated pressure will eventually die of heart disease. Doctors usually list the cause as 'idiopathic' i.e. 'of unknown origin.' Blood pressure is inherited, and it is influenced by our diet.

The most common treatments are diuretics to reduce the fluid volume, and vasodilators to expand the constricted blood vessels.

Part of the relationship between diet and blood pressure is due to excess sodium salt consumption. In earlier eras rock salt was not mined, so sea salt, which is a mixture of magnesium, potassium and sodium salts was used. The prosperity of the city of Timbuktu was due to the yearly camel caravans carrying crude salts from the Sahara desert. This salt was a mixture of minerals, and when refined sodium chloride salts were introduced to Africa, the result was a general raising of blood pressure.

Japanese doctors found that whenever rural areas began to use white rice, the average blood pressure would begin to rise. They found that chief reason was that the pantothenic acid in the rice hulls kept the blood pressure normal. The vitamin increased the urine volume and sodium excretion. Rather than return to brown (unhulled) rice, they recommended that the villagers supplement their diets with pantothenic acid.

Japanese researchers made dogs hypertensive with a prolonged diet of high sodium salts. Then the dogs were given the juice of either carrots, cabbages or apples. Carrot juice had significant blood pressure lowering qualities. The main blood pressure lowering agent in carrots was potassium succinate, which also increased the excretion of sodium salts.

The Vitamin A in carrots is known to have a significant effect on blood pressure. Hypertensive people were given 200,000 units of Vitamin A for a few weeks, and then the dosage was lowered to 25,000 units. In some cases this reduced blood pressure, which had resisted all other forms of treatment. In a study involving 100 hypertensive patients, 25% had a major fall in blood pressure and full disappearance of symptoms, 50% had partial improvement and 25% had no improvement. In one case, which had resisted treatment, the blood pressure dropped from 120/220 to 90/150.

Iodine is present in trace amounts in the body, and until it was added to salt, it was rarely used as a supplement. Iodine has strong effects in arteriosclerosis, and as a medicine it has almost been forgotten. By 1930, doctors knew that iodine supplements prevent deposition of blood cholesterol. When 20 patients with arteriosclerosis were given iodine, 13 were relieved of headaches, dizziness, fatigue and heart palpitation. Five more were partially improved and two were not helped.

Burnham's soluble iodine solution was given to a patient with a blood pressure of 160/300. The heart was enlarged, and there was a murmur and the arteries showed pronounced sclerosis. Taking 25 drops of the tincture before meals reduced the pressure in two weeks to 150/230, and after another two months the pressure was 120/200.

In another case a 59 year-old woman had shooting pain in the head, pain in the heart area and severe fatigue. She was given 30 drops of Burnham's soluble iodine before meals, and in six weeks the blood pressure dropped from 150/250 to 84/170. Iodine is rarely used anymore in medicine, and the use of it to treat arteriosclerosis and high blood pressure raises the question as to whether our diets should contain considerably more iodine.

Garlic is another food remedy with a reputation for lowering blood pressure and aiding the heart. The first scientific study was done in France in 1922. Twenty drops of garlic juice lowered blood pressure up to 80 hours, but 80 drops of garlic juice raised pressure. The strength of the heartbeat was increased by garlic. Studies show varying results from garlic and onions, possibly because of the difference in varieties. The Russians have found that a tincture of red onions is a powerful lymph circulation stimulant.

In Ireland there was an old folk remedy of a mixture of red wine and horseradish *Armoracia rusticana*. It was used to cure headaches and other symptoms of high blood pressure. A study was made of a mixture of one part ground horseradish and five parts of 20% alcohol. A group of patients took a teaspoonful with meals for up to eight weeks. The remedy was quite active in reducing blood pressure, but it did not always lower it to normal ranges. Most people had a drop in pressure of about 40 mm., but there were cases of a 100 mm. drop over a period of three months.

In Russia one of the main treatments for reducing blood pressure is a tincture of a mint called *Lagochilus inebrians*. A test on 82 patients given a 12% tincture of the herb showed that in one to two months, most of them had normal blood pressure. The pulse slowed, the sleep improved, and the vertigo and headaches disappeared.

There are a number of herbs from Southeast Asia which are known to reduce blood pressure. *Morinda citrifolia*, a small tree with an inedible fruit, was brought by the Polynesians to Hawaii, where it was used it mainly to dye bark clothing yellow. In Viet Nam, however, it is used in arthritis, tuberculosis, facial paralysis and depression. The Vietnamese doctor Dang Van Ho found that extracts lowered blood pressure, anywhere from 20-70 mm. within two months. Given to 70 people, the extracts benefited 58. In one case the heart rate dropped from 140 to 70 beats per minute in three months. Nasal obstruction disappeared, and hemorrhoids healed in some cases.

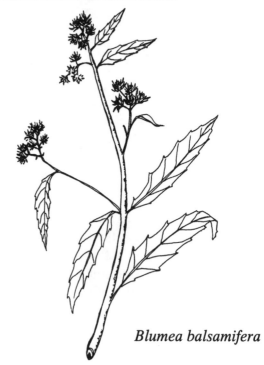

Blumea balsamifera

Blumea balsamifera is now grown as an ornamental flower in the United States. It soothes the nerves and lowers blood pressure. During WWII, French soldiers suffering from shell shock were given a gram a day of the herb.

According to Chinese doctors, one of the most powerful blood pressure herbs is *Coptis teeta*, known commonly as goldthread. When amounts ranging up to four grams per day of the powdered root were given to a series of people, the systolic pressure generally dropped to normal within 59 hours and the diastolic pressure became normal in about 49 hours. Headaches and dizziness disappeared with the drop in pressure. Angina pain usually left on the second day of treatment. In five cases of kidney problems associated with blood pressure, the edema disappeared in one to five days after taking the herb.

Cecropia obtusifolia is a medium sized tree, which grows in the tropical areas of Mexico. In 1905 a French study showed that the leaves were beneficial in the treatment of heart failure. When the leaves were given to rats at a dose of 10 mg./kg., they kept the blood pressure low for long periods of time.

Phaeanthus ebracteolatus is a common tree growing to about 25 feet tall in the Philippines. The inside of the bark is creamy yellow with a bitter taste. Powdered bark made into a tincture is reddish brown. It produces much stronger and more lasting blood pressure reduction than nitroglycerin.

A full description of the herbs used for blood pressure would take many pages. French scientists found that tinctures and teas of the common bedstraw *Galium aparine* reduced pressure, but did not act as a peripheral vasodilator. French doctors investigated *Hunteria elliotii* for its strong and prolonged action. Bulgarian scientists found that *Melissa officinalis* was a good blood pressure herb. In Southern Siberia, scientists isolated salsolin from the desert plant *Salsola richteri* for lowering blood pressure. A tincture of corn silk is useful in scanty urine, urinary retention, and high blood pressure.

Among the many herbs used by Chinese doctors *Phellodendron chinense*, *Morinda officinalis* and *Epimedium macranthum = E. grandiflorum* show effects. A tincture of the Chinese herb *Eucommia ulmoides* has been the subject of several studies. Water or alcohol extracts the hypotensive agent. It is a peripheral vasodilator, meaning that it acts on the vascular smooth muscles that surround the blood vessels. The root of the mint family plant *Scutellaria baicalensis* lowers blood pressure and raises blood sugar. It has long been used in Chinese pharmacies. The old Chinese doctors used thousands of plants and their 'anti-fear' remedy *Uncaria hirsuta = U. formaosana* is now being investigated for reducing blood pressure.

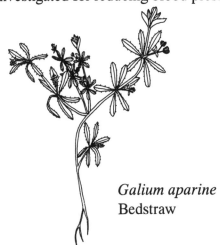

Galium aparine
Bedstraw

SECRETS OF THE BLOOD

"In the blood I observed the serum, in which floated an enormous number of orbicular particles, rejoicing in a very regular shape, seen as an oval when viewed broadside. Moreover these particles themselves are seen to contain another humor within themselves. If I looked upon them from the side, they almost resembled crystalline rods and a variety of figures; and no doubt in the same way; they are rolled around in the serum of the blood.

Biblia Naturae *Jan Swammerdam 1667*

"Thus the water pre-exists in the arteries, although it is not pure and limpid, yet it keeps the state of water here and there. It is seen more pure and clear in the channels of the lymph, because it has percolated through a tortuous route, through the anastomoses of vessels, just as water in wells and streams runs sweet and clearer through sandy earth and stones."

Thomas Bartholin 1653

The ancient Egyptians believed that respiration was the most important fact of life, for they spoke of the 'the breath of life,' but recognized the importance of the blood. In the *Book of the Dead* we learn that when the sun god Rae mutilated himself, the gods Hu and Lia arose from his blood. Mummies were painted red to symbolize the power of the blood and amulets of red stones representing the blood of Isis were used as talismans.

In China, the blood was called 'ke,' and together with the vital substance called the 'tao,' formed the yang (masculine) and yin (feminine) components of the body. Soldiers and wrestlers of ancient times drank blood or ate tiger liver, to increase their courage and vital forces.

The earliest symbol for the blood is a Sumerian 'Y,' which may refer to the branching of the blood vessels. It was from the lower part of Sumeria, which is now known as Iraq, that Abraham migrated to become the legendary father of the Jewish nation.

In the origin story of Adam and Eve, their son Cain, killed his brother Abel. By shedding his blood, he established that the blood was the 'life' of the body. The laws of Moses expressed the idea that the shedding of blood could take away wrongdoing. Later this idea was applied to the shedding of the blood of Christ as a sacrifice. The ritual supper of the Christian church was celebrated with bread, which symbolized the body, and red wine to imitate the blood of Christ.

Occasionally bread and food turns red. The first historic reference dates back to the siege of Tyre by Alexander the Great (-322). His soldiers were eating bread, and they noted drops of blood trickling from it. The soothsayer Aristander said that if blood flowed from the outside, it meant trouble for Alexander, but since it flowed from within, it meant misfortune for the city of Tyre.

In +1169, a priest at Alsen, Denmark, saw blood on the host. He was fearful, so he showed it to the chief priest, who declared that it was a sign of misfortune. Two weeks later an army of the Selini captured the area and enslaved the worshippers. This is the first reference to the red pigmentation of the wafer used for communion services.

It was about this time that the doctrine of transubstantiation arose. This is the idea that the communion wine and bread was transformed into the blood and body of Christ. The church debated if they should hold the "Feast of the Holy Body." In +1364 a priest was celebrating mass, and as he broke the host (bread), he found that it was covered with blood. Pope Urban IV was convinced, and this became the doctrine of transubstantiation. The painter Raphael immortalized this in the painting *Stanze*.

Bread continued to turn into blood and the faithful had their faith confirmed. In 1819 Bartholomeo Bizio investigated a case in Legnaro, Italy. He named the bacteria ***Serratia marcescens***. Scientists found that it made a good dye. In 1920 the Society of American bacteriologists renamed it ***Erythrobacillus prodigiosus.***

Greek and Arab doctors spoke repeatedly about the four humors of the blood. After blood sits for some time, it separates into four layers. The first layer is dark red, then red, a white layer and a layer of clear serum. The idea of the humors may have come from the four layers of settled blood.

The general thinking of all the ancient writers was that the liver generated the blood. In the middle of the nineteenth century, Giulio Bizzorero discovered that the blood is made in the marrow of the bones. Each day the bones generate 200 billion red blood cells, 10 billion white cells, and 400 billion platelets. Maybe William Shakespeare anticipated this when he wrote: "Thy bone is marrowless, thy blood is cold."

Roman doctors differentiated between arteries and veins, but they thought that blood flow was similar to the tides. They distinguished between the oxygen-poor blood of the veins, as carrying the spirit of the liver, and the oxygen-rich blood of the arteries, as carrying the spirit of the heart.

The circulation of the blood is so obvious, that it is a mystery as to why it was hidden so long. The Greek philosopher Alcameon of Croon (-500) wrote, "Animal life is a movement and subordinate to a movement of blood, which even if not always uniform is continuous." In -1270, the Arab doctor Ibn An-Nafi found that the blood circulates from the right side of the heart, to the left lung. Before him, the Chinese had some idea of the circulation of the blood, but they lacked a specific description.

William Harvey

William Harvey was born in 1578. He was nine when Queen Elizabeth had Mary, Queen of Scots, beheaded. He grew up on the southern English coast at Folkestone, on the narrowest part of the Straits of Dover. At the age of ten, he might have seen some of the 132 ships of the Span-

ish Armada come by. The English sea captains Francis Drake, Martin Frobisher and John Hawkins fought them in smaller faster ships off of Gravelines. Then the Armada fled around the north of Scotland, and was destroyed by a storm on the Irish coast. This setting was the start of the age of William Shakespeare, Isaac Newton and William Harvey.

Harvey was not the first man to dissect they body, for Leonardo da Vinci and Andreas Vesalius had already done so. By 1616 Harvey understood the role of the heartbeat, and assigned it the role of propelling nourishment to the rest of the body. As he worked on a book of his observations, it became obvious to him that the blood must circulate. He published this in 1628 in *De Motu Cordis*. The idea originally met resistance, because none of the classical writers wrote about it.

Using the word bloody is particularly British. It first shows up in a play put on in 1606. Swearing in plays was forbidden by law, and there was a heavy fine for it. But bloody was considered a respectable word. Then bloody became a bad word and it disappeared from the written language for nearly two centuries.

In 1892 Rudyard Kipling published *Barrack Room Ballads*, using the real language of the soldiers as they spoke. In WWI "bloody" became the word used by all workers. There was a favorite British marching song sung to the tune of the hymn *Holy, Holy, Holy*. It went "Raining, raining, raining, always bloody well raining. Raining all the morning, and raining all the night. Marching, marching, marching, always bloody well marching; when the war is over we'll bloody well march no more."

Primitive creatures have been studied to try and learn the origin of blood cells. Sponges lack a blood system, but wandering phagocyte amoebocytes take food from the choanocyte food trapping cells, and distribute it throughout the body. Flatworms lack a circulatory system, and they are so small, that the products of digestion and respiration simply pass through the body. The ancestors of the vertebrates are the tunicates, which are sea creatures covered with a tunic. The sea squirts have been studied, for they have blood cells. There are few fossil remnants of blood cells, but blood pigments apparently evolved at different times in ancient forms of life.

The first person to see a red blood cell was Marcello Malpighi, the founder of histology. While looking at a hedgehog's blood vessel, he saw 'fat-globules looking like a rosary of coral.' In 1666 he observed a mass of white fibers remaining after washing a blood clot. This was fibrin, which is the sealing mechanism of the blood system.

In 1674 Anton Leeuwenhoek made an accurate description of blood cells. He could see that they were circular in mammals and oval in fishes and birds. He calculated that 100 red blood cells placed side by side equaled the width of a small grain of sand. He noted that his blood was thicker on nights when he had a big evening meal and thinner on days when he drank four cups of coffee for breakfast.

In 1852 Karl Vierodt devised a method of counting red blood cells. He found that he had five million in each cubic millimeter in his blood. The method of counting blood cells was simplified in 1868 by using a thin glass tube of a known diameter, containing a measured section. Later this was simplified further, by comparing a diluted volume of blood to a prism of red dye. It was moved up and down until the colors matched.

Blood leaves the heart at a speed of about seven miles per hour. Simple mathematics shows that at this rate it would flow 61,000 miles in a year. If you live to the age of 70, your blood would have moved four million miles. Red blood cells make 75,000 round trips in the body to carry oxygen and remove carbon dioxide from the blood, in their 120-day existence.

In 1771 Joseph Priestly discovered the purpose of circulation. When he burned a candle in a closed container, the candle went out. Then he focused sunlight on the mint plant in the container, and after a few hours the candle was able to burn again. The chlorophyll in the mint converted carbon dioxide back into carbon compounds and oxygen. Without oxygen, animals in the container died, and they revived when oxygen was added in time. Our earth is a balanced ecosystem, in which animals release carbon dioxide, and plants convert it back to oxygen.

One of the most puzzling facts about blood is that it is divided into four principle groups. When the early doctors tried to give transfusions, the blood often clotted, and the patients died. Genetic fingerprinting now shows that each person's blood is genetically unique.

The old Chinese had a test known as "ti hsueh" meaning "drop blood." The blood of "blood relatives" will mix when dropped together, but the blood of strangers won't. A drop of blood on the bone of a dead relative will soak in, but a stranger's blood will run off.

Around +1100, Judge Pao Leng Tu, who was famous for his judicial decisions, had a case in which a wealthy man had a daughter who married into another family. In Chinese law, when the daughter marries she becomes part of that family and the inheritance will go to the daughter only if there are no male heirs. In this case the father married late in life and had a son before he died. The son-in-law disputed the inheritance, so the judge ordered the corpse dug up. The disputed son cut his finger, and the drops of blood soaked into the bone, so the son was declared the legitimate heir.

In another of his famous judicial cases, three Buddhist priests murdered a couple and abducted the daughter. They shaved her head, and took her from place to place begging alms. A strange dream caused a man to alert the police and the men were arrested. The daughter begged the police to arrest them for murder. The blood test was used on the bones, and justice was done.

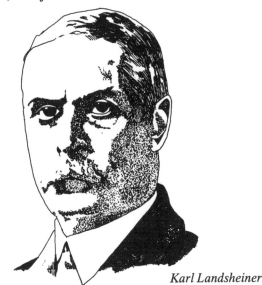

Karl Landsheiner

In 1901 Karl Landsheiner found that red blood cells could be divided into three groups which he named A, B, and C. Type A clumped the cells of type B, and of course B clumped the cells of A. The serum of C (which became known as AB) clumped the cells of both A and B, but wasn't clumped by either. In 1902 a larger study of 155 people found four whose cells were clumped by the other three. This was named type O blood. By 1907 blood groups were recognized as the factor that could make blood transfusions successful.

The frequency of blood types shows where our ancestors came from, and to whom we are related. From the Canadian border to the tip of South America all of the natives were virtually 100% type O blood. There is an island of type A blood in Arizona and New Mexico, from tribes that are assumed to have migrated south out of Canada. Further genetic refinement shows the relationships of ancient peoples in increasing detail.

The surface of the blood is composed of structural units somewhat like shingles on a roof. The genes determine variations of these units. These structural units or antigens are markers that determine our resistance to disease. The best known example is 'sickle cell anemia' which gives Africans resistance to malaria. People with type O blood appear to have 40% more peptic ulcers. Type A persons suffer more often from cancer of the stomach. There are an elevated number of schizophrenics in type A blood, and manic-depressives are more likely to have type O blood. There are many studies of these antigens, and with new techniques more facts are being uncovered.

One of the most curious bits of blood lore comes from Japan where 'blood group psychology' has become popular. Professor Takiji Furukawa first postulated the idea that blood groups determine individual characteristics in 1927. This became a popular fad in 1971 when Nomi Masahiko published the book *Blood Types and Personality.*

Professor Furukawa based his ideas on studies of different groups of people. He noted that 38% of Japanese have type A blood. Military cadet officers had 53% type A blood. Japanese women were traditionally subservient, but women going to an elite school must be strong willed. He found that there was less type O blood among the students.

People with type A blood are supposed to be cooperative and good team workers. Type B people are unconventional and move at their own pace. Those with type O are individualistic, self-assertive and goal oriented. Type AB people are cooperative and conciliatory in public, but they may be irrational and egotistical at home. Factories have even put the blood types on name tags and tried to mix departments according to the virtues of blood types. More AB persons are assigned to the art department, because they are supposed to be more creative.

There has been one recent study of blood groups, but no traits emerged which determined the individual's blood type. Japan is a country where individual initiative is frowned on, so studies in other countries may show different results. But for now, it looks as if blood groups could join astrology. We feel that 'our' sign tells us something, but it is so general that it is meaningless. Blood group traits are probably the same.

During the years of 1651-1653, Olaus Rudbeck described structures emptying milky fluid into the veins. He called this newly discovered system of vessels the "vasaglandularum serosa." In 1651 Jean Pecquet described the thoracic duct emptying into the veins of the neck. In 1661 Marcello Malpighi used a microscope to discover a network of tiny vessels connecting the arteries and veins. This was the step that tied together the lymph circulatory system. It completed William Harvey's work by showing the circulation between the arteries and veins.

A preparation of sweet clover *Melilotus officinalis* was shown to increase lymph flow by 263%. People with angina pain found relief by taking this preparation. Red onions are another strong stimulant of lymph flow.

The mango *Mangifera indica* produces transient skin rashes in the Philippines, and this became the subject of investigation. The mango turns out to be a strong lymph system stimulant. When the juice was injected into dogs it increased the lymph flow by three times. The blood clots more readily, the pressure falls and the lymph is richer in solids.

Canadian researchers discovered that the mucilage from okra could be used to replace blood plasma. Okra plasma has unusual fluid properties. When dried okra powder is added to water at a level of 25 parts per million the fluid friction is greatly reduced. When it is put into the tank of a fire truck, water can be pumped much faster and further, for it has less friction.

If you have a small reservoir of okra in the front of a boat and let it flow into the water it can reduce the effort to move the boat by up to 25%. The U.S. Navy was quite interested in this and they did a great deal of work in attaching slippery coatings to ships and submarines. The problem that naval researchers faced is the difficulty of gluing a slippery agent to a boat. Dolphins require only a quarter as much energy to slip through the water as a man-made object of the same weight and size. The slimy coating on fish must make much of the difference in energy requirements.

In theory, okra plasma would be an excellent substitute, because it would reduce the effort to force the blood throughout the body. It is not known if the slippery agents pass through the intestinal walls. But okra may help your heart slide through its work.

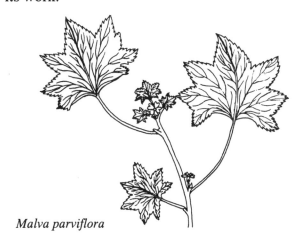

Malva parviflora

One of the great secrets of blood is that when you increase the supply of blood to an area of the body, the healing of that area is accelerated. In 1930 a study was done of the folklore plants of west Texas. The plant that showed the most interesting effects was the Castilian mallow *Malva parviflora*. A solution of this plant had marked vasodilating properties. After about 20 hours, a water extract became inactive. Mixing two pounds of the whole ground plant for a half-hour in five gallons of 95% ethyl alcohol made the best preparation. It is brought to a gentle boil for a half-hour, then cooled and strained.

The herbal extract proved to be highly useful in problems with reduced blood supply. These were problems like Buerger's disease, Raynaud's disease, endarterities, and diabetic gangrene. A soaked cloth in a solution of the extract dilates the blood vessels. An infrared lamp may be used to supply heat to the area.

A woman had diabetes, which resulted in an ulcer and gangrene of the left leg. Diabetic ulcers are extremely difficult to heal. In six weeks of hot malva packs, the ulcer was completely healed over, and the gangrene was eliminated.

A 55 year-old woman had Raynaud's disease. In this disorder, the circulation to the fingers and toes goes down, to the point that they may get gangrene. They become pale, stiff and tingly. All medical treatments failed to work, but hot Castilian mallow packs showed definite improvement in two days. In a month of treatment her circulation was nearly normal.

A woman had a varicose ulcer in her right leg for six years. Ultraviolet light and medical ointments had not produced any results. Castilian mallow packs at a dilution of 1:50 were applied for 3-4 hours at a temperature of 106 F. The severe pain which she had was gone in a week. After six weeks the ulcer showed the first signs of healing. The doctor used undiluted herb packs, and in eight weeks the resistant ulcer was completely healed.

There is one last secret of the blood, which has recently been discovered with genetic probes. Plants have genes for hemoglobin (blood), but the genes are not expressed, so they have sap instead of blood running through their veins. It does suggest that their primitive ancestors had some form of blood for absorbing oxygen. The life of the flesh is in the blood, as the biblical writer suggested, but the life traces behind blood go back to the beginning of multicellular organisms.

✧ ✧ ✧

SECRETS OF THE PULSE

"Often when in the still night I hear, as I lie, the calm continual rhythm of my familiar spirit ever winnowing boon from bane. I am lost in wonder of the long procession of these notes of human time, at this perpetual beat of the manifold tides of life. As I listen to its notes, they seem to fall into the burden. Sixty times a minute, at least; 3,600 times an hour, 86,400 times a day. For us heedful and heedless does this shuttle of life throb to and fro; for us in tireless periods, this pendulum of man's gravitation tells the seconds which can never return."

Clifford Allbutt

The idea that the pulse reveals the secrets of the body might have begun in ancient Egypt. The Ebers Papyrus (-1550) has a passage which reads: "The beginning of the physician's secret: knowledge of the heart's movement and knowledge of the heart. There are vessels from it to every limb. When any physician, any surgeon, or any exorcist applies the hands or his fingers to the head, to the back of the hand, to the hands, to the place of the stomach, to the arms or to the feet, then he examines the heart. Out of his limbs come its vessels; that the heart speaks out of the vessels in every limb."

In legendary history the Chinese Emperor Hoami (-2500) was said to have written a book on the pulse. This is unlikely, because the art of writing was not developed enough at this time. As Chinese medicine developed, the lore of the pulse gained greater significance. The first Jesuit missionaries brought back Wang Cho Ho's *Secret of the Pulse*. It was translated into French, and discussed throughout Europe.

Chinese doctors felt the pulse at three positions on the wrist by using the index, middle and ring fingers. Then they applied light, moderate and firm pressure at three positions on both wrists, to determine the shallow and deep pulses. Their books describe the pulse as either ropy, snakelike, rain on the roof, the jump of a frog and the tail of a fish. Each organ of the body was said to have its own pulse, and the pulse was believed to change during every season.

Hoami, a great Chinese doctor, was said to be able to predict death 35 years in advance from an analysis of the pulse. If the pulse felt like the blunt edge of a sword, death was eight days away. If it was like the pecking of a bird, you had four days; feathers blown by the wind, three days; and if it was like the rapid rolling of peas, you had one day to live.

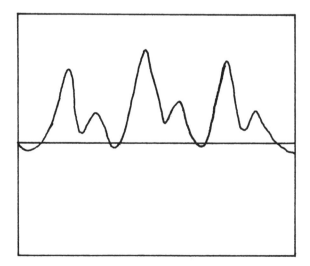

Normal pulse wave

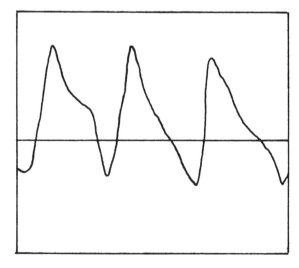

Diabetic pulse wave

One of the old Chinese emperors was said to have tested the pulse theory by having his doctor stick his hand through a hole in the wall, behind which a cow had been carefully positioned. After feeling the pulse for several minutes with the tip of his finger, the doctor announced: "Needs grass."

There have been some recent attempts to determine the arterial waves in the pulse, with the idea that it might confirm the ancient Chinese methods of pulse diagnosis. The pulse waves of normal persons often vary significantly. Many people show large differences in pulse waves corresponding to breathing in and out, but others don't show much difference.

When the artery of the right leg is blocked, it can be detected in the right arm, but not in the left. The difference is small, but it does confirm the Chinese idea that changes elsewhere can change the pulse in the wrist. The idea that the organs can influence the pulse is verified with very sensitive instruments, but the wave changes are so minute, that it is nearly impossible to detect and determine their origin. The study suggests that the changes found by pulse doctors were largely imaginary.

In western literature, Hippocrates mentioned that varieties of the pulse and respiration are the signs of health and disease, but he made no effort to distinguish them. Around -300, Herophilus wrote the first Greek book dedicated to the pulse. He taught that the four characteristics of the pulse were size, frequency, strength and rhythm. He attempted to count pulse beats with a water clock. He is said to have found that diastole and systole (filling and emptying of the heart) were equal in youth, but in old age the systole is up to five times longer.

The pulse is not mentioned in the classical literature of India. It finally arrived as a diagnostic technique from Arab doctors around the twelfth century. The basis of this system was the tridosha, known as vata, pitta, and kappa, which we translate as wind, bile and phlegm. When three fingers were laid on the wrist arteries; the first finger, detects vata; the middle finger, pitta; and the third finger, kappa.

The Roman doctor Galen wrote 18 books on the pulse, which have been lost. He describes variations due to wine, exercise, pregnancy, season and sex. He thought that each organ shaped the pulse, and that it would take an entire life to have a complete knowledge of the pulse.

The quickening of the pulse with excitement, fear, or interest, is a measurement of nervous system excitement. In modern times it is the basis of the lie detector. The *Gesta Romanorus,* one of the most popular storybooks of the Middle Ages, contains the story of a knight who suspected his wife of infidelity. He confirmed his suspicions by mentioning her lover, and "Her pulse immediately quickened to a surprising degree and acquired a feverish heat."

Both Galen and Avicenna believed that the pulse could discern love. There were a number of stories circulating about the detection of love by the pulse. In the stories, various people are named while the doctor continues to examine the pulse for health reasons. Suddenly the pulse increases, and the secret of the hidden lover is revealed. The old accounts provide the historical basis for the reason why we love with our hearts, but use our heads only for cold logic.

The most important medieval work on the pulse was the *Ars Sphygmica* of Joseph Stuthius. He was a Polish doctor, who was a student of classical writers. He studied the pulse by attaching a leaf to the artery on the wrist and watching the pulse rock the leaf. This gave him a better sense of the pulse than feeling could.

Johann Kepler, the astronomer, recorded the first true pulse rate, which he put at 70 in men and 80 in woman. Galileo initially used his pulse to time a pendulum, and when he realized that the pendulum was an exact measure of time, he made

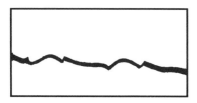

Vasodilator

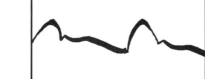

Normal Pulse

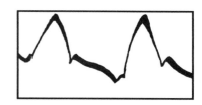

Vasoconstrictor

a pulsilogon. This was a pendulum with a silk cord, which could be shortened or lengthened, to adjust to the rate of the pulse. Since any activity or excitement increases the pulse rate, it is a poor sense of clock time. Galileo did many of his famous experiments by timing them with church song-chants. The meter of these songs is perfectly regular, and this allowed him to do precise experiments without a clock.

There were no secrets of the pulse in any of the old systems of medicine. The real secret was in the nervous system and blood pressure. What the old doctors were doing was practicing lie detection and nervous excitement. Everything else was simply self-deception.

When doctors of the nineteenth century took a new look at the pulse, they made a number of observations. The pulse rate of the fetus before birth is generally about 145 and drops to about 135 at birth. At age one it drops to about 125 and by age two it is 105. It drops to a pulse rate of 70 by age 15. The pulse normally stays at that rate until the age of 50, when it begins to rise again.

The 'Law of Hermann Vierordt' stated, "In all animals independent of their size, 26-29 heart beats are necessary to completely circulate the blood." When this was carefully studied, it was found to be about 48 heartbeats for all animals. This means that all of the blood in the body circulates once in about 45 seconds.

High altitudes and heat speed up the pulse; low altitudes and cold slow it. Generally speaking each 1° F. rise in body temperature during fever increases the pulse by 10 beats a minute.

The first instrument for measuring the wave shape of the pulse was known as the sphygmoscope. The first one in 1837 was made by putting wax on a vein connected to a thread to measure the pulse. The heart sound is described as 'lub-dub-pa' or 'ken-tuck-y'. The interval between the dub and pa is the diastole (relaxation).

The heart discharge and the peripheral resistance determine the contour of the pulse curves. Low heart output means that the curve loses most of its features, because the blood column does not 'jerk.' The pulse taken near the heart shows its sharp features, further away, the curves are more general.

In 1911 Theophil Christen published a "dynamic diagnosis of the pulse." His device was called an "energometer." It described the volume of filling and the "intensity" of the pulse. He was able to tell much more about the health of the body through his device. His device was the last great attempt to make a science out of the pulse, and it was ignored by the medical profession, which was moving in different directions.

However, the hardness of the pulse is a measure of blood pressure and the pulse rate is a measure of the efficiency of the heart. Both diabetics and people with arteriosclerosis have an abnormally shaped pulse wave. A study of the pulse could detect these disorders, but couldn't tell which is which. The pulse doctors could supposedly feel the murmurs, flutter and fibrillation of the heart to a minute degree.

If we look at the tracing of the pulse wave we can tell something about the heart. With each heartbeat we have a strong "n," which tapers off on the right side because of the elasticity of the arteries. Anesthesia or a weak heart reduces the height of the "n." Adrenaline stimulates the pulse and turns it into an inverted "V."

Vasodilatation reduces the height of the 'n,' and vasoconstriction increases it, and makes it more of an inverted 'V' shape. If there is a spike on the top of the pressure pulse, it is due to vibration similar to water hammer. These are the common changes in the pulse that take place with changes in blood pressure.

The strength and flexibility of the walls of the arteries and veins is of interest to us as we age. When there are weak spots, these may form an aneurysm, which bulges out like a balloon. If the aneurysm should break, it is likely to mean death. During the nineteenth century, the most popular treatment was potassium iodide. A poultice over the area was often enough to reduce it to normal in a week or more. From half to five grams of potassium iodide was taken internally per day until the bulge disappeared.

By 1955 a series of careful experiments in guinea pigs established some of the nutritional factors that kept the vascular walls strong. Vitamin C and the bioflavanoids were very important in the strength of the walls. Increased sodium produced spots on the walls and reduced their strength, indicating that a switch to potassium chloride (diabetic salt) would be of value. A low choline diet produced weak walls, and blood easily leaked out. The venules formed a "plumber's joint" and in the ballooned area, red blood cells would flow through the leaks.

If you cross one leg over the opposite knee and allow it to hang loosely, the foot will oscillate with each systole, and you can also see a secondary jerk. The pulse can be seen by bending the edge of a fingernail backwards, and watching the color of the nail alternate between pink and white.

Dr. Arthur Coca was the editor of the *Journal of Allergy*. He discovered a secret that the pulse takers had missed. His wife had several heart attacks. She noted that before each attack, her heart speeded up, apparently due to the foods she had eaten. When she eliminated these foods, she ceased to suffer from heart attacks. Coca published a book advising people to take their pulse after meals. By making a list of foods, they could determine which ones were adversely affecting them, and eliminate them.

Even if the old doctors detected an abnormal pulse, there was little they could do. The pulse slows with digitalis, and the beat becomes more firm. The California Indians must have been aware of the speed of the pulse, because they gave ***Chaenactis douglasii*** to small children to slow down their heart. The heart and blood pressure herbs provided a limited means of altering the pulse.

Two centuries ago Rene Laennec was crossing the court of the Louvre in Paris, when he noted some children communicating by tapping on the ends of a long beam. No sound could be heard in between, but they could hear each other at the ends. In his time, when doctors wanted to listen to the heart, they put their ear to the chest of the patient. Doctor Laennec had an overweight patient, which made this difficult. He remembered the children and he rolled up a piece of notebook paper and listened to the sounds of the heart. This resulted in the invention of the stethoscope, which gave doctors a new outlook on the pulse.

✧ ✧ ✧

SECRETS OF THE HEART

"In all other animals but man, the heart is situated in the middle of the breast. In man alone, it is placed just below the nipple on the left-hand side, the smaller end terminating in a point and bearing outward. It is among fish only, that this point is turned towards the mouth. It is asserted that the heart is the first among the viscera, that is formed in the fetus, then the brain, and last of all the eyes. It is said also that the eyes are the first organs that die, and the heart is the very last of all. The heart is the principle seat of the heat of the body. It is constantly palpitating, and moves as though it were one animal enclosed within another. It is also enveloped in a membrane equally supple and strong, and is protected by the bulwarks formed by the ribs and the bone of the breast, as being the primary source and origin of life."

Natural History *Pliny +75*

Carl Jung, the famous Swiss psychoanalyst, did an extensive study of the relationship of mental problems to primitive images. When he visited New Mexico, he interviewed a Pueblo Indian chief about his traditions. The chief said, "I know you white men think with the brain. That accounts for your shortcomings. We red men think with the heart."

Plato said: "The head is the divinest part of us and lord over all the rest." His pupil Aristotle insisted that the heart was the chief organ of the body. Shakespeare wrote of this dichotomy in *The Merchant of Venice*: "Tell me where is fancy bred, or in the heart, or in the head?"

The ancient Egyptians felt that the heart represented the soul or 'ka,' which was the true inner self. They discarded the brain during mummification because they didn't think it was important, but they gave special care to the heart. Wealthy Egyptians placed copies of the *Book of the Dead* in their sarcophagus, so it would be available for reference in the next world. One of the prayers in this book speaks of the heart in this way:

Stand not against me as a witness among the assessors.
Create not opposition against me.
Do not weigh against me in the presence of the keeper of the scales.

After death, the decreased faced a summary of life, when he was to stand before Maat, the goddess of truth, assisted by 42 demigods. During the ritual of the last judgment, the decreased had to recite the *Negative Confession* while his heart was put on a balance, and a feather was put on the other side. He had to swear that he had not lied, committed adultery, been cruel or committed a variety of common infractions of the moral code. If the heart was burdened by sin, the scales would tip downwards and the 'Eater of the Dead' would devour his heart. If the heart was lighter than a feather, he was led into the presence of Osiris, the Lord of Heaven.

Anatomy was so little known in early times that the Greeks referred to 'kardia' as either the heart or the stomach. Stomach distress is still known in French as 'mal de coer' (bad heart). We get heartburn when we have an acid stomach. The Roman writers referred to stomach ulcers, gall bladder conditions and heart conditions as 'morbus cardiacus.'

The Bible is full of interesting statements about the heart. The heart hears, speaks, walks, falls, stands, rejoices, cries, desires, goes astray, lusts, errs, loves, hates and meditates. The disciples are commanded to "Love the Lord thy God with all thy heart." The head and the brains are ignored.

The heart remains a symbol of love, because of the speeding up of the pulse rate when your lover is mentioned. We wear wedding rings on the 'ring finger,' because of the tradition that a vein from the heart runs to that finger.

Sir Walter Scott described an old Scotch custom in *The Pirate*. You poured globs of molten lead into water, and selected a piece that looked like a heart. When a perfect piece was found it was worn as a talisman, and you were supposed to be cured of heart problems.

The real function of the heart remained unknown until William Harvey discovered circulation. He was given a lectureship by the London College of Physicians, and part of the job was doing a public dissection each year, because a new law gave London surgeons the right to dissect four executed criminals each year.

Harvey noticed that the blood did not pass through the sides of the heart. Each time the heart beat, it could only make room for more blood by circulating the pulsed blood. Galen and the early doctors held to the 'tidal theory of the blood.' They associated the pulse with the heart, but they still thought in terms of the tide, surging in and out. Leonardo da Vinci did wonderful studies of the anatomy of the heart, but even he missed the circulation of the blood.

In order to know that Harvey's theory was right, it had to be proven that there was microcirculation of the blood. Anton van Leeuwenhoek confirmed this with his microscope. He watched the complete circulation of the blood through the semi-transparent skin of a tadpole.

Primitive worms have a simple heart, which is only a strand of muscle wrapped about a tube carrying blood. As we go higher on the scale of evolution the hearts have more chambers. In humans and other vertebrates, there are four chambers. The right side of the heart pumps the carbon dioxide laden blood to the lungs, and the left side pumps 4,000 gallons of blood daily, which is the equivalent of a two to three year supply of gasoline for the car.

It was once believed that strenuous exercise was hard on the heart, but it is now recognized that the heart is a muscle, and muscles need work to remain strong. Most heart specialists now encourage gentle exercises for heart attack victims.

The discovery that the heart is only a muscle comes from Neils Stensen of Leyden Holland. In 1663 he wrote to his teacher and told him that he was examining the heart and the muscles. He was unable to find anything in the heart which wasn't present in the muscles; therefore the heart must be an unusual muscle.

The Tarahumara Indians of northern Mexico are a small Uto-Aztec tribe, living on the high continental divide area. Their main diet is pinole (ground corn), and in lean times they gather wild roots and plants. They hunt deer by running them, until they drop from exhaustion. They run after wild turkeys, until the heavy birds are too exhausted to fly any longer. These people have kick ball races regularly, and 50 miles of running is an ordinary game, and 150 miles is not uncommon. Heart specialists have found that after a 50-mile run, they aren't even breathing hard, and their heart isn't beating very fast.

The real secrets of the heart lie in the blood and the blood pressure. Anemia, which is low numbers of red blood cells, can cause heart enlargement, fatty changes in the cardiac muscle, heart murmurs and electrocardiogram abnormalities. If anemia is treated these changes return to normal.

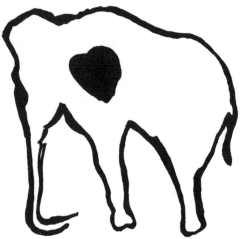

The earliest known drawing of the heart (from the Pindal cave)

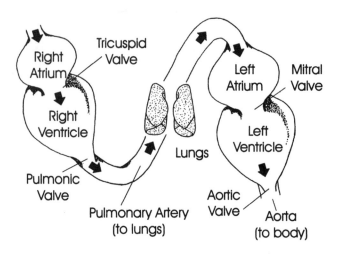

Schematic drawing of the heart

One study involved 34 patients with both anemia and heart problems. Most of them had difficulty breathing, and after the anemia was cleared up, all were relieved. Cardiac pain similar to angina occurred in eight persons, and after the anemia was cleared up, all were relieved. Cardiac murmurs were noted in 30 people, and when the anemia was treated, the murmurs disappeared in 14 people. Twelve people had heart enlargement, and after the anemia was treated, only three had enlarged hearts. Before we attempt to treat major heart problems, we must make sure we have healthy blood.

The heart enlarges at high altitudes to give greater efficiency to move blood with less available oxygen. Hookworms cause anemia, which in turn causes the heart to enlarge. Anemia is now established as a cause of cardiac murmurs, which disappear when the blood is restored by treatment.

In high blood pressure, there are structural changes in the heart and vascular system, which develop as a response to the increased pressure. The blood vessels thicken and the heart enlarges. A study was done of 13 men with high blood pressure. They were treated with beta-blockers to bring the pressure back to normal. When the blood pressure was reduced over a period of time, the bad changes in the heart and blood vessels slowly returned to normal.

There is a strange 'law' that was once discussed. Mammals that accumulate 800 million heartbeats are basically finished living. A shrew that had a heartbeat of 1,000 beats per minute accumulates the 800 million in only a year and a half before it dies. The elephant accumulates the same number in 50 years with a pulse of 30 per minute. We humans live to be three times as old as the heart beat law.

Some of the yogis of India have been able to stop the heart for several seconds, while being medically monitored. This does not seem to reflect any spiritual ability, or have any useful significance. In order to gain control of an organ, it is necessary to stimulate some nerve that controls the reflexes to that organ. This is a point on the neck, which was discovered in 1799, which produces a temporary slowing or stoppage of the heart. This is the reason why a sudden turn of the head or a 'crick' of the neck can leave you dizzy with a palpitating heart.

It is likely that the yogis discovered this during their exercises. After a time, they could simply put mental attention on the point of the neck, and the heart would stop briefly. When the yogis were tested for their ability to stop the heart under scientific observation, they began doing neck contortions, and this exposed their secret.

Before the scientific era, many prominent people believed in the doctrine of signatures. If you had a bad heart you would want the heart shaped herbs to treat the disorder. There is no evidence that this is true, except that many heart herbs do have minerals and vitamins which could have helped in the days of very poor diets. Some of these herbs by name are heart leaf- ***Medicago arabica***, heart wart- ***Aristolochia clematitis***, heart's ease- ***Viola tricolor***, the heart nut- ***Juglans ailantifolia*** and the heart pea- ***Cardiospermum halicacabum*** or ***C. grandiflorum***.

☆☆☆

A MEDICAL DETOUR

"This organ deserves to be styled the starting point of life and the sun of our microcosm just as much as the sun deserves to be styled the heart of the world. For it is by the heart's vigorous beat that the blood is moved, perfected, activated and protected from injury and coagulation. The heart is the tutelary deity of the body, and the basis of life, the source of all things, carrying out its function of nourishing, warming and activating the body as a whole."

William Harvey

It is no surprise to find that two of the biggest medical news stories for the past 25 years have been the heart transplant and the artificial heart. Both of these medical advances focus on a comparatively tiny group of society, older men in poor health. The story began in 1964, when the National Heart Institute drew up a crash plan for the construction of an artificial heart.

There are two types of heart failure. One involves the left side of the heart which pumps blood from the lungs to the rest of the body. The conditions of pulmonary edema, fluid in the lungs and rales (rattling), all refer to this form of heart failure. If, however, the right side of the heart fails, fluid accumulates in the feet and ankles. It is treated by diuretics to get the fluid out, or by inotropic agents such as digitalis, which strengthen the heart and kidneys to remove the fluid.

The first real heart transplant took place at the Mississippi Medical Center in 1964. The heart of a chimpanzee was given to a man dying of heart failure. The man died eleven hours later, and the episode was quietly forgotten. It might have been kept from media attention because of questions about medical ethics.

The first recognized heart transplant was performed by Doctor Christian Bernard in 1967. He replaced the diseased heart of Louis Washkansky at the Grorte Schur Hospital in South Africa. The recipient died 18 days later, but public interest turned Bernard into the best known doctor in the world. It launched attempts at heart transplants throughout the world.

The medical media event of the century was the transfer of a completely mechanical heart into the body of a Seattle area dentist. Barney Clark's heart transplant took place on December 2, 1982. Before the operation he was given an eleven-page consent form which was signed by a psychiatrist, a social worker and his heart doctors. The fine print at the bottom read: "I understand that subsequent to signing this form, I could not be deemed not acceptable for any reason whatsoever, including, but not limited to, death resulting from any cause or other medical complication."

Each of us has a time to live, contribute, and a time to die. This idea is present in religious and secular tradition, but doctors find it hard to allow death to take place, even when it is clear that it is natural process, and there is no way the person can return to a normal life. This seems to be true of Barney Clark, for before his operation, he repeatedly expressed his wish to be allowed a peaceful death. A member of the heart transplant team called his requests "a form of suicide," and therefore unacceptable. This begins the dilemma of whether the heart transplant team was merely a group of medical vultures or heroic scientists.

Barney Clark finally died after 118 days of being on page one of the newspapers. The president called to tell the family what a brave and courageous man he had been, even though he was so sick most of the time he hardly knew what had happened. The relatives held a public funeral, so hundreds of people who didn't know him, could attend. The leader of the organization that made the heart was named 'inventor of the year.' He had no patents on the mechanical heart, and it was developed as a group effort.

The second mechanical heart was installed in William Shroeder. The device kept him alive for 20 months. During this time he had little vitality, and required constant medical monitoring. Days after the transplant, he had a multiple stroke that left him paralyzed with impaired speech and memory. The high point of his medical story was a press conference with Shroeder drinking beer, and Dr. William De Vries talking about the great medical success. Allowing a seriously ill patient to drink at a news conference says something about the circus aspect of the transplant and the ethics of the doctors. Schroeder lingered for months in the twilight zone of consciousness.

William Shroeder became despondent and privately raised the possibility of suicide. Doctor De Vries began to keep his patient from reporters, and to speak for him. This was apparently done to conceal the failure of the artificial heart program. Medical success doesn't just mean keeping the patient barely alive, it means restoring them to a relatively normal life. When a CAT scan showed that most of his brain had been destroyed by the stroke, the heart was shut off.

These attempts at mechanical heart transplants aroused the interest of investment capitalists on Wall Street. Newspapers reported that corporate leaders were talking about 15,000 mechanical heart transplants a year by 1992. The minimum cost of an artificial heart was $100,000, and the hospital care could easily reach a half million dollars, if prolonged medical complications were involved. The amount of money to give a heart to one aging person could provide more than a hundred dollars of necessary health care to a thousand needy young people. We are bankrupting the medical piggy bank to provide heroic care for those at the end of their useful life.

The newspapers reported that more than $200 million was spent to develop the artificial heart. During that period of time, little or no money was spent to investigate the nutritional causes of heart failure. Our bodies are built from the foods we eat, and the heart is no exception.

In the accounts of mechanical heart transplant patients, nothing is mentioned about dietary or physical therapy. The doctors might have been ignorant of this, for surgeons don't study nutrition. The surgical feat of transplanting a mechanical heart, is an achievement worthy of climbing Mount Everest. As a matter of practical endeavor, it is similar to sitting on a flagpole for a year. Did the doctors ever consider the real questions? Is this step good for society? Where will the money come from? And, most importantly, could we help the body to repair itself?

Heart transplants are now acceptable, and they increase the average lifespan by five years, but there is a heavy price to pay. The doctors talk about how successful the operation was, but the patient has his family uprooted and his financial and career plans are wrecked. There is a high rate of divorce, suicide and psychosis among the transplanted. Their faces are puffy and moon shaped from taking heavy doses of steroids, and often the heart flutters. The body is constantly trying to reject the organ that must keep it alive, and if immunosuppressive drugs aren't taken, the immune system will destroy the new heart.

In 1969 Walter Schmittammer was taken to a hospital in Bonn, Germany, to get a heart transplant. Doctors told him it was his only chance to live. When a heart was available, the luckless man had an infection, so someone else got it. When another heart became available, he was too ill to operate, so it was given to somebody else. Both of the heart transplant patients died, but Schmittammer got better on his old heart, and was able to live a relatively normal life.

When someone's heart is failing, the doctors can say that they will be dead in a few hours. The doctor then plays the 'savior role,' and puts in a new heart. We love the drama of life and death, and the heroic doctor who snatches the patient away from death's door. We can say, "The surgeon saved him from certain death." Of course we don't say: "For a quarter of a million dollars, he's been given another five years of an uncertain and painful existence."

Medical literature contains a number of hints that simple therapy can cure congestive heart failure. When the body begins to retain water, and diuretics don't work any longer, this is recognized as the terminal phase. Fasting often produces a marked loss of water. When five patients with congestive heart failure fasted for five days, four of them had marked improvement. There was one failure, possibly due to jaundice.

The strongest diuretics are mercurial, and when the patients fail to respond to these, it's often over for them. When a group of heart patients were given supplements of 20 grams of the amino acid lysine, most of them improved.

In 1938 an attempt was made to treat heart failure with Vitamin C. Nine people with severe edema were given Vitamin C. Three had good results, and four had moderate results. The urinary output increased more with Vitamin C than with digitalis.

In 1966 Russian physiologists noted that cases of heart failure were critically low in the B vitamin pantothenic acid. A trial was made by treating a group of patients with chronic heart failure by giving them 100 mgs. of calcium pantothenate three times a day. The blood pressure, heart beat frequency and respiration were restored to normal levels in this group. The control group was treated with strophanthin, and they did poorly.

What would have happened if Barney Clark had a 'real doctor'? He would have started out with a short fast. He would have taken supplements of the vitamins known to strengthen the heart. The mineral supplements of silicon, selenium, magnesium and manganese would have been added. He would have drunk kidney bean pod tea, ginkgo leaf extract, nettles, hawthorn and cherry bark with ribose supplements. He would have had electronegative supplements like potassium citrate put in these drinks. There would have been no life and death drama, and in six months he might have been back to work.

There wouldn't have been press conferences by surgeons, and newspapers wouldn't have headlines. His supplements and therapy bills would be only a few thousand dollars at most, instead of a quarter of a million dollars. But what is news doesn't become news. What passes for the latest in medicine is sometimes just scientific quackery.

In 1957 the bypass operation for the heart was developed. Coronary bypass rapidly gained in popularity, for it created new channels to give the heart extra oxygen. In 1970 a study was done on 1,400 patients at London, Ontario. It compared bypass surgery to aspirin therapy. There was no change in the incidence of strokes. The operation does give relief from pain, but it does not change the death rate. There is a chance of death from the surgery, and thousands of people suffer complications from the surgery each year.

We have 28 times the number of coronary bypass operations in the US as in Europe. There are some 100,000 operations per year, with a minimum cost of $25,000, and an actual cost that is generally double that. Bypass surgery is used to correct

The main reasons for doing the surgery is to relieve pain, but it doesn't increase the length of life. About 1% of the patients die from the operation and another 1% suffer brain damage. There are herbal cures for angina pectoris.

The problem that created the 'need' for surgery is arteriosclerosis. If we could find a solvent for the wax-like cholesterol, we could dissolve this buildup in our blood system, and we wouldn't need bypass operations. Rabbits were fed high cholesterol diets, until they developed severe arteriosclerosis. When they were given one gram of choline a day for six months, 74% of the rabbits became free of arteriosclerosis in six months.

The idea was extended to people who had coronary thrombosis. A test was made by comparing 52 patients taking choline, to an equal number taking nothing. During the first year, the choline patients had three deaths, compared to seven deaths in the untreated group. Through the duration of the study, the untreated death rate was more than doubled.

The doctors found that the best therapeutic results were 32 grams of choline a day. This had striking therapeutic results when taken over a two to three year period. People quickly became free of all signs of heart failure, and some lost all anginal pain.

Lecithin is a solvent containing choline, which dissolves water and oils. Egg yokes are rich in cholesterol, fats and lecithin. Lecithin is extracted from soybeans and sold at health food stores. Lecithin is generally easier to take than choline.

A Canadian man helped in his wife's health food store. While packaging lecithin, he began to sample it and soon he began eating several spoonfuls a day. When his blood pressure was taken sometime later, it was found to be unusually low for his age. He thought that the lecithin had removed the cholesterol from the arteries, and lowered the heart pumping pressure.

One of his friends had a massive heart attack, and was retired from work with a full pension. The doctors told him that he would never walk again, and soon he would need a heart bypass operation. After a few weeks of eating three tablespoonfuls of granule lecithin a day, he didn't need the operation. This happened to two other people that doctors recommended for heart bypass operations. By eating lecithin for three to six weeks, the cholesterol deposits are cleared out of the arteries.

Many people want surgery – it is the quick fix of the problem. Few people want to change their lifestyle; surgery is the easy way out. Surgery doesn't cure the problem, which is arteriosclerosis, but it relieves the pain, tightening and heaviness of the chest. The problem remains, and comes right back to haunt these people over a period of time. Many other alternatives are discussed in my chapter on arteriosclerosis.

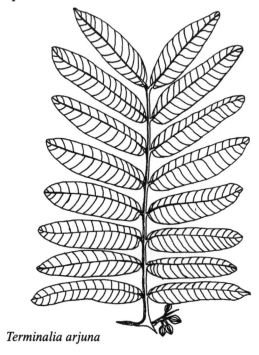

Terminalia arjuna

Of the many herbs used for the failing heart, several appear to be quite active. The old Sanskrit writings in India refer to the bark of **Terminalia arjuna** for heart problems. The herb was given to healthy volunteers, but it had no effect on the heart rate, output or on the blood pressure. The bark was ground to a powder and extracted with strong alcohol. Twelve patients with congestive heart failure took either a placebo or the herbal extract. All of those taking the herb showed signs of recovery, with a weight loss of about five pounds. The stimulation of the heart probably casued the loss of excess fluid.

We should remember the story of the Swiss missionary in Zambia, Africa, who was ill from a serious heart condition. He had been sick for four years, and his doctor advised him that he had perhaps six months to live. He said to himself: "God has a remedy for me, I just have to find it." He resolved to journey through the bush country and ask everyone and try every remedy that he came across. One day while walking, he brushed against a bush, and walked a little further, and then wiped the sweat off of his forehead. It smelled like coffee, but it wasn't, and he hadn't had a good cup of coffee for a long time.

He walked back and picked the seeds, roasted them in his frying pan and ground them. Then he made "The finest coffee I have ever tasted." He decided to camp there and pitched his little tent. He had been unable to sleep more than 30 minutes at a time, because his heart was so bad that he would be gasping for breath. After drinking the 'coffee,' he got five hours of unbroken sleep. Then he picked all the seeds he could get and drank three cups a day. When he returned home, his doctor pronounced his heart condition cured. The cure was the seeds of **Senna occidentalis = Cassia occidentalis**. This is not a rare plant, for it grows wild in Texas and parts of the south. The plant is related to the herb which furnishes the laxative 'senna.' It should be noted that the raw seeds are toxic, and must be roasted to remove the toxicity.

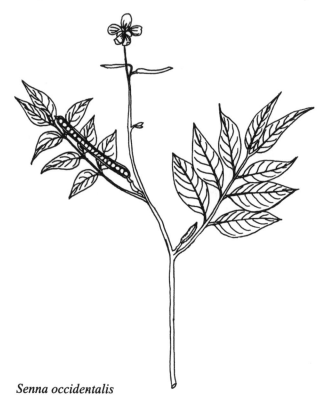

Senna occidentalis

A study was published on the active compound of **Senna tora = Cassia tora**. These seeds are used in Asia to treat asthma and improve eyesight. Glycosides were isolated that had a strong effect on damaged livers. They may be the same as the heart curing principle. These compounds could easily be isolated and used in cases of heart and liver failure.

There are other varieties of this plant, which may be of interest. Coffee weed is **Senna tora**. In Trinidad wild coffee is **Senna occidentalis = Cassia occidentalis**.. In the Amazon basin, the native healers use retama flowers **Cassia loretensis** and retamilla **Cassia marginata** to cure damaged livers and hearts. The beans of retamilla make an excellent coffee substitute.

This story ought to make people aware that there are alternatives to surgery and transplants. Surgery is the darling of medicine. It often achieves miracles, but the surgeons forget that the health of the organs depends on the nutrition that they receive.

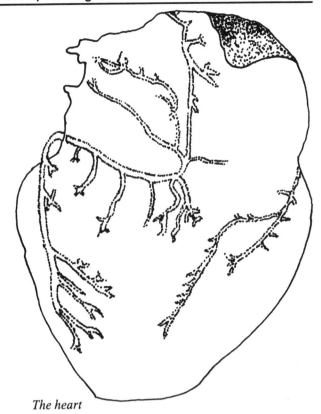

The heart

✿ ✿ ✿

HERBS OF THE HEART

"True is it, my incorporate friends," quoth he, "that I receive the general food at first,
Which you do live upon; and fit it is; because I am the store-house and the shop
Of the whole body. But, if you do remember, I send it through the rivers of your blood,
Even to the court, the heart — to the seat o' the brain, and through the cranks and offices of man.
The strongest nerves and small inferior vein from me receive that natural competency,
Whereby they live."

Coriolanus *William Shakespeare*

In the last decades of the nineteenth century Doctor Michael Green had a reputation as a wonder worker for failing hearts. People from all over Europe came to him at Innis, Ireland, and his pills and tinctures worked wonders on failing hearts. After his death in 1894, his daughter revealed that the secret of his practice, was the ripe hawthorn berries from ***Crataegus curvisepala = C. oxyacantha***

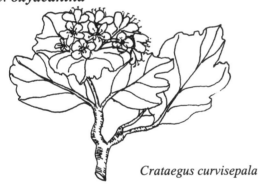

Crataegus curvisepala

Most hawthorn species are inactive, but the leaves and berries of ***Crataegus curvisepala*** and ***C. monogyna*** are quite active. The leaves and berries contain the bioflavanoids vitexin, hypersoide and epicatechin. Epicatechin is a strong coronary dilator, and increases the flow of blood around the heart by as much as 50%. It is also found in ***Pterocarpus marsupium***, which is used as an antidiabetic herb in India. When the insulin-producing cells of a rat's pancreas are destroyed with alloxin, they can be regenerated with 30 mg/kg. of epicatechin, when given for four days.

A water extract of hawthorn leaves and fruits was administered to 42 German heart patients, for periods up to six months. In 36 cases there was an improvement of heart function, anginal pain, vertigo and headaches. The extract does not act in the same way as digitalis, but in many cases it can eliminate or reduce the need for digitalis. It does enable many diabetics to reduce or eliminate the need for insulin. Its main action on the heart seems to be due to dilation of the coronary vessels.

In 1867 Clifton Allbutt reported that he was successful in using cherry bark in heart murmurs and disturbed heartbeats. It was forgotten in England, but it was revived by an American doctor in 1894, and then forgotten again. In 1969 Hungarian medical researchers found that the flavanoids from cherry stalks, had a powerful effect on frog hearts damaged by quinine and posterior pituitary extract. The flavanoids stopped vasoconstriction and decreased coronary resistance by 30%. In an amount of 2 mg./kg., it did not change blood pressure, but it slightly decreased it at 10 mg./kg. The positive effects of cherry extract on the heart are due to dilation of the coronary arteries, and modifying the metabolism of the heart muscle.

The stigma and styles of the ***Crocus sativus*** provide the spice known as saffron. It is a very expensive spice, because it requires so much labor, and the yields are so low. It was traditionally used as an emmenagogue, carminative and diaphoretic. Crocetin and alpha-crocin chemically re-

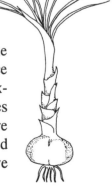

Crocus sativa

semble prostaglandins, which control many of the vital functions of the body. These chemicals also control the fertilization of algae in the ocean.

In Valencia, Spain, saffron is consumed almost daily, especially with rice dishes. Although the general diet is high in fats and calories, the incidence of cardiovascular disease is low. When crocetin was added to the diets of rabbits, it almost completely prevented arteriosclerosis, and it increased the oxygenation of the tissues. Saffron has been suggested as a help for mountain climbers, and people with breathing difficulties, because it increases the oxygenation of the tissues.

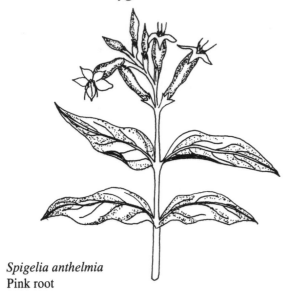

Spigelia anthelmia
Pink root

One way of testing the active heart herbs is to artificially damage the heart, and then test things to see which restores heart functions. A tincture of **Spigelia anthelmia** increases the amplitude and volume in hearts poisoned by a variety of agents. It increases the amplitude and coronary flow in isolated human hearts, and increases physical performance in laboratory animals.

Indian scientists damaged rat hearts with isoproterenol, to produce myocardial necrosis. The chemical duplicated the damage taking place in heart disease. Then alcoholic extracts of two herbs used in Indian medicine for heart complaints were given to rats. **Embelia officinalis** decreased the levels of free fatty acids, and showed a significant rise in blood sugar levels in the heart. It could be used to regenerate damaged hearts. The other herb didn't accomplish anything.

A flavone glucoside in the fruit of the Osage orange **Maclura pomifera** is one of the strongest

of all heart-affecting chemicals. At a dilution of one part to twenty million, it increased the strength of the systole and diastole in laboratory hearts. The rate of heartbeat stayed the same, but the irregularities disappeared. Its utility has never been tested in people.

It has long been known that the common nettle **Urtica dioica** lowers uric acid and blood sugar, and raises the level of red blood cells. In anemia the heart enlarges and gets weaker. The heart is dependent upon oxygen supplies from the capillaries around it, and lowering the amount of oxygen available causes it to enlarge. The old medical reports indicate that nettles can treat the same heart conditions that would make the doctors of today begin thinking about heart transplants.

Helenium microcephalum has helenalin, which increases the levels of cyclic AMP in the heart muscle. The action of the muscles is based on this chemical. It increases the force of the rested heart muscle.

Coleus barbatus

Another herb which increases the levels of cyclic AMP is **Coleus barbatus = C. forskolii**. It has a significant effect in lowering blood pressure, and it increases the coronary blood flow. It is being extensively investigated for its strong effects on the cAMP. At a small amount, it increases the left ventricular pressure by 30%, and it increases the heart rate.

Among the drugs now used to treat heart disorders are beta-blockers. The leaves of *Jatropha curcas*, which is a small shrub in tropical America, has a strong beta blocking effect. A small dose of the leaves increases the amplitude of the heart.

An alcohol extract of the common edible onion has a heart stimulant, which increases pulse volume, frequency, systolic pressure and coronary flow. The extract stimulates smooth muscle, increases bile production and reduces blood sugar.

Another class of heart drugs is calcium antagonists. They decrease the heart rate and dilate the pulmonary vascular beds. The roots of *Ligusticum chuanxiong* increase the plasticity of red blood cells, so that they flow more easily. It takes about five days before the heart begins to improve when it is used. An investigation of the flora of Japan showed that *Boenninghausenia albiflora var.japonica* contains chalepensin, a calcium blocker. The lignins in *Boerhavia diffusa* reduce the heart rate and lower the blood pressure by the same mechanism.

The common store mushroom *Agaricus campestris* was once used to treat hay fever in France. Argentine scientists discovered that it has something that stimulates the heart. It increases the strength of contraction of a toad's heart, and changes the rate of a dog's heart. Do we have healthier hearts after eating this mushroom?

Many of the traditional heart herbs were based on the doctrine of signatures, so anything that was shaped like a heart was good for the heart. Hilda Leyel compiled a book of traditional heart herbs under the name *Heart's Ease*. Another list of heart herbs was compiled by a German doctor. It included *Althaea officinalis*, comfrey, caraway, oat blossoms, agrimony, rue, *Bellis perennis, Rorippa nasturtium-aquaticum* and *Viola tricolor*.

Violets were once commonly known as 'heart's ease.' The pansy, which is a violet, got its name from the French word pensee, meaning 'good thoughts.' These plants contain rutin and bioflavanoids, which improve the circulation. Good circulation means clear mental processes, so the meaning may be more than folklore.

✿✿✿

THE IRREGULAR HEART

"Love, my love, lay your small hand on my heart, hear every second a beat and a start
There dwells a carpenter, —evil is he, —always at work on a coffin for me.
He hammers by night, and he hammers by day, long he has driven my sleep far away.
Hammer, old carpenter, hammer your best! So that I quickly, may go to my rest."

Heinrich Heine c. 1840

The doctor who listens to your heart is listening for a good solid 'lub-dub-pa.' Occasionally, there is an irregular sound or murmur. The heart has a pacemaker, which sends out the signal to the entire heart to contract. Sometimes, another bit of heart tissue will independently act as a separate pacemaker, and cause irregularities of the heartbeat.

At the top of the heart is a spot known as the sino-auricular node, or more commonly called the pacemaker. During the life of the heart, it will send out two to three billion signals. Occasionally, it sends out extra signals, which disturb the rhythm of the heart and disorder the regularity of the pulse.

Fibrillation is one of the major causes of sudden cardiac death, and is the least understood of all cardiac problems. In 1887 John McWilliam found that in some cases of sudden death, the heart didn't just stop, it became completely disordered. He called this 'delirium corditis,' but it later became known as fibrillation. Instead of a coordinated effort at beating, the heart becomes much like a can of writhing worms, with muscular contractions occurring at random all over the heart muscles.

A single electrical shock at just the wrong time in the heart cycle can completely disrupt the rhythm. In 1914 George Mines hooked up an electrical shocker to his chest. He was studying the phenomenon of fibrillation, and was trying to find if a sudden brief electrical shock could make the heart fibrillate. The janitor found him dead on the floor, surrounded by his electrical equipment.

The heart condition known as paroxysmal auricular tachycardia is characterized by a rapid pounding heartbeat. The sensation is extremely upsetting to those who have it. The heart begins to beat at nearly double its normal rate, and the usual heart remedies don't work.

One way of stopping this frightening condition is using ipecac syrup to produce vomiting. In 1910 a patient with this condition took wine of ipecac, and it promptly restored the heartbeat to normal. He told his doctor, and the doctor used the treatment on others.

A surgeon had increasingly frequent attacks of rapid pounding heartbeat. Quinidine, digitalis and other medicines failed in his condition. Ipecac produced vomiting, and within two minutes the pulse fell from 160 to 80. The treatment worked on 11 other patients plagued with episodes of pounding heartbeat.

An irregular heartbeat is normally not serious, and most people with it go on to lead a normal life. If the beat becomes severely irregular, it interferes with the filling and squeezing action, and lowers the capacity to do work. It is this problem we are interested in correcting.

In 1749 Jean-Baptiste de Senec found a remedy for auricular fibrillation. This was during a time when quinine was just coming into popular use in France as a treatment for malaria. Senec noted that quinine cured 'rebellious palpitation' of the heart.

Senec was using a quinine tonic for people with digestion problems, when he discovered the effect on the heart. He wrote, "Of all the stomachic remedies, the one whose effects have appeared to me the most constant and the most prompt in many cases, is quinine mixed with a little rhubarb. Long and rebellious palpitations have ceded to this febrifuge, seconded with a light purgative."

His observations were forgotten for 170 years, until they were rediscovered in 1918. The rediscovery came because a malarial patient with auricular fibrillation took quinine. The bark of the **Cinchona succirubra = C. pubescens** tree contains up to 3% quinidine in addition to quinine. Both compounds act on the heart, but quinidine is more active and less toxic. Quinidine slows and regulates the electrical impulses to the heart. It takes a dosage of about 200 mgs. taken several times a day, to control an irregular heart beat.

Cinchona succirubra
Peruvian bark

When the heartbeat becomes normal, the capacity to pump blood increases by a third. Congestive heart failure is often reversed. The patient feels strong and ready to return to work, with the fatigue removed and the breathing easier.

There are several herbs that have a similar action to quinidine. Horehound **Marrubium vulgare** has been studied by French researchers, because it has a strong action on irregular heart rhythms. The active agent is marrubium, which gives horehound cough drops their characteristic taste. The effect is strong, but of short duration. In 1927 French researchers noted that *Lycopus virginicus* gave good results in extra systoles. It

Marrubium vulgare
Horehound

stimulated the smooth muscle fibers and shortened the QRST complex on the electrocardiogram.

One of the curious discoveries in heart herbs is that the roots of chicory **Cichorium intybus** are nearly as active as quinidine. Chicory leaves have been used in salads and the roots are roasted and mixed with coffee. This produces a pleasant bitterness, which some people prefer to straight coffee.

Cichorium intybus
Chicory

Egyptian researchers studied chicory as a substitute for coffee. The climate was suitable for raising it, and coffee had to be imported for hard currency. They sliced the roots and extracted them with hot alcohol. The extract had a quinidine-like action on the heart and was useful in tachycardia and arrhythmia. The samples were variable in action; the most active types were the large rooted Rohness chicory, and 'a cafe de Magdebourg' chicory.

Motherwort is sometimes known as heartsease, but botanists know it as **Leonurus cardiaca**. It controls heart palpitations and slows the heartbeat. The herb was first mentioned in 1540 in the

Leonurus cardiaca

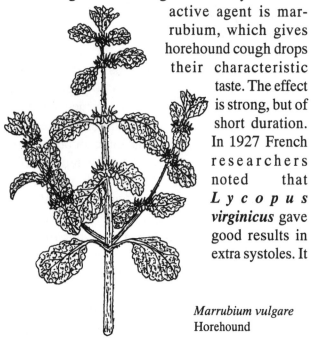

Botanicon of Theodore Dorstensius. He called it 'cardiace,' because it relieved palpitation and pain in the area of the heart. The old French, German and Dutch popular names all have the meaning of 'heart tonic.' It does not stimulate the heart, or have a digitalis-like action.

Ventricular tachycardia is a heartbeat of 180 to 250 beats per minute, which can degenerate into ventricular fibrillation. One curious old remedy, which slows the heart, is creosote. The word comes from the Greek words 'I save flesh,' Today it is made from coal tar, but the original form of creosote was made from the fractional distillation of beechwood *Fagus grandifolia*. It was originally used as a cough cure. One doctor kept awakening in the middle of the night with his heart racing at 130 beats per minute. When he took beechwood creosote his cough cleared, and to his surprise the tachycardia disappeared. He used a drop of this three times a day. The effect may be due to the guaicol in the beechwood.

Stone root *Collinsonia canadensis* was named in honor of botanist Peter Collinson. It is found in the damp woods from Canada to Florida and westward to the Mississippi River. It is traditionally used for urinary problems and water retention. The fresh roots are usually grated and mixed with water for kidney stones and diuretic conditions.

A doctor had a young woman who couldn't walk any distance without experiencing heavy breathing and alarming heart palpitations. She took about 10-15 drops of the fresh stone root three to four times daily. In a few weeks all traces of her heart irregularities were gone.

A young man had a "bellows murmur" and his disability was so great that he couldn't continue in business with his fluttering heart. After taking 20 drops of stone root tincture several times per day, his heart returned to normal. The property of this plant had not been explored further.

The roots of the desert plant *Pteryxia terebinthina* contain pteryxin and several other substances. Rat hearts were made to beat irregularly with aconite, and then the potassium chloride in the blood plasma was reduced. If the heart continued to beat irregularly, the rat was used as a test animal. It took seven times more quinidine sulfate, than the extract from *Pteryxia* to bring the heartbeat back to normal. Another test showed that water extracts from four different plants stopped aconite fibrillation but only one was active in fibrillation. This suggests that there are great differences between individual plants.

Uncaria rhynchophylla has been studied in Japan, because it can reduce irregularities in heartbeat. The alkaloids hirsutine, hirsuteine, and rhynchophylline reduce the irregularities. *Sophora flavescens* is another eastern herb with strong antiarrhythmic effects. An alcoholic extract decreases the incidence of irregular beats. The tranquilizer plant *Rauvolfia serpentina* has the alkaloids ajamaline and serpentine which make the heartbeat more regular.

The leaves and bark of several species of hawthorn have potent, long lasting antiarrhythmic activity, which is present in both water and alcohol extracts. Rabbits were given a small amount of aconite, which made their hearts beat irregularly. Then extracts of *Crataegus curvisepala, C. pentagyna* and *C. monogyna* were used to normalize the heartbeat. The active substances are a mixture of bioflavanoids.

The leaves and twigs of a tree *Zanthoxylum coco* growing in northern Argentina have alkaloids which act on the heart. During WWII quinidine was in short supply in Argentina, and pharmacists tried to find an alternative medicine. They tested a number of plants on dogs, and then tried them in humans. When six persons with heart irregularities that quinine did not control were given fagarine alkaloids, five of them developed a normal rhythm. In one case a single dose of the alkaloids caused an irregular heart to return to normal four weeks later.

Cherry bark *Prunus virginiana* was once considered to be a great heart tonic when taken as a tincture or a tea. Doctor Clifton Allbut would listen to the heart with a stethoscope, and when he heard the thin slapping sound which is called a 'heart murmur,' he prescribed cherry bark. When it was taken for a few weeks the murmur usually disappeared, and a solid lub-dub sound took its place.

The salts in the blood help the tissues to act normally, and an addition of potassium abolishes ectopic beats caused by digitalis. In 13 cases of paroxysmal tachycardia (irregular fast heart), an addition of magnesium sulfate stopped it in five persons, provided temporary relief in four and didn't help in another four.

One nutrient which health food stores stock is coenzyme Q10. This coenzyme maintains ATP production and more efficient oxygen usage. It decreases or eliminates the irregular beats in about one out of four people.

Another nutrient that helps regulate the heart is Vitamin E. Tests showed that alpha tocopherol normalized the activity of the heart enzyme systems and reduced the irregularity. The antioxidant properties are believed to help the arrhythmia and the wandering pacemaker.

In large areas of China, selenium is lacking in the soil. This causes a heart muscle degeneration disease called 'Keshan disease.' It often leads to congestive heart failure in children under 15 years old. A test of the benefits of selenium for the heart was made in this area. A study of 10,000 children on regular diet showed 53 deaths from Keshan disease. When 37,000 children took selenium as a supplement, there were 3 deaths. Selenium reduced the rate of failure of the heart muscle by seventy times.

The great biochemist Albert Szent-Gyorgyi developed a marked arrhythmia, and was treated with traditional heart remedies. He began to wonder if there was a nutritional basis for an irregular heartbeat. He started taking 100 micrograms of selenium daily, and three days later the arrhythmia was gone. His heartbeat remained normal two months later.

☆ ☆ ☆

ANGINA PECTORIS

"The attack is very short like a storm. It usually ends in an hour. I have undergone all bodily infirmities and danger; but none appears to be more grievous. Why not? Because to have any other malady is to be sick; to have this is to die. I, in the midst of suffocation have not omitted to indulge in cheerful and resolute reflections."

Seneca c. +60

"They who are afflicted with it, are seized while they are walking, more especially if it be up a hill, and soon after eating with a painful and most disagreeable sensation in the breast, which seems as if it would extinguish life, if it were to increase or continue: but the moment they stand still, all this uneasiness vanishes."

William Heberdeen describes angina pectoris in 1768.

John Wesley called the mysterious disorder "quinsy of the breast." It didn't have an official name until William Herberden read a paper before the Royal College of Physicians of London in 1768. Angina pectoris has the literal meaning of 'choking of the chest.'

The cause of this painful disorder was not completely associated with the heart for more than a century later. The first doctor to do so was Edward Jenner, the discoverer of smallpox vaccination. From his studies of autopsies of patients, he deduced the relationship between their symptoms, and the narrowed coronary arteries he found. He wrote: "As the heart I believe, in every subject that has died of the angina pectoris, has been found extremely loaded with fat, and as these vessels lie quite concealed in that substance, is it possible this appearance may have been overlooked?"

We now know that the fat is really cholesterol. The walls of the arteries contain muscular contractile tissue, and are capable of changing their size. This explains why sudden movements, emotional happenings, indigestion and bad dreams may bring on angina attacks. The nicotine in tobacco also contracts arteries and can bring on angina attacks.

Mark Twain died of angina pectoris at the age of 74. He remarked: "This is such a mysterious disease. If we only had a bill of particulars, we'd have something to swear at."

John Hunter suffered from it and wrote: "My life is in the hands of any rascal who chooses to annoy and tease me." During a meeting he angrily left the room, and fell down dead in the hall. Charles Morgan used the disorder in the novel *Sparkenbrooke*. An illicit love affair develops, but angina pectoris intervenes to stop it.

Chest distress, heaviness, squeezing, tightness, and a burning mark this painful disorder. It isn't a heart disorder; it is coronary artery disease, caused by plugged arteries.

The air we breathe is a mixture of 21% oxygen, 78% nitrogen and 1% rare gasses. An understanding of the mechanism of angina pain may be gained by looking at experiments in which the oxygen concentration was slowly dropped. Nearly all volunteers developed the symptoms of angina

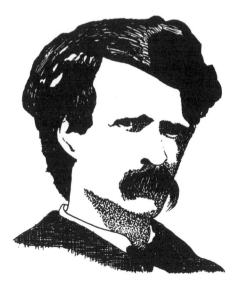

Mark Twain

pectoris when the concentration of oxygen dropped to 12%. The clogging of the arteries reduces the ability of oxygen to supply the heart, so angina can be described as an oxygen deficiency disorder. In a curious way, simply breathing in a paper bag can often stop angina pain. The increase in carbon dioxide dilates the blood vessels, and allows more oxygen into the heart.

One of the best descriptions of angina pain was published by "Dr. X' in the journal *Heart*. He was eating breakfast when he "became conscious of a dull aching pain at the chest. Afterwards for a few seconds only, did my mind continue centered in the news. For the pain, at first felt in the midline beneath the upper part of the sternum, was now extending upwards to the throat, finally to reach the molar region of the jaws. The pulse was irregular; its rate was rapid enough to be beyond my powers of computation. Objects seen at a distance across the room, seemed to stand in a dark field surrounded by mist, which rolled in eddies from the center towards the circumference."

Doctor X relieved his angina pain by crushing a capsule of amyl nitrate, and relief from the pain spread over his chest. He tried to remove the problem with a diet of vegetables, fruits, milk and eggs. The problem grew worse, and he switched to a diet of high protein and low carbohydrates. In ten days he lost nine pounds, and was able to walk about 500 feet without pain. In two months he lost 28 pounds, and was able to walk two miles without pain. His blood pressure continued to drop, and soon he no longer needed nitroglycerin.

In 1846 Christian Schonbein developed guncotton by dipping cotton in a mixture of nitric and sulfuric acids. In 1847 the Italian chemist Ascanio Sobrero discovered nitroglycerin in the same way. Being a curious chemist, he wetted the tip of his finger and tasted the new explosive, and experienced a strong migraine headache, which lasted for hours. The Italian government attempted to determine the value of the new explosive but found that it was too dangerous to use, because it could spontaneously explode. Alfred Nobel made a fortune by mixing the unstable nitroglycerin with porous silica, and created the safe new explosive known as dynamite.

The story of Sobrero's headache came to Constantin Hering, a professor at a homeopathic college in Philadelphia. He experienced the same headache even with a tenth of a drop. Using homeopathic doctrine, of like curing like, nitroglycerin became the remedy used for headaches, sunstroke, epilepsy and inflammation of the heart. It was not used for angina pains; that was left to a British pharmacist to discover. Thomas Brunton had angina pain, and he constantly experimented on himself. Eventually he found that nitrates cure angina pain. Then nitroglycerin became his remedy of choice, 33 years after Ascanio Sobrero developed his first headache.

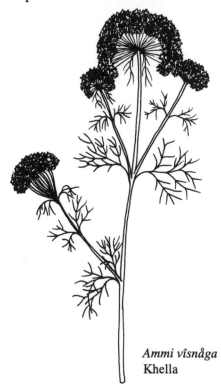

Ammi vîsnåga
Khella

Most of the known botanical remedies act the same way that nitroglycerin does, i.e. they dilate the coronary blood vessels and increase the blood flow to the heart. The ancient Egyptians might have been familiar with at least one remedy, which was rediscovered in 1948. The Arabs called it 'khella,' but botanists know it as **Ammi visnaga**. The seeds of this umbelliferous plant have a powerful ability to vasodilate the coronary arteries, and it has a wide margin of therapeutic safety. Since the plant also dilates the sacs of the lungs, it is useful for bronchial asthma attacks. The extract of the bitter seeds were made into tablets, and given to 14 people with angina pectoris. A placebo produced no relief, but the real thing produced improvement in eleven cases. In four people, improvement continued after the preparation was discontinued. It produced nausea in three people and insomnia in two.

In one case a 66 year-old man was taking up to 40 nitroglycerin tablets daily to control angina pain. While awaiting surgery, he took an extract of the herb, and thereafter was able to live a relatively normal life. Other members of the carrot family may contain substances which act on the heart. The Talmud states that those taking black cumin *Cuminum cyminum* won't suffer from heart pain. Carrot seed extracts are also known to oxygenate the tissues and relieve angina.

Saint Hildegaard, the great early medieval healer, suggested the first remedy known in Europe: "When your heart troubles you, take one, two or even three tablespoons of parsley-honey wine everyday. All pains in the heart will disappear as if blown away. You need not be anxious or afraid, because it cannot do any harm. Not only for slight heart pains, but also for cardiac weakness and real heart trouble, this parsley-honey will do you a great service, and perhaps bring about a recovery."

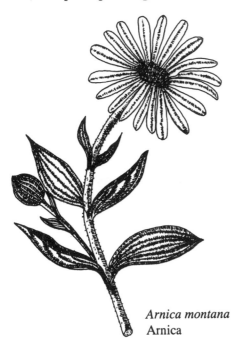

Arnica montana
Arnica

Johann von Goethe (1749-1832) is considered to be German's greatest literary figure. He became a national celebrity by age 24. More than 3,000 of his drawings and 12,000 of his letters survive. Nietzsche called Goethe an "entire culture."

Late in life he suffered from angina pain. He tried many remedies but nothing worked. Then a friend brought him some arnica flowers *Arnica montana*. Three spoonfuls were added to two cups of boiling water. The tea was then strained and drank. Goethe was quite surprised to find that this eliminated the pain.

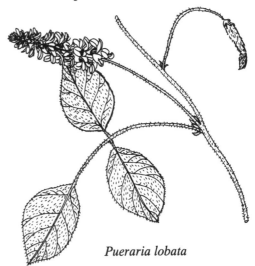

Pueraria lobata

China has two plants known to be coronary vasodilators, which have received some attention. A tincture is made of the roots of the kudzu vine *Pueraria lobata* with 95% alcohol to obtain a bioflavanoid known as puerarin. Five minutes after 20 mg./kg. was injected into dogs, coronary blood resistance fell 25% and blood flow increased by 36%. Blood pressure, heart rate and oxygen demand also fell. The kidneys quickly eliminate it, so the action is short.

A tincture made from the roots of *Salvia miltiorhiza* has similar effects. The extract contains chemicals known as tanshinones, which improved heart problems in 86% of those studied. The chemical prolonged the survival time of rats and mice, when put in conditions of low pressure. It could be of use to mountain climbers and people with lung damage.

Extracts from hawthorn berries and leaves are completely safe and can be taken in any amount. In 1915 a heart doctor reported that he was successful in treating angina pectoris using *Crataegus curvisepala*. He had tried using nitroglycerin, but it gave him no relief for his pain. Two days after taking a tincture of hawthorn, the intervals between his angina attacks were longer. He was able to get more sleep, although he still had to sit up. In four weeks he was able to walk up and down stairs, and resumed some work. Six months later he was able to resume his surgical practice.

A 45 year-old woman had arrhythmia, mitral murmur and aortic stenosis, with a heartbeat that went up to 190 beats a minute. At the slightest exertion she had pain, but after taking hawthorn tincture, she was able to do light housework three months later. In about five months she was essentially cured.

Cratagtus curvisepala is called a 'digitaloid,' because it works on the heart, but it has no cardiac glycosides. The active substance is 1-epicatechin, which increases the strength of the heart contraction. It increases the flow of blood by up to 50% in the arteries that feed the heart. It can reduce digitalis, but it usually does not substitute for digitalis.

A double-blind test was done in China of *Crataegus pinnatifida*. The leaves were made into 100 mg. tablets, which were taken with meals. A third of the patients in the placebo group reported improvement, but 85% of those in the hawthorn group showed improvement. There was a marked difference in the need to take nitroglycerin tablets, and there was an improvement in the electrocardiogram. The active ingredient is a bioflavanoid known as vitexin rhamnoside.

In 1885 a Russian medical journal described two successful cures of angina pectoris, using the dried leaves and berries of the snowball bush *Viburnum opulus*. In one case a 40 year-old woman had been treated by castoreum, lily-of-the-valley and many other things without results. An infusion of two tablespoonfuls of dried snowball berries to a glass of hot water was divided into three portions, to be taken each day. In two months her anginal attacks were reduced from one every two to three days, to one every four to six weeks. After six months of drinking the tea, there were no further angina attacks.

A test was done in Mexico with selenium and vitamin E. Twenty-four patients took either a placebo or a mixture of selenium and Vitamin E. After five weeks, those on the placebo and the vitamin were switched. In 5 cases out of 24, patients reported that the placebo improved. In 22 of 24 cases patients reported that the selenium vitamin mixture reduced angina pain and made their life easier.

One of the most curious remedies for angina pain is an ounce of castor oil and a tincture of iodine. After a few days of taking this, angina pains are said to be reduced enough to get a good night's sleep. Castor oil has a different structure from the normal oils, which are converted to prostaglandins. These control the muscular contractions of muscle cells.

Injections of Epsom salts (magnesium sulfate) were used by one doctor in 200 angina cases. He chose to study 50 cases in detail and found that half of the patients had essentially complete relief from pain after a course of 12 injections. It is possible that taking magnesium supplements may help, although magnesium is poorly absorbed into the body.

The remedies known to reduce arteriosclerosis should be considered for the long-range benefit of angina pain. In many cases the arteries are clogged with cholesterol, and the heart isn't getting enough oxygen. This is why iodine, silica and the other remedies dealt with the cholesterol chapter may permanently cure the condition.

THE DIGITALIS STORY

"I have heard of some experiments you have made on the action of digitalis, and other poisons on yourself. I hope you will not indulge in trials of this kind. I cannot see any useful result that can arise from them. It is in states of disease, and not of health, that they are to be used; and you may injure your constitution without gaining any important result."

A letter of Sir Humphry Davy to a medical student.

The most famous plant in botanical medicine is ***Digitalis purpurea***, not necessarily because it is the most useful, but because it fulfills a need which had not been filled by modern medicine. The plant was called foxglove, which is derived from the Anglo-Saxon word 'foxesglow,' i.e. 'fox music'; a reference to ancient musical instrument consisting of bells hung on an arched support.

The plant is mentioned in several old English herbals. John Gerarde wrote in 1587, "It doth cut and consume the thick toughness of gross and slimy phlegm and naughty humors." The 'consuming of the bad humors' could be a reference to the edema of heart conditions. In 1650 foxglove was included in the London Pharmacopoeia, but it seems to have been a relatively unknown plant. Few doctors from these early times mention it, except with reference to nausea and vomiting.

In 1644 a manuscript of medical recipes says: "Against ye falling sickness take purple foxglove, two handfuls of the leaves with four ounces of polipodium [probably mistletoe] of the oak. Boil them in beer or ale and drink ye decoction. One that had this disease 26 years so that he fell with it two or three times in every months was so cured by ye use of the decoction that he had not a fit for 16 months after."

William Withering was born in Wellington, England, in 1741. His father and his mother's father were doctors, so it was natural for him to study medicine at the University of Edinburgh. He graduated in 1766 and began his practice of medicine at Stafford, England. He was a man of wide accomplishments, who analyzed mineral waters with the crude knowledge of the chemists of the time. He studied minerals and translated Torbern Bergmen's book *Outline of Mineralogy*. As a result of his interests, the mineral barium carbonate was named Witherite after him.

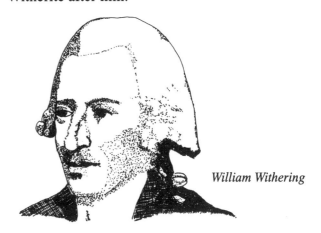

William Withering

His interest in botany became much greater when he met Helena Cook as a patient. She painted flowers; and they were married in 1772. He began a study of botany, which led to a book: *Botanical Arrangement of All the Vegetables.*

He had such a poor medical practice that he moved to Birmingham. He became friends with many of the noted English scientists of the time. An old herb lady in this area possessed a remedy known for its power in curing dropsy. Withering was impressed by the fact that the woman cured dropsy after the regular doctors failed, and he was determined to learn the secret. Old Mother Hutton's medicine was composed of some twenty herbs, and it proved easy to determine that the active one was foxglove.

Withering began his experiments with foxglove in 1775, dried a large quantity of leaves and gave them to his fellow doctors in order to establish the usefulness of the medicine. By 1785 he was able to publish a book titled: *An Account of the Foxglove and Some of Its Medicinal Uses, With Practical Remarks on Dropsy and Other Diseases.*

The book summarized the results of medical experiments on 163 people and reports from other doctors. He gave complete instruction for other doctors desiring to use the remedy. This book is considered a classic in medical literature. Withering had to do a careful job, because foxglove is quite toxic, and it is easy to poison patients. During this time, most doctors paid little attention to dosage, but in using foxglove it was absolutely necessary.

Withering used small doses twice a day and mixed them with opium to control nausea and vomiting. He claimed a success rate of 72%, with side effects in 18%. Digitalis therapy became popular in England, but doctors began to use it for a whole series of illnesses for which it had no benefits. Then it went through a period of decline, until James MacKenzie re-established its value as one of the great remedies in 1910.

Erasmus Darwin included the foxglove in his poem: *The Botanic Garden:*

Digitalis purpurea

Divine Hygeia from the bending sky,
Descending listen to his piercing cry:
Assumes bright digitalis dress and air;
her ruby cheek, white neck and raven hair.
Withering himself had written:
The foxglove's leaves with caution given,
another proof of favoring heaven.
Will happily display,
The rapid pulse it can abate,
the hectic flush can moderate.
And, blest by Him whose will is fate,
may give a lengthened day.

The secret of the foxglove captured the imagination of George Eliot. In *Silas Marner* Eliot wrote: "Marner had cured Sally Oates and made her sleep like a baby, when her heart had been beating enough to burst her body for two months or more. Recalling the relief that his mother had found with a simple preparation of the foxglove, he promised Sally Oates to bring her something that would ease her."

Pharmacists have used cats, dogs, goldfish and frogs to standardize digitalis. Different animals react quite differently, and even frogs from different sources are unreliable. One 'cat unit' is enough to stop the heart of a cat in systole. In 1933 a number of "standard tinctures" of digitalis were tested. It was found that the strength varied by twenty times from the weakest to the strongest. The tinctures deteriorate, but the dried leaves don't, which is a good reason for returning to Withering's original methods.

Most medicines are made from *Digitalis purpurea* but *Digitalis lutea* is often used. Many doctors believe that *D. lutea* produces less nausea and vomiting. The foxglove has been tried for nearly everything, but only the treatment of the heart remains.

In the 1930's Dr. Israel Bram operated the Bram Institute for Goiter and Glandular Diseases in Philadelphia. He noted that too many square meals make round figures, and sought a simple way to break the cycle of hunger, which leads to overweight. Heart patients often react with nausea when taking foxglove and this gave him the clue for an effective treatment.

He tried using foxglove on 140 overweight patients. The oldest patient was 67 and the youngest was 6 years old. Patients were given from 30 to 120 mgs. of powdered digitalis leaves. An average of 60 milligrams was taken before meals to produce a slight nausea, but no vomiting. The amount was raised or lowered to produce nausea without vomiting.

The nausea produced by digitalis reduced the amount eaten, so most patients were quite comfortable on less than a thousand calories a day. During the first two months the average weight reduction was 11 pounds per month and 7 pounds per month thereafter. After the first 30-40 pounds the amount of digitalis could be reduced or discontinued and the weight reduction would continue.

A 14 year-old boy lost 84 pounds in six months. A 50 year-old woman lost 70 pounds in ten months. In many cases the digitalis could be discontinued and the patients would not gain weight, or would continue to lose until they reached their normal weight. A normal weight was reached by 83% of the patients in an average of 16 weeks.

Despite its great success the method didn't catch on, and it was forgotten. Careful medical supervision is needed to follow such a regimen. Foxglove is an extremely dangerous plant in overdoses, but it is safely used by millions of people under standardized conditions.

Two centuries have passed since the time of Withering, but scientists do not fully understand why digitalis produces the effects it does. When muscle fibers pull together, ions travel from the outside of the walls of the cells to the inside. The four ions that are important in muscular contraction are sodium, potassium, calcium and magnesium. With each pull and relaxation of the heart muscle, the sodium and potassium ions change place. It is now believed that when digitalis is taken, some of the sodium ions exchange with calcium, and this produces a stronger and slower heart beat.

This effect on the calcium balance seems to indicate why calcium can sometimes substitute for digitalis. Experiments with calcium lactate at a level of three grams a day showed it acted like a diuretic during heart failure. Calcium salts strengthen the heart, slow its rate and lower blood pressure. Calcium by itself has a limited value in treating hearts. When it is given with digitalis, it augments the strength of the heart.

Maurice d'Halluin noticed this effect in his work with heart patients. He recommended alternating calcium salts with digitalis. The heart performed better, and there was less toxicity from the digitalis.

DIGITALIS SUBSTITUTES

*"The poison used here is called kombi [**Strophanthus glabra**] and is obtained from a species of strophanthus and is very virulent. Dr. Kirk found by an accidental experiment on himself that it acts by lowering the pulse.I n using his toothbrush, which had a bitter taste, he attributed it to quinine on the handle. Though the quantity was small, it immediately showed its power by lowering the pulse, which at that time had been raised by a cold, and next day he was perfectly restored. Not much can be inferred from one case, but it is possible that kombi may turn out a valuable remedy".*

Travels *David Livingstone*

Birds feed on insects, so it would be easy for a fast-moving bird to catch a slow-moving Monarch butterfly. When a young bird catches this kind of butterfly, it begins to vomit, and from then on, it won't touch another butterfly with the same markings. The monarch caterpillar feeds on milkweeds. It absorbs cardiac glycosides from the plant, which makes it poisonous to birds. The chemical structure of the milkweed glycosides closely resemble digitalis.

There are several species of grasshoppers that protect themselves in the same way. A species of grasshopper than feeds on *Calotropis procera,* absorbs the cardenolides, and birds will ignore it. The grasshoppers advertise their immunity by being brightly colored, and are left alone. The European hedgehog is insensitive to cardenolides and eats grasshoppers with impunity.

The first of the classical heart remedies is mentioned in the Ebers Papyrus of ancient Egypt. This is the squill or sea onion *Scilla maritima*, to which they gave the name 'Eye of Typhon'. They probably did not recognize heart aliments the way we do, but they did know that it was a diuretic. Traditional lore held that Pythagoreas or Epimenides introduced it into Greek medicine.

The use of squill was forgotten until it was revived around +1700. It does two of the same things that digitalis does: produces a heart block, particularly in cases of auricular fibrillation, and it changes the T wave of the electrocardiogram. Most preparations of squill are about a sixth as active as a similar preparation of digitalis. The good point is that it rarely produces toxic symptoms, even in large doses. The bad side is that is usually does not improve heart patients the way digitalis does. Squill is poorly absorbed orally and that makes digitalis the preferred treatment.

In 1883 Doctor See advocated sparteine from Scotch broom in cardiac disease. It strengthens the pulse as well as digitalis and regulates the rhythm. It lessons the frequency and increases the force of the heart. The alkaloid sparteine is useful in postoperative suppression of urine, for it restarts the stalled kidneys. Sparteine is also found in *Lupinus luteus* and *Anagyris foetida*.

In 1892 *Lynchis vavia* was claimed to be superior to digitalis. One person had an enlarged heart and could not take digitalis. This herb acted dramatically in reducing heart palpitation, hard breathing and irregular heartbeats. One woman couldn't work at all, but after taking the tincture for eight days she was nearly normal.

The lily-of-the-valley *Convallaria majalis* has long been used in Russian popular medicine for ailing hearts. The plant was extensively investigated around 1885, and was found to be a useful heart remedy. It is about five times stronger than digitalis when injected, but it is poorly absorbed through the stomach walls, so it does not give consistent results orally. The flowers are about twice as strong as the roots and stems.

The room of the old fortress of Frausenberg in East Prussia where Copernicus spent so much of his time,

Convallaria majalis Lily-of-the-valley

is preserved with his belongings. He is known as an astronomer, yet he was educated as a medical doctor and graduated from Padua, Italy, in 1499. Near his portrait is his medical insignia with his favorite plant, the lily-of-the-valley, painted on it. The room also contains his only preserved prescription, a mixture of 21 substances, including this plant.

Since the cardiac glycosides are so toxic, they were used as arrow poisons. Most of the species of **Strophanthus** trees in Africa have been used in arrow poisons, for the sudden dose of alkaloids stops the hearts of animals. The most important glycoside is 'ouabain' from **Strophanthus glabra**. It is used in acute dilation of the heart. In many cases of advanced heart failure, it is a better remedy than digitalis, and it is still used as a heart medicine.

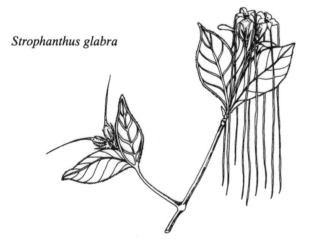

Strophanthus glabra

The poisonous aconites were gathered in India and China as heart medicine. When the roots were gathered in the summer and early fall, they disturbed the heartbeat. When they were gathered in the months of November through March, they acted as a useful heart stimulant.

In 1948 newspapers carried the story of a Sarasota, Florida, man who died from a heart attack after inhaling smoke from a brush fire. The fire was consuming a thicket of oleander plants **Nerium oleander**, and the smoke was rich in oleandrin. This alkaloid acts like digitalis, and small quantities produced heart stoppage.

The Star-of-Bethlehem **Ornithogalum umbellatum** is a useful substitute for digitalis. It won't work by mouth, because the secretions of the stomach attack it. If it is given as a coated tablet, it works very well, and is a good substitute for

digitalis. It is less nauseating and has greater strength than digitalis. The reason why it is not marketed is due to the cost of bringing a new drug to a market dominated by a long established effective product.

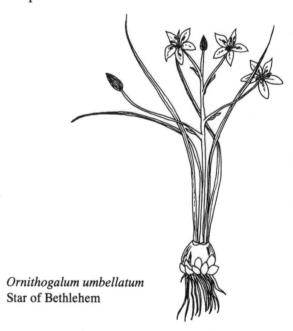

Ornithogalum umbellatum
Star of Bethlehem

In 1829 Doctor Walker had a heart patient who was unable to help with digitalis, mercury or iodine. As a last resort he was directed to drink daily a half-pint of woodruff tea **Galium odoratum**. In a few weeks the patient was almost completely cured.

Apocynum cannabinum is called Canadian hemp because the tough fiber was once used to make rope. It was first used as a digitalis substitute in 1826. A doctor taking a small amount of the extract found that his pulse fell from 70 to 50 in the first hour, and then dropped to 45 before slowly climbing back to normal. The active substance was isolated in 1910, but it causes more nausea and vomiting than digitalis, and it isn't used.

The Japanese and Chinese have a long history of eating seaweeds as a normal part of the meal, and this could be why they have such a low incidence of heart problems. An alcoholic extract of the 'kobu' **Laminaria japonica** strengthens the heartbeat of laboratory animals and reduces edema. The cardiotonic substance dissolves in alcohol, but is relatively insoluble in water.

In Mexico the heart flower yolete-xochitl **Taluma mexicana** was first mentioned in an herbal in 1552. It has diuretic and digitalis-like effects. The Ayurvedic doctors of India used *Achyranthes aspera* for cardiac dropsy. A list of all of the other plants with digitalis-like properties could go on and on.

There are plants that are claimed to be cures for the conditions which digitalis treats. Around 1850 Doctor Themont had heart patients put two handfuls of unprepared oats boiled in three quarts of water for 15 minutes. Regular drinking of oat tea was said to cure cardiac dropsy. The hulls of oats contain interesting chemicals that have been used in allergies.

A century ago Doctor August Ramm published a little booklet on the effectiveness of kidney bean pods in curing cardiac dropsy. One of his heart patients had a severe case of dropsy. She stopped coming to him, and when he saw her, he was surprised to see that she had no sign of dropsy at all. She told him that she had tried a variety of herbs. One day she drank a tea of kidney bean pods and began passing large quantities of water. To make sure that it was not just a coincidence, she drank another glass and again she had profuse urination. After drinking the kidney bean pod tea for three weeks, she was cured and there was no sign of dropsy or heart disease.

Ramm tried the remedy on all his dropsy cases and on all cases of heart disease. In every case there was large quantities of urine voided, and the patient was cured. The albumin disappeared from the urine, and the dropsy showed no signs of returning. It not only cured the dropsy, but kidney stones disappeared from the kidneys and kidney problems were cleared up. In some cases of diabetes, the sugar disappeared from the urine. Many cases of cystitis cleared up, and kidney bean pods looked like a real wonder drug.

If the remedy was not completely forgotten, Ramm might have achieved the fame of William Withering. The fresh ripe pods of the kidney bean

Phaseolus vulgaris are picked, shelled and made into tea. An ounce of the pods are put in four quarts of water and boiled. The mixture is strained, cooled and drank, for it is said to lose its activity upon sitting. When a popular health magazine printed a summary of Ramm's work, a number of readers wrote in to say that it had cured their problems. The beans have no activity, and only the fresh pods are active.

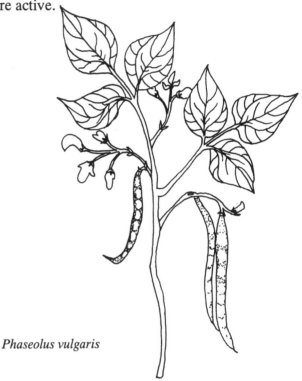

Phaseolus vulgaris

Kidney bean pod tea is more than just a remedy to remove the fluid from the body, when the heart is failing. Ramm used it in gout, rheumatism, kidney stones, gravel and gallstones. In cases of diabetes, it takes about three weeks before the sugar disappears from the urine. In kidney disease the albuminuria quickly disappeared. Ramm noted that five cases of bleeding from the kidneys were cured after prolonged use of the tea. He also believed that it was useful in the albuminuria, or uremic states that occur during pregnancy.

BEYOND THE HEART ATTACK

M. Macroton: "To such an extent, indeed, that to draw, detach, wrest, expel and evacuate the said humors will require a vigorous purgation. As a preliminary step, I think desirable, and there is no contraindication, to employ some minor anodynes, that is, some slight emollient, detersive and refreshing draughts which can be mixed with her ptisan."
M. Bahis: "Afterwards, we will come to the purgation and the bleeding, which we will repeat if necessary."
M. Macroton: "With all this it is still possible that your daughter may die; but at least you will have done something, and you will have the consolation, that she died in due form."
M. Bahis: "It is better to die in accord with the regulations than to survive in defiance of them."

From the French satirist Jean Baptiste Moliere

The term "heart attack" is actually a young expression dating back to the 1930s. Before this time there are numerous expressions such as heart anguish, heart agony, and in older English "the heart smote him." The person who first focused attention on the heart as a cause of death was Giovanni Lancisi. Pope Clement XI asked him to report on the causes of death in Rome. He found many oversized and undersized hearts and aneurysms in those who died suddenly. His book *De Subitaneis Mortibus* (On Sudden Death) was published after his death in 1720.

During the years 1925 to 1945, Italian bread was made entirely from whole fiber wheat. Benito Mussolini prohibited refined bread to save on importing wheat. Bakers prefer to use the starchy part of the wheat grain and throw away the live part of the seed. During those years, the ratio of heart problems between men and women stayed relatively equal. In 1947 the laws against refined flour were lifted, and heart conditions in men rose rapidly, but they rose only slightly in women. Vitamin E was probably the factor in whole wheat, which kept Italians healthier.

Vitamin E was initially tagged as the fertility vitamin, because it was needed for fertility. Evan Shute was a Canadian obstetrician who used Vitamin E for habitual abortion. He found that it delayed the clotting of blood. One of his patients was so ill, that he couldn't have an operation, so Schute tried Vitamin E and the man quickly improved.

Shute's mother was dying of edema, high blood pressure and an irregular heartbeat. She could only sleep a few minutes at a time sitting up. She had chairs in the middle of every room and in every doorway. She refused to give up her house and lived by moving from chair to chair. She was given 200 units of Vitamin E daily. Three weeks later, she was outside spading up her flower garden. She died nine years later of an unrelated infection.

The work of the Shute brothers attracted attention from popular health magazines. One woman wrote, "About two years ago I began having some pretty gruesome rheumatic fever symptoms; chest pains, extreme heaviness in the chest, difficulty in taking a deep breath, extreme weakness and undefined fear, such as I'd never known."

Her doctor said she'd just have to live with it. She went to the Shute Clinic and began taking 300 units of Vitamin E a day. Two months later she wrote, 'I was breathing normally and gasping every time I did more than walk straight! I suddenly realized that I didn't have that terrible feeling on my chest and that those vague aches and pains in my chest were gone."

Vitamin E received a great deal of attention and numerous cases of help were reported. The governing body of Ontario doctors heard the testimony of those who were helped and put out a report saying that all of the cases were simply "faulty diagnosis." The report ended: "The committee is convinced that Vitamin E has no place in the treatment of cardiovascular disease."

Seven baboons died in an animal park in Georgia. Autopsies showed that they died of heart failure, for they all had white or pale patches on the heart muscle, and anemia was present. It was finally determined that the baboons were suffering from a lack of Vitamin E. When the diet was supplemented with the vitamin, the other animals remained healthy.

In 1983 five Mongolian wild horses at the Bronx zoo in New York City had to be destroyed. A pathological examination showed destruction of the myelin sheaths of the nerves. During the winter the animals were fed hay, and grass in the summer. A comparison of wild animals with zoo animals, showed different levels of Vitamin E. With extra Vitamin E, heart disease in captive animals disappeared.

From the time that Vitamin E was put on the market in the 1930s, its use was surrounded by medical controversy. In 1993 the *New England Medical Journal* published a study of thousands of men and women, that finally removed medical doubt.

The study of 51,000 men showed that those taking the highest amounts of Vitamin E had lower risk. In order for the vitamin to be of benefit, men had to take at least 100 units per day for two years. A study of 87,000 women showed a major difference between the lowest amounts of Vitamin E and the highest amounts. Those who took larger supplements for several years had 40% less risk of coronary heart disease.

Hans Selye studied the effects of stress and cardiac toxicity. He found that both Vitamins E and K would prevent cardiac muscle death in bad diets. In his studies, Vitamin K often proved to be more important than Vitamin E. In Russia, it was found that Vitamin B6 prevents heart attacks. With extra B6, it took a greater dosage of toxic agents to stop the heart.

The worst things that we can include in our diet are high levels of saturated fats and processed sugars. When rats were fed a diet of 15% corn oil and 50% cornstarch they gained 1.72 grams. When the starch was replaced by sugar they gained 3.56 grams. The combination of oil and sugar produced a body proportion of 33% fat, compared to 22% in the other diet. High intakes of sugar and oils are linked to heart disease.

When the chest tightens and searing pain radiates from the center of the chest, what can you do? Until recent times people felt helpless without the presence of a doctor, for there was no way to revive the heart. The beginning of artificial heart stimulation took place in 1878, when Carl Boehm showed that rhythmic forceful compression of an intact chest wall of a cat could raise the blood pressure by 50 to 120 mm. of mercury.

CPR or 'cardio-pulmonary-respiration' has been around for about 50 years. Three doctors who spent time working on cadavers in the morgue developed it. They had to experiment within 45 minutes of death before rigor mortis set in, and the chest became immobile. Too much pressure could crack the ribs, and too little pressure wouldn't do anything. The techniques they discovered have become the standard Red Cross techniques for giving first aid to those with heart attacks.

Another method of treating heart attacks developed in Japan. Jujitsu was the old Japanese method of self-defense, used by the samurai. During their training, these people would throw blows at each other, which had the potential to kill, if not skillfully deflected. If a student was hit in the wrong place and knocked unconscious, he might not revive, unless he was treated promptly.

Each of the vertebrae of the spine has pairs of nerves, which lead into the chest and control the organs. 'Kuatsu' consists of propping up the unconscious person, and striking the seventh cervical vertebra, with regular rhythmic blows. The seventh cervical vertebra is on the middle of a line between the upper shoulder blades. The rescuer puts one hand over the vertebra, and the other hand, pounds it like a hammer and nail. The jujitsu student would usually recover consciousness quickly, and then his arms were rotated several times. Then he was helped to his feet, and taken for a short walk. If these steps weren't followed, he might lapse back into unconsciousness.

The nerve pairs of this vertebra lead to the heart area, and sharp blows strengthen the heartbeat. Albert Abrams was able to show that many patients with weak, declining hearts would regain a forceful beat in several minutes. He used the method to revive people suffering from sunstroke, drowning and heart attacks. It seems to have been forgotten, although it could be used to revive some people in comas as well.

The late John Christopher was an extraordinary herbalist, who followed directly in the steps of Samuel Thomson. He traveled widely through the Northwestern U.S. and lectured. The police frequently interrupted his meetings, for the AMA sent them to arrest him for practicing medicine without a license. He was a naturopathic doctor, and practicing herbalist. He talked like a combination of a revival preacher and a soapy old politician. He often got his facts twisted in his lectures, and as a historian, I often winced! He used and absolutely believed in the power of herbs to heal any disorder, and his words deserve careful study.

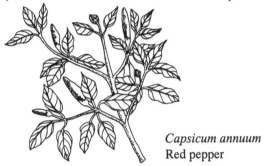

Capsicum annuum
Red pepper

Doctor Christopher spoke of how he treated hundreds of cases of heart attacks with cayenne pepper without ever losing a patient. Then he would pour a large spoonful of red hot pepper *Capsicum annuum* into a glass of water and drink it, while remarking that it made 'smoke pour out of his ears.' He told stories of people who had been incapacitated for weeks after a heart attack. When the next heart attack began they used a heaping tablespoonful of red pepper in water, and they were well in minutes.

If you are not used to taking red pepper, and you take a spoonful, you will begin to sweat profusely in about a minute. Experiments with dogs show that the veins dilate, the blood pressure drops rapidly, and the heart slows. Blood flow in the mesenteric, renal and femoral arteries decrease, but blood flow increases in the cardiac artery. The immediate effect is to reduce blood pressure, and take the load off the heart. If there is a clot, the widening of the arteries allows it to pass through.

Capsaicin acts on the primary afferent sensory neurons by interacting directly with a cell membrane receptor. It opens the ion channels; so more calcium can enter the cells. Capsaicin stimulates the uptake of calcium into the neurons. Calcium intake is important to the operation of the heart muscle fibers. There is some interest in treating heart conditions with capsaicin and resiniferatoxin.

This is found in *Euphorbia* species and is some 10,000 times more potent than capsaicin.

Fibrin is the material in the blood which causes clots, and in 'thrombosis' clots are the reason for the damage and the heart attack. A study in Thailand showed that the average man had a fibrinolytic activity time of 167 minutes, but a similar group of American men had an average time of 254 minutes. The basic difference seems to be the consumption of cayenne pepper. When experimental subjects held red pepper in their mouth for two minutes, the fibrinolytic time fell from 165 minutes to 145 minutes. Red pepper would act to aid in clearing the blood clots. In addition, it dilates the blood vessels and allows the blood to pass before the areas become damaged by lack of oxygen.

Ginger *Zingiber officinale* is known primarily as a seasoning spice, but it is used as a medicine in China and Japan. Japanese researchers extracted dried ginger roots with alcohol and isolated three gingerols, which proved to have powerful heart stimulation effects. These substances are chemically similar to the same compounds in red pepper. Ginger is a potent inhibitor of thromboxane synthetase, and it inhibits platelet aggregation. It would be very useful in preventing and dissolving blood blots.

Zingiber officinale
Ginger

The blood contains a natural enzyme that degrades blood clots, which occur naturally in the blood in an active form called plasminogen. If the levels of this clot-degrading enzyme are low, blood clots persist and their effects last. Heart attacks become more likely.

Bromelain (pineapple enzyme) stimulates the conversion of plasminogen to plasmin, which breaks down fibrin clots. There have been two small trials using bromelain to treat heart attacks. In one trial of 140 people less than 2% died over a two-year period, whereas 20% would have been expected to die. In another trial of 76 heart attack patients, less than 3% died while 35% would have been expected to die in the four-year period after the heart attack.

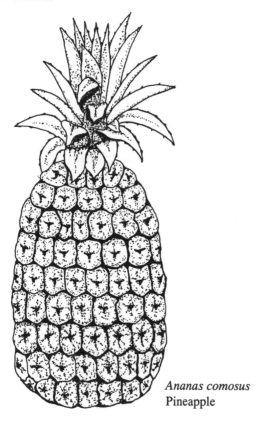

Ananas comosus
Pineapple

Ribose is a sugar which is a powerful heart stimulant. When experimenters using rats constricted the abdominal aorta and depressed the heart function with isoproterenol, the rats would usually die. When they gave them ribose, the biosynthesis of muscle-acting adenine nucleotides was stimulated so much, that soon the heart action became normal. These are muscle-acting compounds, which provide the energy for ATP to contract the heart muscles. An injection of ribose increased the rate of biosynthesis by more than five times. Ribose is a cheap simple form of sugar present in small quantities in plants, which was once studied for use by diabetics. The use of ribose to regenerate the heart was given U.S. patent number 4,719,201.

Calcium is a necessary ingredient of the contraction of the heart muscle. In 1904 Doctor Maurice d'Halluin was giving intravenous injections of potassium chloride to stop ventricular fibrillation. He wrote a book about his experiments in using salts to aid heart conditions. He found that the addition of calcium chloride produced a marked improvement in the heartbeat.

In 1933 doctors found that cardiac massage, electrical defibrillation and ephedrine had little effect on cardiac arrest. When they injected a solution of calcium chloride into the left ventricular cavity, the heart began to beat, and with continued massage it developed a strong beat. Calcium has a direct effect on the heart, and is a major aid in restoring a normal beat.

A new picture of heart disease began to emerge around 1990. Fifty years before this, it was found that capillary fragility was due to lack of Vitamin C. Our capillary system is somewhat like a car's radiator, and in older cars we use solutions with particles which plug the leaks. The body plugs the leaks with a special lipoprotein. Lp(a) begins the process by depositing in the weak areas of the capillaries. These patches become sites for cholesterol deposits and begin the clogging of the arteries.

In 1941 a study showed that four out of five coronary heart patients suffered from Vitamin C deficiency. In 1954 a study by C.G. Willis showed that a daily supplement of 500 mgs. of Vitamin C reduced leg artery deposits by 30% within six months. A similar group of patients who didn't take supplements had no changes in artery deposits.

In 1991 Mathias Rath discovered that the amino acid lysine detached the sticky Lp(a) from the blood vessels. He found that supplements of Vitamin B3 in the form of nicotinic acid (but not nicotinamide) lower the levels of the lipoprotein. The amino acid proline was found to be nearly as active as lysine. A combination of 500 mgs. of lysine, 500 mgs. of proline and 500 mgs. of Vitamin C helped to remove the deposits from the arteries. Linus Pauling found that angina pectoris patients would gradually return to normal after months of taking this combination. Many heart patients were able to return to normal.

SECRETS OF THE LIVER

"Liver, liver little liver, once so light upon my chest;
Then I needed to question, wherefore comes this indigestion,
Like a nightmare's nest.
Liver, liver, swelling liver, secret source of many an ill,
Naught can still thy sad commotion, blister, lotion, poultice, potion,
No, nor Cockle's pill.
Liver, liver, swollen liver, so the chained Prometheus felt.
When the bird of evil omen, fattening on his fat abdomen,
Pecked beneath his belt."

Anonymous poem c. +1880

Carl Jung, the great Swiss explorer of the primitive mind, had a series of dreams that gave him clues to the operation of the inner self. In one vivid dream he saw "Liverpool," a great circular city, with a square inner center. In the middle was a pool, which had an island, with a great flowering magnolia bursting into reddish flames.

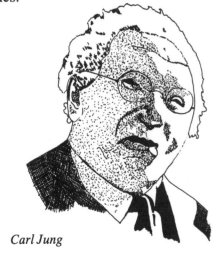

Carl Jung

Why Liverpool? Jung recognized that the "liver" in ancient times was felt to be the source of blood, and consequently the life. "Pool" conveys the image of water, signifying the unconscious being that shapes our outer thinking. The city was the place, where self voyaged to the inner world, and gathered the images of life, so spirit could operate.

In the expressions of language, a timid person has a weak liver. The secretion of the liver means the opposite, because people with lots of gall are said to be overly bold or forceful. When Hamlet does not take vengeance on his father's murder, Shakespeare records: "But I am pigeon livered, and lack gall to make opposition."

In America when we have headaches, we take aspirin, and our troubles and trials are solved. In France an upset stomach is "un rhume de foie," meaning a "cold of the liver," and a backache is "un foie congestionne." When a French athlete has a off day, he has a "crise de foie." A sick child suffers from a tired liver, and "le foie de reveillons," is a hangover from too much French wine. A man of courage has a hot liver, and a coward has a white liver.

In both France and Italy liver trouble is a disease with class, for it is an indication of too much good food, sauces and fine wine. In Italy, people with liver trouble just raise their eyebrows and gently tap the fingers below the right ribs. Everyone understands that the good life has gotten to their liver.

When Napoleon and his army were in the midst of the bitter Russian winter of 1812, he wrote this letter back to Paris, "We will soon attack Moscow, but my liver is troubling me due to strange food. I cannot wait to return when mamma and I take the cure at Vichy."

Vichy is a resort town south of Paris devoted to putting bad livers back in working order. Crowds of somber Frenchmen talk in low tones, about their "mal au foie," at the mineral water spa. It is dominated by a large glass and bronze building called "Le Grande Grille." Three mineral springs gush from the earth, and the sufferers bathe and drink of the mineral waters.

The same situation exists at Chianciano and Montecantini in Italy. At the latter, it is common knowledge that the great poet Dante Alighieri cured his ailing liver there, after too much rich food, wine and his love affair with Beatrice. Julius Caesar is said to have stopped there, as well.

Capillaries surround the intestinal tract, and the first passage of blood from the intestines is through the liver. The liver enzymes break down any foreign material, before the blood reaches the heart and the brain.

Low blood sugar is a mark of liver disease at any stage. As the carbohydrates come from the intestines, they are converted to the stored sugar form of glycogen. When the level of blood sugar drops, glycogen sugar is released. The tiredness, fatigue, and mental confusion, known as hypoglycemia, is an indication of liver trouble.

When liver function is poor, night vision goes. In diseases of the liver such as hepatitis, the sharpness of day vision suffers in accordance with liver damage. There is some evidence that links liver function with near sightedness.

There is a theory that schizophrenia and mental illness may be due to an inactive liver. The enzymes of the liver detoxify chemicals, and there may be a chemical factor which they have failed to detoxify. When the blood of mentally ill patients is treated on dialysis machines, the patients improve. If we could improve the performance of the liver, we might be able to cure some forms of mental illness.

Not only does the liver act as a detoxification center for poisons, but it also acts as a storage center for them. When 0.02 grams of silver was injected into the blood of rats, the liver captured 66% in 15 minutes. Similar experiments resulted in the liver capturing 60% of selenium, 42% of the copper and 67% of platinum in 15 minutes.

Part of the action of the liver herbs may be to reduce the effects of toxins in the liver. *Withania somnifera* is a shrub used in medicine in India. Mice were poisoned with the toxic metal cadmium, which accumulates in the liver. Then an alcoholic extract of the root was given to them. This increased the activity of liver enzymes, and protected the animals against the toxic metals.

Selenium was once believed to be a dangerous metallic toxin. By 1941 nutritional researchers were finding that animals fed purified casein died of liver degeneration. A search for the unknown vitamin brought about some important nutritional discoveries. Vitamin E protected the liver against degeneration, but it didn't provide the final answer. Eventually it was found that trace amounts of selenium protected the liver against a poor diet.

Those who believed that they had a bad liver protected themselves with the old liver herbs. These plants were named from the resemblance to the liver. Liver weed was *Hepatica triloba*, ground liverwort was *Peltidea canina*, marsh liverwort was *Ricca* species, water liverwort was *Ranunculus aquatilis* and just plain liverwort was usually *Marchantia polymorpha*.

In November, Japanese fishermen catch thousands of porcupine fish. They have spines all over their bodies and are known as blowfish. Restaurants and chefs of Japan must be licensed to prepare the fish. "Fugu" is the caviar of Japan, but the liver of this fish concentrates poisons, and an ounce of the liver could theoretically kill 65,000 people. Each year about 20 people die from eat-

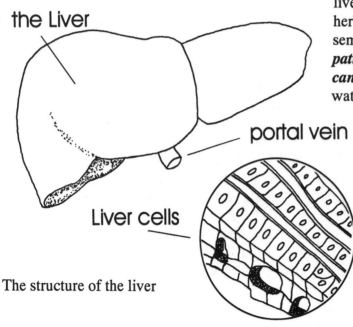

the Liver

portal vein

Liver cells

The structure of the liver

ing fugu, but this is a small price to pay in Japan for the supreme fish delicacy.

Liberace, the glittering piano player and entertainer, used to clean spots on his suits with carbon tetrachloride before performing. He didn't know that it was a powerful liver toxin. Scientists use it to poison the livers of rats, when searching for liver protective agents. Liberace used too much on a suit in 1963 and became sick during the concert. He was rushed to the emergency ward of the St. Francis Hospital in Pittsburgh, Pennsylvania.

He was hooked to an artificial kidney and remained in critical condition for many weeks. After being given the last rites, he was visited by a nun who asked him to pray to St. Anthony. That prayer released an inner feeling that he was to live and perform again. He began to recover at that time.

George Washington Crille spent years studying the structure and function of the body. He concluded that the liver and brain form opposite electrical poles. The body fluids act as an electrolyte, just as acid forms a circuit between the poles of a car battery.

When any trauma happens to the body the voltage of the brain decreases, and the voltage of the liver increases. Here are several of Crille's examples:

Ether	brain -20%	liver +26%
Strychnine	brain -6%	liver +30%
Fright	brain -7%	liver +65%

When the liver is surgically removed there isn't any influence on the heart, kidneys or any other organs of the body. However, the brain and nerve cells begin to die. If the body is truly a battery, then removing one pole destroys the ability of the other pole to function.

The earliest models of the liver were of clay, and were used for instructing in liver divination, at the Babylonian temple schools. The model on display at the British museum is divided into squares and covered with cuneiform writing. Similar models were found in bronze, covered with Etruscan writing, at Pianze, Italy. These models were superior to the known anatomical concepts, until dissection began in the sixteenth century.

When an animal is sacrificed a large part of the blood is found in the liver. This observation led to the belief that the liver was the source of the blood, and hence was the seat of the soul. By look-

ing at the liver, you looked at the soul, and then you knew the mind or will of God. The science of divining with the liver was called heptoscopy, from the Babylonian word 'hep,' meaning liver.

Julius Caesar was once said to have his augurs sacrifice a sheep, to foretell if he should go to battle. Each liver kept telling him "no," but he was determined. After fifteen sheep were sacrificed, the next liver finally gave directions to go ahead with the battle, and it was won.

Chinese medicine recognized the liver as the storage area of the blood, and they felt it must contain the soul. In the Chinese medical classics, the liver was spoken of as the father and general of the heart, and the king and director of the body.

The custom of eating raw liver is common among the Arabs and tribes of the Sudan, for it is supposed to increase virility. The natives of Darfur in the Sudan eat liver to increase the health of the soul, for they believe the liver is the seat of the soul. Their wives are forbidden to eat liver, because they have no soul.

The Arctic explorer Vilhjalmur Stefansson was interested in the Eskimo custom of not eating the liver, since these people don't waste any part of the their food. He explored the taboo by eating some liver, and suffered no ill effects. Later it was found that some polar bear livers contain about 10 million units of Vitamin A per pound, which could make you very ill.

Maybe the reason why the French had so many terms denoting liver complaints is due to their habit of eating pate de fois gras. This dish is prepared by force feeding geese in small pens, where they cannot exercise. The liver becomes very tender and fatty, and can reach two pounds in weight. When prepared by French chiefs, it is said to be one of the greatest meat dishes of the world. The clerical wit, Reverend Sidney Smith, once defined heaven: "Eating pate de fois gras to the sound of trumpets."

Rats were divided into three groups. The first group received normal rat food, the second had added B vitamins, and the third group had 10% liver powder added. When they were put into cold water and forced to swim, the first group lasted 13.3 minutes, and the second group lasted 13.4 minutes. In the group supplemented with liver, only three of the 12 rats lasted less than two hours when the experiment was terminated. There was no difference in warm water swimming time, but something in the liver made a big difference in cold water.

The liver remains a paradox to medical scientists, just as it was to the ancient thinkers. The Hebrew prophet Jeremiah identified the liver with the soul, when he wrote: "My liver is poured upon the earth, for the destruction of the daughter of my people." The Greek philosopher Democritus regarded the liver as the center of lust and greed. The followers of the ancient religious teacher Mithridates believed that the soul existed in three parts of the body, but the negative part was in the liver.

Maybe this is true, but only when the liver isn't working right!

LIVER REGENERATION

"A healthy liver is our life."
                    Galen +150

"According to the views of the ancient physicians, the liver is the seat of the natural powers, being the grand organ of blood generation and the blood being the food that nourishes the whole body."
                    Paulus Aegina

"So long as a man imagines that he cannot do a thing, so long is he determined not to do it, and so long is it impossible for him to do it."
                    Ethics *Baruch Spinoza*

Ancient people believed that the liver was the seat of soul. It is far larger than the heart, and since it was filled with blood when an animal was butchered, it must be the source of the blood. Furthermore, it was the source of bitter gall, and a person with a 'lot of gall' was someone who couldn't control his temper.

Since the liver was the seat of soul, it reflected the will of God. The liver has all sorts of anatomical variations much like the lines in our hands. The Biblical prophet Ezekiel wrote, "The king of Babylon stood at the parting of the ways, at the head of the two ways, to use divination. He made his arrows bright and consulted with images and looked into the liver."

We say, "How are you?" but there are several tribes who said, "How is your liver?" The key to the heart is the sound, but when something goes wrong with our liver we turn yellow, or our urine turns a muddy yellow. When the red blood cells in our bodies have reached 120 days, they are broken into bilirubin and excreted. If the bile duct is blocked, the pigment gets into the blood and we turn yellow.

If alcohol or drugs damage the liver it will swell up like a small pillow. Overeating will turn it into a mass of fat, and the force feeding of geese makes the fatty livers known as pate de fois gras. In the case of alcoholism, it is generally fairly easy to regenerate the liver if it has not been damaged too badly. A careful diet and vitamin supplements with herbs will speed up the regeneration.

The liver is one of their most easily healed parts of the body. If two-thirds of the liver is removed, the remaining third will easily take over. The cells will multiply until they reach their former volume, and no other organ of the body will do that.

The biggest news in medicine in the early 1980s was the ease of liver transplants. By 1983 doctors performed 417, and it was estimated that 5,000 people per year could get them if everything was perfect. But transplants involve some six months of intensive care, and they are very expensive.

If we could do liver transplants on a mass production basis, the cost is about $100,000. If complications arise, the cost can double. If doctors did all the liver and heart transplants they would like to do, the family insurance bill would more than double. This raises social questions, for one person in 10,000 receives the benefits that the other people are paying for.

The pressure is already on the insurance companies and politicians to pay the bills. Desperate parents appeal for funds to radio and TV stations. Newspapers print heart-rending stories about little children, who will surely die, if they do not receive transplants.

If General Motors sold cars whose engines needed 'transplanting' at 30,000 miles, nobody would buy cars from them. The buyers know that mechanical care and maintenance will make the engines last far longer than that. There is every reason to believe that the regeneration of the liver is dependent on the raw materials it receives. Instead of spending thousands of dollars, a few dollars of raw material might do the same job.

Most of the regenerative experiments with the liver have been done by giving rats a dose of carbon tetrachloride, which causes liver damage and possible death. Half of the rats receive the supplement and they are compared to the others who have to struggle to recover on their own.

Experiments like this have shown that quite a few herbs and amino acids help the liver to regenerate. Among the herbs with regenerative power are the berries of *Schisandra chinensis* and the leaves of *Thjuopsis dolabrata* in Japan. In China the best protective plants are *Bupleurum chinense* and *Elephantopus scaber* var. *oblanceolata*. *Chionanthus virginicus*, *Bauhinia variegata*, *Eclipta prostrata*, *Echinops grilisii* and *E. latiifolius* are known to be strongly liver protectant. *Artemisia capillaris* protects the liver against carbon tetrachloride damage. An alcoholic extract used during flu epidemics gave good protection.

Culpepper mentions that our lady's thistle *Silybum marianum* was able to open obstruction in the liver and spleen and would help jaundice. An extract of *Eupatorium cannabinum* is just as active as *Silybum*, when 30-60 grams are given a day.

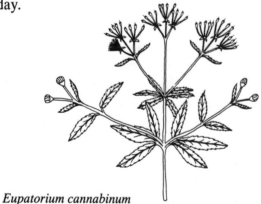

Eupatorium cannabinum

Scientists in Sri Lanka damaged the livers of rats with carbon tetrachloride. They found that *Osbeckia octandra* was very active in restoring liver function. Russian scientists studied the effects of toxic hepatitis on the livers of white rats. They found that *Odontites vulgaris = Bartsia odontites* stimulated the regeneration of the liver and the microsomal oxidation system, which is the cellular detoxification of the liver. There are many others which may aid in regenerating the liver.

A bioflavanoid from *Acacia catechu* known as (+)-cyanidol-3 was first crystallized in 1821, and the chemical structure was determined in 1902. This bioflavanoid comes from the gums known as Nauclea gambir, from *Nauclea junghuhnii*, and *Acacia catechu*. When added to the diet it increases ATP levels, which is the energy active substance of muscles. This bioflavanoid protects the liver against the mushroom poisons alpha-amanitin and phalloidin. It increases the speed of healing in hepatitis, and returns the liver to its normal size in cirrhosis.

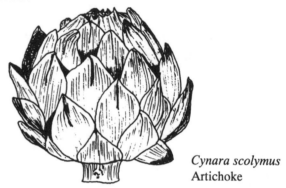

Cynara scolymus
Artichoke

A chemical present in the leaves of the edible artichoke *Cynara scolymus* has a powerful regenerative effect on the liver. It has a strong effect on liver problems, and is used as a medicine in Italy. German scientists surgically removed the lobes of the livers of a group of rats. Then they were given either distilled water or cynara extract. The rats with artichoke extract regenerated 20% faster.

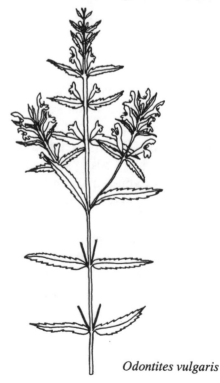

Odontites vulgaris

The livers of rats were partially removed and their regeneration was studied with injections of spice oils. The most active oil in increasing the regeneration was nutmeg, and the next most active was sassafras oil followed by parsley seed oil.

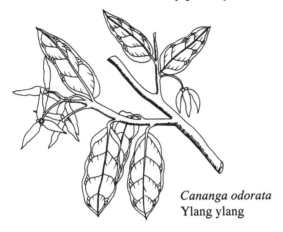

Cananga odorata
Ylang ylang

When the liver was intact and oils were injected; parsley seed oil and tarragon oils caused marked increases in the ratios of wet and dry liver weights to body weight. The most active chemical was 4-allylanisole, which is found in fennel, anise and tarragon oils. Isosafrole from the oils of *Ligusticum acutilobum* and *Cananga odorata* has been shown to stimulate liver regeneration. Other compounds produced a marked increase in liver weight, but some similar chemicals had no stimulation.

Two Italian scientists collaborated to see if the hormones that speed up the growth of plants could speed up liver regeneration. Gibberellic acid is a powerful plant growth stimulant, but it had no effect on liver regeneration. Kinetin had weak liver regenerating properties.

The powerful plant growth hormone known as IAA or indoleacetic acid had a marked effect on the lipids in the liver. It stimulated the cytokinetic and mitokinetic process of the regeneration of the liver. The amounts used were 50 mg./kg. of liver weight.

The National Institute of Health funds and gives direction to medical research in the United States. They have allocated millions of dollars of tax money for liver transplants, but virtually no money for research and trials in liver regeneration. If we put as much money into regeneration as we put into transplantation, it is likely that most of the people who need transplants wouldn't need them.

I listened to a doctor on a talk show who was promoting the medical wonders of transplants. One caller asked the logical question: "Why aren't you trying to rejuvenate the liver?" The doctor remarked that they really hadn't done any work on that.

Then a Texas nurse called to say that she was disgusted with the whole liver transplant program. She worked with transplant patients for years. Most of these people had destroyed their livers with drugs and alcohol, and the transplants were paid for with public funds. The nurse was angry, because many of these people were back into drugs and alcohol again.

When triple bypass operations were successfully commercialized, doctors made no attempts to correct the causes that created the condition. The problem is cholesterol buildup; an operation is a mechanical way of dealing with it. A whole series of discoveries had been made since 1912 of ways to deal with the problem. But these solutions are ignored in place of surgery!

Like the mechanical heart, liver transplants make big news. The surgeon is the master of life and death. In one moment, a child is dying, and in the next moment the child is given a new liver, and a new chance to live. Liver transplants are not without risk, for there is a high rate of death in the first year.

I have little doubt that inexpensive alternatives exist for most victims of liver problems. If we are going to be exploring cost-effective medicine, we must start working with alternatives. This means looking at the herbs and combinations of herbs, which I have listed here and elsewhere. Doctors and politicians have not had the courage to say: "Transplants must be the last resort, not the first resort of the suffering." I look forward to the day when most liver transplants are recognized as another form of medical superstition.

✿ ✿ ✿

CIRRHOSIS OF THE LIVER

"Liver n. A large red organ thoughtfully provided by nature to be bilious with. It was at one time considered the seat of life; hence its name liver, the thing we live with."

The Devil's Dictionary *Ambrose Bierce*

Surgeon: "Now I must tell you his principal dolor lies in the region of the liver, and there's both inflammation and tumefaction feared; nary, I made him a quadrangular plumation, where I used sangquis diaconis, by my faith with posers incarnative which I tempered with oil of hypericon, and other liquors mundificative."

Fair Quarrel *Thomas Middleton c. +1610*

In 1817 Samuel Black of Newry, Ireland, published a paper titled: "Dissection of Two Habitual Drunkards." He did an autopsy on an alcoholic and noted, "The only very striking morbid appearance was in the liver, but the state of that viscous was very remarkable. It certainly was not one-half its natural size, perhaps not much more than a third. Its substance, when pressed between the fingers, felt perfectly hard and rigid, and was throughout full of small hard tubercles, of the size of a garden pea, some of them larger; and they were of a dark brown color."

In 1826 the French doctor Henri Laennac studied 'atrophic nodular livers' produced by drinking. He named this condition 'cirrhosis.' Cirrhosis affects about 8% of those who drink heavily over a long period of time. When dogs are given a well balanced diet and all the alcohol they can be made to drink they don't get cirrhosis of the liver. If the diet is deficient in protein and vitamins, cirrhosis is quickly produced. Toxins such as tars and carbon tetrachloride also produce it. A diet of high fat and alcohol readily produces cirrhosis. It is not what one eats, but what one fails to eat that produces cirrhosis of the liver.

Alcoholic drinks are measured by "proof" instead of percentile and 200 proof is 100% alcohol. In an earlier era there was no easy way of testing the alcohol to see if the trader had dumped water in it to make a bigger profit. The old way of testing whiskey on the frontier was to wet gunpowder with the drink and touch a match to it. If it would burn, it was 100% proof, that is at least 50% alcohol. The Indians would pour a little of the whiskey on the fire, before paying for it. If it had enough alcohol in it to burn it was 'firewater' and worth paying for.

The results of hard drinking make the liver swollen and yellow with fat. It develops strands of fibrous connective tissue much like scar tissue. Generally it takes from 5 to 25 years of heavy drinking to produce cirrhosis of the liver. The liver is normally about three to four pounds and about the size of a small loaf of bread. When cirrhosis affects the liver, it may reach 15 pounds and be the size of a small pillow.

Most people who develop cirrhosis of the liver have a nutritional deficiency of B vitamins. In fact, whiskey makers once considered adding B vitamins to their product to preserve the health of their customers. The FDA blocked this on the grounds that they were adding medicine to the whiskey. The distillers weren't particularly health conscious. They just wanted customers to live longer, so they could continue to drink, and buy their products.

There are a number of plants that have toxins that can produce cirrhosis of the liver. *Amsinckia intermedia* grows throughout Washington, Idaho and California. The seeds have a nut-like taste and are readily eaten by animals. After they become ill, they avoid them. Cattle and pigs develop a 'hard liver' from the toxic plants, and horses get 'walking disease.' As the liver is destroyed, the horses tend to wander aimlessly.

The *Senecio* genus is the worst of the cirrhosis-producing plants. Groundsel. *Senecio vulgaris* and tansy ragwort *S. jacobaea* were once commonly used herbs by women for dysmenorrhea and amenorrhea. The senecios have been widely used in folk medicine in Africa. They cause all sorts of health problems, such as headaches, dizziness, nausea, etc. The pyrolizidine alkaloids in the plants poison the liver.

When sheep eat senecios, they get a sort of facial eczema. Could eczema be due to a nonfunctioning liver? Some of the liver stimulants are known to cure skin problems. Doctors have not considered this idea in treating eczema.

In Saudi Arabia, there was a study done on the high rate of cancer of the Bedouin people. These people used a local member of the senecios *Senecio glaucus* for wounds and snakebites. It caused liver damage, and it was believed to be responsible for the increased amount of cancer.

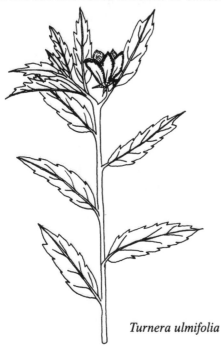

Turnera ulmifolia

There is a high rate of cirrhosis in Jamaica from the use of 'bush tea.' Rats were given a cirrhosis-producing diet and fed Jamaican herbs to see which plants protected the liver. *Picramnia antidesma* and *Turnera ulmifolia* protected the liver and kidneys against injury. The fresh leaves of *Picramnia* species were the most active in treating cirrhosis.

Cirrhosis has the effect of making the legs as smooth as ivory and the soles of the feet tender. The appetite for food vanishes, and if thiamin is lacking the condition is much like beriberi. The heart enlarges and there is edema. In Germany this is known as "Bierharz" or beer drinkers heart. Cirrhosis can lead to congestive heart failure and circulatory collapse.

Brewers yeast protects laboratory animals against cirrhosis, and this was a good treatment before B vitamins were available. The amino acid methionine gives considerable protection to liver injury and cysteine gives moderate protection. One of the best treatment for cirrhosis combines multiple vitamins with two grams of methionine and two grams of choline daily. In a short time the enlarged liver returns to normal, and most of the cell damage is repaired.

When rats were fed a diet of torula yeast, it damaged the liver and the cells began to die. The condition could be prevented by Vitamin E, cystine or a substance from another yeast known as factor 3. The mysterious liver protection factor turned out to be selenium. When rats were fed torula yeast with sodium selenite added to the diet, it resulted in complete protection.

Nearly every year inexperienced mushroom pickers eat the dangerous amanita mushrooms, which destroy the liver unless treated immediately. In about 24 hours after eating them, there is nausea and vomiting. Death is almost certain if the liver is destroyed.

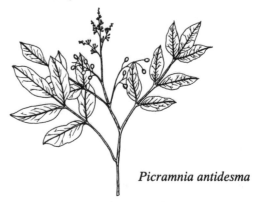

Picramnia antidesma

German researchers tested four herbs used in folk medicine to help the liver. Rats had their livers damaged with carbon tetrachloride. Researchers checked the amount of damage, by measuring the amount of p-hydroxy phenylpyruvic acid that the liver secreted. The only herb with significant results in restoring normal liver function was the blessed thistle *Silybum marianum*.

In 1949 it was found that a tincture of *Silybum marianum* protected the liver against several known liver toxins. The silymarin in the seeds stimulates the manufacture of RNA and speeds up healing of hepatitis. It is one of the few things that will cure amanita poisoning, but full protection is only possible if it is given a half hour after the toxic mushrooms are consumed. The purple flowered plant is active; the white flowered plant is inactive. Silymarin is no longer curative about 12 hours after the mushrooms have been eaten, because the liver damage is too far gone by that time.

In 1991 Oregon newspapers reported that a group of people picked and ate poisonous mushrooms. Four liver transplants were done at once, which was a new record. They did not report that a fifth person had gone to a naturopathic doctor. He took an extract of blessed thistle and didn't need a liver transplant.

In 1989 a study of treating cirrhosis of the liver with silymarin was published. During a four-year period, 170 patients were studied with a blind test. Half received 140 mgs. of silyamarin three times a day. The survival rate increased from 39% to 58%. Those suffering from alcoholic cirrhosis did better than those suffering from other forms of cirrhosis.

There are many reports on the liver and kidney regeneration chemical in the leaves of the artichoke ***Cynara scolymus***. It is sold as a drugstore medicine in Italy. When guinea pigs in France were given a combination of arsenic and artichoke leaves, the herb protected them from liver damage, and most of the arsenic was eliminated in the urine. Geese are force fed to produce fatty livers for a gourmet delicacy. If they are given artichoke leaves, the liver won't enlarge and they remain normal.

In India ***Eclipta prostrata*** has been found to provide significant protection against carbon tetrachloride poisoning. When laboratory animals were pretreated with the herb, most of them lived. Most of the control animals died. This herb is part of a registered herbal treatment of the liver known as Liv 52. This combination of herbs has proved to be so successful, that some western doctors use it in liver conditions.

With real cirrhosis of the liver, survival time is generally short. Mexican doctors tested the theory that colchicine from the autumn crocus ***Colchicum autumnale*** could help patients. The survival time of a group of patients with cirrhosis with a placebo was 3.5 years before half of them died. The group given one-milligram of colchicine daily had a 50% survival rate of 11 years. The extract was a major factor in extending the quality of life as well.

☆☆☆

JAUNDICE

"The liver is the root of many diseases. It is a vital organ on which many, nay, almost all organs depend."

Paracelsus

"Supposing that you can make nothing of your patient's case: tell him confidently, that he has obstruction of the liver. Should he reply, that it is his head or any other part that ails him, say boldly that the pain comes from the liver."

Arnold of Villanova

"The mumps are raging in the army and every other disease known to human beings. I have the jaundice and am as yellow as a Yankee pumpkin and am so bilious. I cannot keep anything down that I eat, and oh how sick I am."

From the 1862 Civil War diary of Cyrus Boyd during the battle of Corinth.

The term "jaundice" comes from the French word for yellow. It is not necessarily a disease, for the yellowness of the skin can be due to hepatitis, malaria, yellow fever or the blocking of the bile passages by gallstones. There is also false jaundice from the eating of carrots, when carotene builds up in the blood and colors the skin.

When the bile passages are obstructed, bile is forced into the blood, making the skin yellow. Bilirubin is the main coloring component of the feces. It is formed in the reticulo-endothelial cells of the spleen and bone marrow. The liver excretes it, and if it is obstructed it goes into the blood. When the liver is diseased the cells don't eliminate the bile pigments. This produces anorexia, itching and pain in the right side, and the skin becomes yellow. The urine becomes more yellow and the feces become clay colored.

At first, we may not know that we are sick, until our skin begins to yellow. We become tired, irritable and itchy. In cirrhosis of the liver from alcoholism, or hepatitis, the initial signs may be nausea, vomiting and weakness. The bitter bile was once associated with forcefulness, but the yellow in jaundice was linked with retiring and cowardly acts. In medieval paintings Judas Iscariot is always clothed in yellow. Under Hitler, Jewish people were forced to wear yellow.

Jaundice is really an incomplete medical term for infectious, obstructive or hemolytic conditions. The presence of gallstones causes a lot of pain, which isn't associated with other conditions. Diarrhea is another sign of jaundice, and as the liver heals, the bowel movements become normal.

Most cases of infectious jaundice are now classified under the name of hepatitis, but investigators are still searching for unknown infections. Hemolytic jaundice is marked by excessive destruction of red blood cells, which result in a large increase in bile pigments, and pigment stones may form in the gall bladder. This condition is marked by severe anemia, which is cured by removing the spleen to stop the destruction of the blood.

The Biblical writers used the word 'yerakon' to refer to jaundice. This means 'greenish,' referring to either coloring, fungus, or the skin. Yerakon is mentioned six times in the Bible, but only in Jeremiah 30:6 does it mean real jaundice. It is usually translated as blasting and mildew. In ancient belief 'yerakon' was a disorder of both men and plants. Yerakon was synonymous with gall, which in Hebrew was associated with hatred. Jaundice was considered to be divine punishment for hatred.

The writers of the *Talmud* recommended such remedies as the urine of an ass, or the flesh of a donkey. Among the improbable remedies are salted fish, salted locusts, Persian dates and purple aloes. Beets were recommended, for the red juice would cancel out the yellow color. The Hebrews claimed that the cures to diseases were lost when the herbals of Solomon and Noah were lost. The *Talmud* contains little practical medicine.

Any damage to the liver is associated with anorexia, and we just don't want to eat. Since the liver acts first on the blood coming from the capillaries surrounding the intestinal tract, anorexia is the body's reaction to potentially toxic materials which haven't been broken down. Anorexia can potentially be cured by being treated with liver herbs. There is some information indicating that anorexia nervosa may be curable with liver tonics.

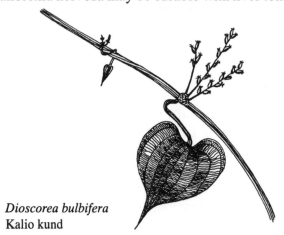

Dioscorea bulbifera
Kalio kund

In 1965 Indian newspapers published a story on the 'secret' of the holy men, who live in caves and fast for long periods of time. Many of the men would drink a tea of 'kalio kund,' which are the roots of ***Dioscorea bulbifera***, because it decreased the desire to eat.

When kalio kund was tested in dogs, it decreased the appetite, but the effect soon wore off. The steroids in the root decreased liver function and produced temporary anorexia. Prolonged fasting to gain attention was just another spiritual con game, although fasting can be remarkably beneficial over a short period of time.

Perhaps the most famous liver tonic of the nineteenth century was boldo. It comes from a small tree in Chile known as ***Peumus boldus***. It was said to have been discovered when a flock of sheep with liver disease was herded into an enclosure, which had just been repaired with boldo branches. The

sheep ate the leaves and cured their problems. The value is considered doubtful today.

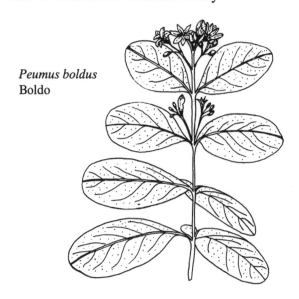

Peumus boldus
Boldo

An herbal clinic in Nigeria found that patients with hepatitis had a remarkable improvement in liver function in two weeks after taking extracts of ***Garcinia kola*** seeds. Extracts of the seeds were tested in mice using phalloidin toxin from the death cap mushroom ***Amanita phalloides***. The kolaviron extract completely protected the mice from the lethal effect of phalloidin.

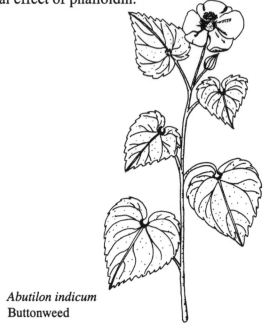

Abutilon indicum
Buttonweed

In India, Ayurvedic doctors use ***Abutilon indicum*** to treat jaundice. It is said to cure the problem in three days. This plant is a common weed in the cornfields of the American Midwest. The farmers call it buttonweed and spray it with chemicals to get rid of it. As an Iowa farm boy, I eradicated my share of this weed from the cornfields.

Ayurvedic doctors in India made a paste of the fresh root bark of ***Moringa pterygosperma = M. oleifera***. A 33-year-old man had jaundice, and an unpleasant taste in his mouth. He took 3.6 grams of root paste three times a day. By the third day the stools changed color and his taste was improving. By the fifth day most discoloration of the skin was gone. In another instance a retired military officer was treated for jaundice for a long time without improving. After six days of taking the herb, he felt much better and within two weeks all of the yellow color disappeared from his skin.

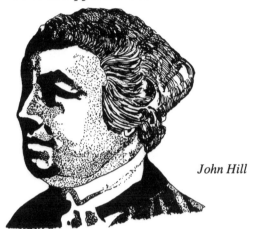

John Hill

The English herbalist writer John Hill tried to support himself by writing medical booklets. In 1768 he published a booklet on curing jaundice with agrimony ***Agrimonia eupatoria***. He divided jaundice into three stages and noted that gallstones weren't always the cause of jaundice.

Weakness, weariness, and a pale yellow skin color marked the first stage of jaundice. Hill claimed that it was easily cured with a half pound of chopped agrimony leaves. Boiling water was poured over them, and a glass of strong tea was drunk every eight hours. Four glasses were said to cure it.

The second stage was marked with white stools

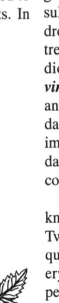

Agrimonia eupatoria
Agrimony

and yellow eyes. A tea of six ounces of chopped roots of agrimony to a quart of boiling water was used. Hill recommended taking a vomit of ipecac and adding this to the agrimony. Medical literature suggests that vomiting spasms stimulate the gallbladder and help to expel gallstones. Ipecac is also strongly antiviral.

The third stage of jaundice was marked with a weak pulse, vomiting, thirst and swollen ankles. Hill added dandelion roots and chicory to the tea. He believed that this would give considerable relief, even if the jaundice couldn't be cured.

In 1967 researchers published a report on a screening of 130 plants for possible antiviral use. Six plants were selected for further studies. The plant which looked most promising, was an alcoholic extract of agrimony. It reduced the death rate of a normally fatal virus of mice by 50%. Perhaps John Hill was right: agrimony really could cure jaundice caused by viral hepatitis.

Andre Michaux was one of the early French explorers in North America. In 1795, he wrote in his diary that ***Celtis occidentalis*** mixed with the leaves or roots of sarsaparilla ***Smilax*** species was an excellent remedy for curing jaundice. It was said to take about eight days.

In 1843 Doctor Isham Gross was salivated, i.e. given lots of mercury to cure a disorder. As a result of mercury poisoning, he was swollen with dropsy and yellow with jaundice. Several doctors treated him, but they were unable to cure his jaundice. In despair, he finally tried ***Chionanthus virginicus***. He made a tincture of the roots in gin and took a tablespoonful three times a day. In five days his jaundice began to disappear, his appetite improved, and his digestion became normal. A few days after his cure, he met someone with the same condition, and cured them with the same remedy.

Chionanthus virginicus was commonly known as the "fringe tree" or "old man's beard." Two ounces of the fresh bark were mixed with a quart of gin. A half-ounce of the tonic is taken every three hours. The treatment worked wonders in people with jaundice from mercury poisoning. In one case a woman suffered with liver and stomach trouble for two years. She took half teaspoonful doses of fringe tree tonic three times a day and was cured in a few days.

In 1933 a Texas doctor wrote about a popular

Mexican cure in southwest Texas. He had a case of jaundice in a ten year old girl, which experience taught him would last at least four weeks. One of the girl's neighbors stated that she had a tea that would clear up the jaundice in a few days. The doctor was surprised when it cleared up in three days.

The Mexicans called the shrub cenizo, but the botanical name is *Leucophyllum frutescens*. It has ash-colored leaves and purple flowers. The leaves are made into a tea and three to six glasses are drunk daily. The taste is good and there are no side effects. The doctor treated 16 cases of catarrhal jaundice and all cleared up in less than ten days. He even treated another doctor who had suffered from jaundice for two weeks and was bedridden. The second day after drinking the tea, he felt markedly improved.

In Northern Nigeria, herbalists were successfully treating jaundice with the roots of *Cochlospermum planchonii*. The herb had no special chemical; the active portion was zinc formate salt. Rats were given carbon tetrachloride to produce liver damage and jaundice. Synthetic zinc salts quickly healed the jaundice. This suggests that anyone with jaundice should take a supplement of zinc salts in addition to herbs.

One of the old time tonics that achieved folklore status was "Carter's Little Liver Pills." These were a mixture of aloes and podophyllum resin *Podophyllum peltatum*. The combination was tested in 1942, but it failed to increase the bile or help the liver.

The viral disease of hepatitis, which causes a major part of jaundice, is studied further in my book *The Fighting Herbs*. Jaundice is an undefined word in older medical literature. I have discussed these herbal discoveries under this name, but we don't always know if it was hepatitis, some other disorder, or if gallstones were involved. The herbs should be studied further, for it is almost certain that there are several important medical discoveries to be made.

✵ ✵ ✵

THE FUNCTION OF BILE

"These passageways end in a single channel, which comes from the hollow of the liver and extends to the gall bladder. This is like a long pear in the concavity of the liver arising in the middle. It is provided with a body adapted for distending and relaxing. The anatomy professors are convinced that the bile is preserved in this bladder, until by the action of the special duct, it is thrust forth into the duodenum. The bile must be carried along with the refuse of the stomach. Its biting quality irritates the intestines for propelling this refuse, and frees them from the phlegm, which clings to the refuse."

The Epitome of Andreas Vesalius *c. +1550*

"If the bile is driven out of the body like an exile out of an insurgent state, it causes diarrhea and dysentery, and all sorts of similar disorders."

Timaeus *Plato*

The Hebrews named the liver 'kabed,' which meant 'heavy,' for it is the largest organ in the body. Attached to the liver was the gall bladder, which was called 'mara' or 'bitter.' There was a good deal of philosophizing over the meaning of the organs. Sweetness was associated with love and good feelings, while bitterness was associated with anger. The gallbladder with its bitter bile was the organ of anger, but the liver, which stored sugar in the form of glycogen, was believed to be the source of love. Roman mythology represented Cupid as the God of Love. When his arrows pierced the liver, the person had a fatal attraction for someone.

The Egyptians viewed the heart as the center of love, as opposed to the Babylonian view of the liver for this function. The Hebrew sacrificial rituals and the statements made by Biblical writers show a good deal of confusion about the meaning of the organs. There is little doubt about the gallbladder; and in Hebrew literature, bile, poison, and bitterness are the same things.

A gall bladder

There is a legend in the Talmud that the angel of death stands at the sickbed with a drop of bile on the edge of his sword. If the dying individual opens his mouth in fear, the drop of bile falls into his mouth and he dies. His face turns greenish-yellow like bile, and after death the body takes on the odor of bile.

The Rabbis interpreted the passage in Deuteronomy 7:15: "And the Lord will take away from thee all sickness [choli]" as God's prevention of the 83 diseases due to bile. The word 'choli' is the same in Greek. Liver disorders in modern medical language are derived from this word, so terms like cholecystic, and cholangitis, refer to bile disorders.

The old English word for bile was 'gall' which meant 'yellow.' Associating bitterness with anger and yellow, was part of the popular Greek theory of the four humors. If you had too much black bile, you were melancholy. An excess of yellow bile produced a choleric disposition, meaning that you were angry or overexcited.

Bile dissolves fat and country people used it to wash grease spots out of clothing. Painters used it to mix colors. During the nineteenth century dried ox bile was used as a laxative. It stimulates the motor activity of the large intestine. During hibernation, bears produce ursodeoxycholic acid in the bile. This dissolves gallstones and is of medical interest.

In the animal world, deer have gallbladders, but horses don't. Giraffes and antelopes may or may not have them. The hawk has a gall bladder, but the pigeon doesn't. This was the ancient explanation for the gentleness of the pigeon, and the fierceness (gall) of the hawk.

We never have "tired" blood, because every 120 days our red blood cells are completely regenerated. The iron is recycled, but the broken down blood cells become the bile pigments. The pigments are excreted into the intestinal tract, and they give the feces its characteristic brown color. When the liver fails to excrete bile, the feces become clay colored.

The bile acids prevent bacterial growth in the small intestine, since bacteria here prevent the body from absorbing fats, protein, and B12. The bile pigments have no effect on the normal bacteria flora, which inhabits the large intestine. Researchers have shown that bile kills or inactivates harmful stomach bacteria, but it does not affect the normal bacteria. Olive oil stimulates bile, and it can cure dysentery. A lack of bile is associated with stomach gas.

The most important function of bile is to render cholesterol soluble. This wax-like steroid is almost completely insoluble in water, but bile allows it to mix in and be excreted. The broken down red blood cells from three main bile acids, which are cholic, chenodeoxycholic and deoxycholic acids. If gallstones block the bile duct, or if the liver fails to excrete bile, these acids accumulate in the blood and produce a yellow skin.

The effects of bile can be understood by an experiment in feeding bile to patients. After bile was taken by mouth it produced hunger and often overcame anorexia. This suggests that bile stimulants could be a useful medicine for disorders like anorexia nervosa. The bile produced an increase in tone of the digestive tract, and intestinal contractions began to mix the food. Bile could help cases of poor digestion.

The Lahu tribesmen of northern Thailand used bear gall in sprains and arthritis. It is dissolved in a little water and rubbed on the area. Sive Namasondhi was an astrologer and editor of *Thai Prediction* magazine. He had a bad knee, which bothered him for months. He went to a doctor who said that he needed an operation. He wanted to wait until after hunting season, so he limped through the backcountry. He stopped at a Lahu village and a medicine man rubbed it with bear gall. In a week

he could walk without pain. After a few more treatments, the painful knee never bothered him again.

The Lahu use crow gall when they want to grow a mustache. It is rubbed directly on the skin to simulate hair growth. In emergencies when they want to stay awake, a solution of bitter bison gall is drunk. It is said to keep men awake for days.

Agents that increase the flow of bile are known as cholagogues. When 14 popular drugs were studied for their ability to stimulate bile and the emptying of the gall bladder, the only thing that worked was olive oil. The active portion is oleic acid. When olive oil was mixed with bile salts and taken by mouth, it helped 72% of the people taking it overcome gastric problems caused by lack of bile.

A Japanese study of the traditional bile stimulants found that bearberry *Arctostaphylos uva-ursi* was a strong bile stimulant. *Coptis teeta, Scutellaria baicalensis* and *Phellodendron amurense* produced moderate increases in bile secretion. In a curious way, the bile stimulants are true blood purifiers, for they increased the breakdown of 'old blood,' and the body must generate new red blood cells or it will become anemic.

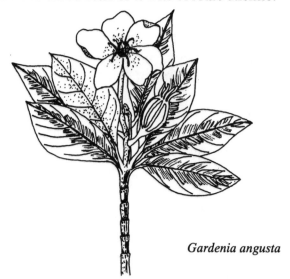

Gardenia angusta

These liver herbs may stimulate the cells which gather the bile and excrete it into the gall bladder. Chinese herbalists used *Gardenia angusta*, which gives big increases in bile secretion for an hour after it is taken. It is usually mixed with other bile stimulants such as *Salvia haematoides* and *Artemisia capillaris*.

In the southern US, Culver's root *Veronicastrum virginicum* was mixed with quinine to treat malaria. When it is used regularly the stools turn dark brown or black, indicating that the production of bile pigments is increased.

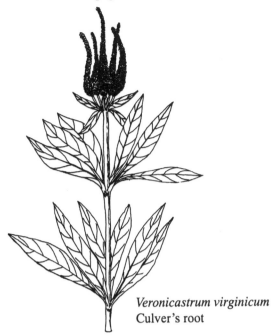

Veronicastrum virginicum
Culver's root

Another southern herb used to treat liver troubles is the fringe tree *Chionanthus virginicus*. It was used for both jaundice and diabetes. One southern doctor claimed that a tea with added Epsom salts helped every case of diabetes in which it was given.

Berberine-containing herbs have along history of being used to heal the soreness of gall bladder walls in inflammatory conditions. Goldenseal, goldthread, and Oregon grape root have all been used. The Asian mint *Orthosiphon stamineus* is also known to clear up jaundice and inflammation of the bile tract. The herb increases the sugar storage of the liver, and it apparently acts on the bile-producing cells of the liver.

Teucrium marum is a strong smelling and bitter tasting mint, known for attracting cats. In former Yugoslavia, Karl Radonicic used this plant in thousands of cases of liver and gall bladder problems. He had such good results that the herb was added to the official pharmacopoeia.

The berries of the mountain ash *Sorbus aucuparia* are used as a spring tonic in Lapland. A medical test was made to see what properties the berries had, and it was found that they increased the level of prothrombin. This increased the ability of the blood of clot.

An extract of mountain ash berries produced good results in gall bladder trouble. When a gram of the extract was used per day (=2grams of the berries), it took seven to ten days to get noticeable relief. Complete relief of symptoms was obtained in 36% of the group and partial relief in 36%.

The kitchen spice turmeric *Curcuma longa* has a powerful effect on the gall bladder. If sodium curcumin solution is injected, the gall bladder rapidly empties. Curcumin is easily absorbed from the digestive tract and the pigment is eliminated through the bile ducts within fifteen minutes. Fat intolerance is a sign of gall bladder trouble and taking turmeric by mouth can cure this. People generally feel better in about three days, and there is relief in a week. Turmeric tea or a spoonful of turmeric before meals is used.

A 37 year-old teacher suffered from a full sensation after meals, and had a great deal of discomfort. There was slight jaundice with severe unilateral headache. After taking turmeric for three days she felt much better. The jaundice began to disappear in six days, and the tenderness of the abdomen left in two weeks.

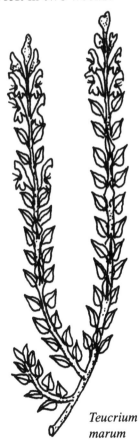

Teucrium marum

☆ ☆ ☆

GALLSTONES

"Horrible and stupendous calculi coagulate in the gallbladder, their shape, color, number and wonderful effects producing vomiting, nausea, heaviness, low spirits, tearing of the stomach and hypochondrium, atrophy, tabes, obstruction of the viscera, inflammation, incurable jaundice, sleeplessness, lassitude, sadness, melancholic affections, inclination to anger, difficulty and heat of urine, lepra of skin, fever, sudden death by a hidden and generally unknown seminary and foment of disease and symptoms."

Lithogenesia *Johannes Schenck*

The gall bladder is a pear-shaped organ about the size of a hen's egg. Half of its surface is fastened to the liver directly above it. Most animals living on the direct products of the soil have gall bladders, but animals such as elephants, living on leaves do not have them. There are at least a dozen known cases of human who have no gall bladders and a similar number of cases with two of them.

The first mention of gallstones is by the Greek doctor Alexander Tralianus, who described them as "dried up humors, concreted like stones." In +1400 Benivenius of Florence wrote, "A certain noble lady had been suffering from pain in the liver region and although she had consulted many doctors, she had not been able to get rid of the malady.... When she departed this life, we opened the body, and there were found small stones differing in shape and color, which had collected in the lower part of the membrane of the liver. Some were round, others angular or quadratic, as position and accident had affected them."

Gallstones form in about 10% of all adults over 40 years of age, although they are not serious enough to cause trouble in many cases. The French chemist Ferdinand Chevruel discovered that they are made of cholesterol. This acts like a lump of wax, and plugs up the bile ducts. They may be 'mulberry stones,' which are a mixture of cholesterol and minerals. In rare instances the stones may be made of minerals or the pigment bilirubin.

The first attempt to dissolve gallstones was in 1782 when Doctor Durande recommend a combination of three parts ether and two parts turpentine. Lawson Tait in England performed the first gall bladder operation in 1879.

Gallstones are part of a body of foreign materials that form in the alimentary canal or the bile ducts. Pearls are the 'gallstones' of oysters. Bezoars and enteroliths form in the alimentary canal of birds, reptiles and fishes. They are common in goats, calves and horses. We can have both gallstones and true stones – kidney stones.

Gallstones are directly related to the diet. The natives of South Africa have an incidence of 2%, but the white settlers have an incidence of 14%. The Chinese and Japanese diet produce few gallstones. People adopting a Western type of diet have higher incidences of gallstones.

Bile is made up of lecithin, bile salts and water insoluble cholesterol. In medieval times solutions of bile from animals were used to clean grease and stains from wool and linen, and to mix the colors in paint. Bile and lecithin enables water and oil to mix.

Bile salts by themselves are not sufficient to hold all the cholesterol in solution. Sodium cholate was the most effective of the three main bile salts in dissolving cholesterol. An increase in bile helps to dissolve cholesterol. Lecithin also acts to dissolve fats and water.

I once visited an old Polish aeronautical engineer, who dug out a medical folder and began to talk. A hospital x-ray showed that his problem was gallstones, and the doctors advised an immediate operation. He delayed the operation and called his sister who was a doctor in Hungary. She sent him a gallstone remedy used in Eastern Europe. He took the mixture of oils and herbs, and the pain left immediately.

He went to the Group Health Clinic of Seattle for a checkup. The doctor took x-rays and wrote on his medical form: "The patient thinks he was cured by taking an herbal medication." Weeks later he received a call from one of the doctors who said: "My wife has to have a gall bladder operation, and I'd like to borrow some of your medicine." He replied, "Why don't you send for the medicine and use it on a regular basis."

"We'd lose our medical licenses if we did," the doctor replied.

He came into the clinic and put a bottle on the table. "You know that it's illegal for you to take this medicine, but I'll turn my back, and you can swipe it." The doctor's wife took the medicine and was cured. The writing was in Polish and Latin, but I believe that it was similar to an old German mixture of essential oils known as 'cholify,' developed more than a century ago.

Gallstones are much like lumps of lard in the dishwater. If we didn't have a detergent to emulsify it, fat will remain on the dishes. Lecithin keeps cholesterol in solution, and it is believed to prevent gallstones. If lecithin is taken by mouth, a third of it will pass into the bile.

Turmeric contains a terpene known as 'curcumen.' It dissolves cholesterol, and gallstones brought into contact with it disintegrate. Experiments indicate that from 100-200 mgs. taken three times a day are sufficient to be active.

Olive and cottonseed oils, lecithin, essential oils, and the mixture known as cholify operate on a slow basis, by dissolving the waxy cholesterol. Tests show that olive oil opens Oddi's sphincter through which the bile and stones must exist. Olive oil is the basis of a number of folk remedies for the removal of gallstones. One remedy calls for drinking two cups of olive oil mixed with lemon juice, and then lying on the right side (the gall bladder is on the right side). Since a large portion of olive oil is immediately secreted by the gall bladder, the oil helps to remove the cholesterol stones.

The first use of olive oil to dissolve gallstones dates to around 1890. In a recent case written up in medical literature, a man was diagnosed with multiple gallstones. He declined the operation and consulted an herbalist. He was told to fast 12 hours, and then take a pint of olive oil and ten lemons. Every 15 minutes he was to take four tablespoonfuls of olive oil and a tablespoonful of lemon juice until it was gone. The next morning the patient had diarrhea and abdominal pain. He sieved the stools and recovered four large gallstones and twenty pea sized stones.

The gallbladder is made up of muscular folds that are capable to making rhythmic contractions, given the proper stimulus. These contractions are much-like kneading bread, and serve to mix cholesterol with bile. The herb known as jaborandi *Pilocarpus jaborandi* contains pilocarpine. It produces powerful gallbladder contractions. It was once used to treat jaundice, due to gallstones.

One doctor treated 30 cases of jaundice with injections of 10 mgs. of pilocarpine. The injections were made once or twice a day for up to three weeks. All of the cases of jaundice disappeared. By stimulating the muscular contractions of the gallbladder, the contractions either dissolved the stones or eliminated them.

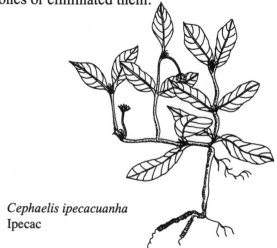

Cephaelis ipecacuanha
Ipecac

Ipecac, which comes from the Brazilian plant *Cephaelis ipecacuanha*, probably works in the same way. A syrup is sold in drug stores principally for use in treating poisoning of children. It probably works by stimulating the muscular contractions of the gallbladder. The ipecac is given in levels just below the amount needed to cause vomiting. In the tropics ipecac is used in dysentery, liver abscess, and hepatitis.

A 50 year-old woman had gall bladder pain with jaundice. Ipecac was taken several times a day, and there was some vomiting initially. The pain was relieved, the jaundice became less, and in three weeks the constipation disappeared. Soon her eyes were clear and the gallbladder could no longer be felt.

A 24-year old man suffered from white stools and black urine. There was intense pain and profuse sweating. He was given pulverized ipecac at levels below that which caused vomiting. In a week he was better, but it took five weeks until he was cured. The emetine of ipecac fights infections of the bile ducts. These may become infected with *Escherichia coli* and in this case 30 mgs. of emetine will remove an infection that penicillin won't.

Over a century ago a Hudson's Bay trader was traveling through the north of Canada bartering for furs. His suffering came to the attention of an Indian medicine man. When the medicine man found the area of pain, he went out into a swamp and returned with gold thread *Coptis trifolia*. The man took the herb and it removed the gallstones and he had no further suffering.

Coptis trifolia
Gold thread

An English doctor reported on a case of a 70 year-old woman who suffered from gallstones for years. He was told that an operation was the only thing that would relieve her suffering, but she didn't want an operation. Having heard that a friend was relieved by parsley tea, she made a tea of a double handful of freshly chopped parsley in a pint of water. After boiling and drinking the tea, her gallstones left. This may be due to the apiol in parsley, which promotes uterine

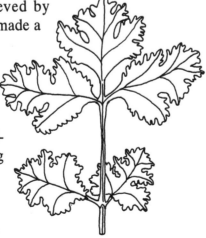

Petroselinum crispum
Italian parsley

contractions. It may also stimulate the muscle folds of the gallbladder.

This property of parsley is mentioned in the old herbals. In 1764 *James's Dispensatory* says: "Parsley is attenuating, opening, detergent and diuretic and is principally used in obstruction of the liver, kidneys and the gall bladder." Culpepper mentioned this in his books: "Parsley openeth obstructions of the liver and spleen... An excellent medicine to help the jaundice, the dropsy and stones in the kidney in this manner."

The correspondence on parsley in the *British Medical Journal* uncovered another interesting remedy. A patient suffered from jaundice and colic from a gallstone, and refused an operation. When the doctor met him three months later, he found the old man was quite well. He had found an herb woman in the village, who prepared a tea of the Scotch broom *Cytisus scoparius* that relieved him of his gallstones.

Cytisus scoparius
Scotch broom

In 1757 the Scotch broom was the subject of several reports at the Academy of Sciences in Stockholm, Sweden. A wine made of it had a remarkable healing effect on a catarrhal epidemic in the Swedish army. The spartenine in the herb has heart tonic effects, but is is different from digitalis. It is a stimulant of the smooth muscle fibers, so it acts on digestion.

Experiments in Rumania showed that it had strong stimulant effects on the contraction of the gall bladder. It was given in amounts of 80 mgs. up to three times a day to 13 people with malfunctioning gall bladders. It did not work in all cases, but it was a major help.

In 1936 a German report was published on the use of the juice of the black radish *Raphanus sativus* for gallstones. The black radish is a cultivar of the common radish. Patients began taking 2-3 ounces of fresh juice a day and increased this to 5 ounces. A Swiss pharmaceutical company produced a concentrate of radish juice mixed with bile salts. A tablet was taken after meals generally three times a day. The juice worked just as well, but there was a taste problem and people wouldn't drink it.

After the first week, the patients were generally free of pain, and the constipation was gone. X-rays showed the stones slowly being dissolved and eliminated. After five weeks, all symptoms of 26 of 37 patients were completely eliminated. Most of the others received relief, without side effects.

In 1940, there was a German study on using red pepper to stimulate the gall bladder. This acted as a bile stimulus by increasing muscular contractions of the gall bladder. Using red pepper along with other remedies may be an excellent way of removing gallstones.

In the Amazon, the native healers use an herb known as "chanca piedra." This is generally **Phyllanthus niruri** or **P. stipulatus**. The leaves are said to be a highly effective cure for gallstones, kidney stones and urinary inflammation. The herb is exported to Germany, where a number of doctors use it.

During the winter of 1873-4 one person in Doctor Goldsmith's family suffered from gallstones. Eventually the patient was taken to Carlsbad, Czechoslovakia, which is 70 miles west of Prague. The Sprudel is the largest and hottest spring. The patient drinks a glass of water from the spring every 15 minutes. After three glasses of water and a half-hour wait, breakfast is eaten. The waters are a strong bile stimulant.

An artificial treatment was done by dissolving 1.1 grams of the salts in three glasses of hot water. The water is drunk warm and slowly at intervals of fifteen minutes. It is said to be just as successful as going to Carlsbad. A six-week course is said to cure nearly all patients of gallstones.

In 1903 Dr. Robert Glaser reported that his "chologen" mixture of mercury, podophyllin, **Melissa**, camphor and caraway was highly successful. He did hundreds of experiments and prepared three different mixtures. He claimed that gallstone colic was quickly relieved.

A 48-year-old woman had many gallstone colic attacks with headaches and constipation. Morphine had to be used to control the pain, and the patient refused an operation. She took six tablets of chologen a day. Her yellow skin began to clear up, and there were no more gallbladder attacks.

A 72-year-old man had distress after eating. He was confined to bed for four months with chills, fever, constipation and backache. He was in such bad condition, that the doctors didn't want to operate. He was put on chologen, and in five months was able to lead a normal life.

In order to x-ray the gall bladder, doctors used to use a fat meal with barium. The barium produced a shadow under x-rays. French doctors found that a mixture of egg yokes and glycerin reduced the size of the gall bladder. The lecithin in the egg yolk was the active substance that diminished the size of the gall bladder. This may offer help in treating gallstones.

A simple gallstone treating remedy was available in Denmark more than 60 years ago. It was 300 mgs. of peppermint oil made into tablets. Two pills were taken three times daily. It was said to be a good inexpensive way of treating gallstones.

In 1960 a gallstone dissolving remedy known as Rowachol was introduced in Europe. It is a mixture of 32% menthol, 17% pinene, 6% menthone and 5% of camphene and borneol each. The main ingredient is peppermint oil, the source of the menthol. It dissolves small gallstones in a few weeks, but it may take up to a year to dissolve large ones. It leaves a strong peppermint taste in the mouth.

The Hippocratic oath for doctors was developed 2,500 years ago. The early Christian doctors added the statement: "I will not operate for stones." These doctors believed that the body was the temple of God, and entering it was to defile it. The death rates from the crude operations were high, so they probably feared sending their unbelieving patients to hell, should complications develop. We operate because we don't know what else to do. Experiments may prove that most operations could be avoided by using simple herbs!

✫✫✫

DIURETIC HERBS

"On limbs enormous, but withal unsound, soft-swollen and wan, here lay pale hydropsy,
Unwieldy man; with belly monstrous round, for ever fed with watery supply,
For still he drank, and yet was ever dry."

Castle of Indolence *James Thomson*

"He [the doctor] trusteth not the single witness of the water, if better testimony may be had. For reasons drawn from the urine alone are as brittle as the urinal. Sometimes the water runneth in such posthaste through the sick man's body, it can give no account of anything memorable in the passage, though the most judicious eye examine it."

The Holy State *Thomas Fuller c. +1650*

When Thomas Addis wrote, "All we know for certain about the kidney is that it makes urine," he was expressing the real knowledge of the ancient doctors. Four hundred years before the time of Christ, Hippocrates made a few statements about the urine and kidneys. "Bubbles appearing on the surface of the urine, indicate disease of the kidneys and prolonged illness." "Those whose urine during a fever is like that of the beast of burden, either suffer from headache or will do so." "Colorless urine is bad." "Diseases of the kidneys and of the bladder are difficult to cure in old age."

The kidneys are bean-shaped organs located above, and on either side of the urinary bladder. They consist of a million tiny tubes, which filter out the waste materials in the blood. If the kidneys aren't working, the eyes get puffy, and the ankles may swell. The blood pressure rises and albumin is present in the urine. The body swells with extra fluid, and the person becomes tired. The brain senses the change in fluid, and sends out ADH (antidiuretic hormone), which regulates the amount of water. The kidneys also produce a hormone called erythropoitin, which regulates the formation of red blood cells.

There were three general conditions of the kidneys, which had been described by the end of the eighteenth century. The first was known as 'acute nephritis,' which occurred after an epidemic of scarlatina in Europe around 1750. Dropsy and bloody urine mark it. Acute nephritis is a streptococcus infection of the kidneys. It is now uncommon because of sanitation, and it is treatable with penicillin and other antibiotics.

In 1765, Domenico Cotugno reported that he found a solider who had coagulatable urine after it was heated. He noted that the albumin of people suffering from fluid retention was also coagulatable. This gave him the idea that blood fluids were being discharged into the urine.

Richard Bright found a way to distinguish phosphates in the urine from albumin (proteins) by adding acid to it. He heated the urine in a spoon with a candle flame, and noted if it became cloudy. Bright wrote: "When the albumin is proved to exist, however slight a tendency to this condition may be, I always look upon it with anxiety, and the confirmed derangement I always view with dread." The third condition was called 'nephrotic syndrome.'

It has recently been discovered that many cases of kidney disease are an autoimmune disorder. The immune system fails to recognize kidney cells as part of the body. It attacks the kidney cells and destroys them. This results in an antigen-antibody complex, which forms clumps of cells in the kidneys. Another curious immune system disorder, connected with kidney failure, is systemic lupus erythematosus. Butterfly-like red patches on the face mark it.

'Chronic nephritis' is the condition in which the kidneys are failing. Richard Bright described the symptoms of added headaches and urination during the night. As the kidney condition deteriorates, the healthy color of the skin fades, and the patient becomes weary and depressed. A hard pulse and an enlargement of the left side of the heart mark the final stages of the disease. The kidneys shrink in size. The mind becomes confused and sentences are shorter. There is difficulty in doing mental arithmetic.

Bright received the highest honor a doctor can have by having a disease named after him. He didn't have much advice for the victims of kidney failure except to say: "Don't get chilled, don't over exercise, don't drink wines, and eat light meals." He does not seem to have used diuretics, but he mentions a person who took gin to promote the flow of urine. Gin is made from juniper berries, which is a strong diuretic.

Paulus Aegina described 'hardness of the kidneys' in the middle of the seventh century. He used a compound mixture of spikenard, cassia, cumin, licorice and other ingredients. He did use the effective diuretic squill, and as a last resort he had his patients take a dry spoonful of ox dung every day! Cattle manure is a rich source of Vitamin B12, and the lack of this vitamin is implicated in many cases of water retention.

Kidney bean pods are a strong diuretic, and they also help diabetes. The active ingredient has not been isolated, although it is known that the kidney stimulant ingredient of the fava bean *Vicia faba* is calcium glycerate.

Edema or water retention often occurs as a result of bad nutrition during wars. In mild cases the legs become puffy, and in severe cases the stomach and body swells. In 1528 when the French army was laying siege to Naples, Italy, poor nutrition destroyed the army. The soldiers had pallid skin color, swollen legs and bloated bellies. The first sign was puffiness around the eyes, which spread to the ankles.

During WWI, there were many cases of nephritis in hunger stricken Germany. Most of these people had edema and blood in the urine. During the spring of 1916 doctors found that asparagus was able to clear up the nephritis.

The old Russian expression "swollen from hunger" is true, and in both war and famine this syndrome is common. The lack of protein and vitamins in the diet causes fluid retention. 'Prison dropsy' was common in nineteenth century prisons, but with better food it disappeared. During WWI, German medical literature had many articles on edema. It was common in the famines of India and China, and British doctors tried to isolate the mysterious germ that caused it. Many of the victims had symptoms of glaucoma; with dim vision, rainbow-like halos, and steamy sight. Glaucoma is edema of the eyes.

The missing ingredient of the diet that causes fluid retention seems to be choline. When nine rats were fed a diet without protein, four of them developed edema. If the rats were given extra choline, they didn't develop edema. In 1949 doctors found that lecithin (which contains choline) produced striking relief from edema in patients when given orally.

Oxydendrum arboreum
Sourwood

One of the best diuretics that the old doctors discovered in the United States was sourwood *Oxydendrum arboreum*. The leaves and bark were an effective diuretic, when everything else failed.

Ajuga chamaepitys increases the excretion of urea. A group of test people were kept on a constant diet and given 250 mgs. tablets of the powdered herb. It was an effective urea excretion stimulant. Urea is a waste product of the body, which builds up in kidney disease.

The most common diuretic of the old European doctors was the bark of elderberry *Sambucus nigra*. A handful of the inner bark or root bark was put into a liter of water and boiled. A 13 year-old girl had scarlet fever, and her body was swollen with excess water months later. She drank the tea for a month and was fully recovered. In four cases of edema of two to three months standing that had resisted all other remedies, elder bark tea was a success.

A Polish study of popular diuretics showed that the best were the strawberry *Fragaria vesca* and the bark of the birch *Betula pendula*. In America the arbutin in the leaves of ***Arctostaphylos uva-ursi*** and ***Chimaphila umbellata*** are active diuretics. French doctors tried ***Chimaphila*** in 13 cases of kidney insufficiency, and found that it more than tripled urinary volume.

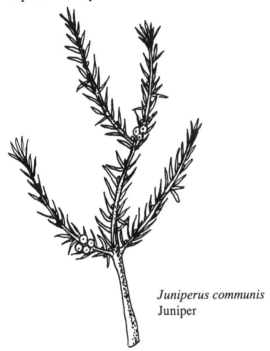

Juniperus communis
Juniper

German pharmacists tested a variety of popular diuretic herbs on rats. The two strongest diuretic herbs were juniper berries ***Juniperus communis*** and the rest harrow ***Ononis campestris***. The juniper had the advantage of increasing the excretion of waste nitrogenous products. Both herbs increased the salt elimination by more than 100%. They tried combining the herbs in hopes of producing an even more effective mixture, but the combination was less efficient.

In 1868 many of the residents of the alms (poor) house of New Hanover County of North Carolina were troubled with obstinate dropsy. The superintendent offered to cure them with a secret remedy. It produced a striking improvement in diuresis, and often by the second day the swelling in the limbs went away. The tea was drunk either warm or cold. The superintendent lost his job due to politics, but before he left he showed Adam Wright the secret herb. It was ***Vaccinium crassifolium***, which grew in upland savannas in moist places with a carpet of black berries.

A shipsmith was troubled with asthma and great swelling of the ankles and abdomen. A tea resulted in profuse diuresis and clear urine. His breathing became much easier, and he remained in good health.

A woman suffered from jaundice with scanty urine. She was given the herb, and her urine became clear and plentiful. The yellow hue of her skin quickly disappeared.

One doctor used the herb on a patient with severe general swelling and the woman passed eight pints of urine a day. It was the first thing that worked on her. Other doctors wrote to say that it was a miracle cure, and they would continue to use it.

In 1946 a Pennsylvania newspaper told the story of a woman who was near death when her kidneys failed to work. As a last resort, the doctor made a tea of three tablespoons of watermelon seeds ***Citrullus lanatus*** in a quart of water. This stimulated the kidneys and she recovered.

In 1686 the Oxford Philosophical Society reported that Sir William Room was in deplorable condition from dropsy. He was advised to steep four cloves of garlic in every quart of ale. He drank this at meals, and in a month was restored to perfect health.

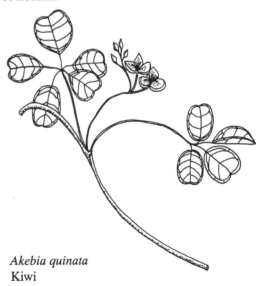

Akebia quinata
Kiwi

When Japanese researchers studied the diuretic action of some popular herbs, they found that the best diuretic was ***Akebia quinata***. ***Sambucus racemosa*** and *S. sieboldiana* had mild increases in urine as a tea, but strong increases as a tincture.

In Sri Lanka ***Aerva lanata*** is grown as a diuretic and preventive of urinary infections. It is a very active diuretic and a small amount causes marked increases in urine.

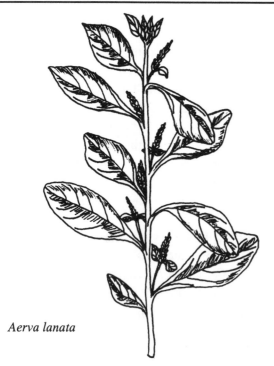

Aerva lanata

In Jamaica the root of ***Moringa pterygosperma = M. oleifera*** is used as a diuretic. This is known as the horseradish tree. It grows up to 20 feet tall. A tincture of the root has a cherry color and an agreeable taste.

Doctors were unable to relieve a case of cardiac edema with drugs. Digitalis, diuretics and mercurial compounds weren't working and the woman's lungs were filling with fluid. Someone in the hospital suggested that pineapple juice was good for reducing the swelling of sore throats. As a last resort it was given to her. The glass of fresh pineapple juice increased the urinary output by four times in the next day. The water was eliminated from the body, and the lungs returned to normal.

This was known in Malaysia, and Chinese patients with dropsy always asked for pineapple. The British doctors used their traditional diuretics but added pineapple juice. The enzyme of pineapple juice is bromelain, and this is the active ingredient.

Another type of edema is hydrocephalus, when the brain swells with water. The disorder can re-

sult in confused thinking and can cause mental disorders and movement problems like Parkinson's disease. The disorder was found in infant rats after their mothers received a diet of casein, which is an unbalanced protein. Folic acid reduced the incidence of the disorder, and a combination of folic acid and Vitamin B12 always prevented it, in situations of bad diet.

The signs of hydrocephalus in children are irritability, hostility, insomnia, cold extremities, and crying. One child was treated with six injections of nicotinamide for six days. By the second injection sleep and appetite returned. Then he was put on 50 mgs. of nicotinamide a day by mouth.

Hydrocephalus may be caused by food allergies, particularly wheat. Sometimes this happens to children, and they seem mentally retarded. The brain swells with fluid, which inhibits thinking. Other side effects of the allergies can be migraines, vertigo, which results in poor balance and even jerky movements like epilepsy. Removing the food allergy results in great improvement.

Poisoning of the liver can result in hydrocephalus. Eating ***Gyrometra*** mushrooms causes cerebral edema. When the livers of rats were poisoned with galactosamine, the rats developed hydrocephalus. The disorder is benefited with choline and methionine, which aids in liver function. The liver herbs would probably produce beneficial results.

A deficiency diet and salt produced severe edema in seven of 15 rats. When another group of deficient rats was given a supplement of 50 mg./kg. of bioflavonoids, five out of 15 developed mild edema. Bioflavanoids don't act as a diuretic. They strengthen the membranes of the cells, so they don't absorb water.

I have dealt with edema as a kidney disorder, but the hydrocephalus which is brain edema, and the edema of the eyes known as glaucoma, might be helped in a similar way. Since most cases of edema seem to be due to dietary factors, the first step in fighting it is through diet, vitamins and food factors. It is clear that many discoveries of effective herbs offer help to needy people.

✤ ✤ ✤

KIDNEY REGENERATION

"But we could not live if these substances were allowed to accumulate. The kidneys filter the excess water in the following manner. When we allow Sumi ink to remain overnight in an unglazed earthen pot, a clear water filtrate seeps through the vessel, while the black material remains within it. Similarly, the kidneys filter and separate blood to form the urine, which in turn is expelled from the bladder."

Oranda Iji Mondo
(Discussion of Dutch Medicine) K. Sugita, +1795

"I have never yet examined the body of a patient dying with dropsy attended by coagulatable urine, in whom some obvious derangement was not discovered in the kidneys. In all the cases, in which I have observed the albuminous urine, it has appeared to me that the kidney has itself acted a more important part, and has been more deranged both functionally and organically, than has generally been imagined."

Richard Bright 1827

The kidneys and the liver are the cleaners of the blood. When drugs are added to the body, the liver converts them to a form that is recognized and excreted by the kidneys. If the kidneys don't work, unexcreted urea and toxins in the blood poison the entire body.

The kidneys are composed of a vast number of tiny filtration tubes known as glomeruli. A normal kidney contains from 800,000 to 1,000,000. There is a decrease in glomeruli in old age and the number can go down to 600,000.

Kidney activity is related to the health of the body. A protein deficient diet leads to small kidneys. If the thyroid is removed or is inactive, the kidneys shrink. When thyroid extract (thyroxine) is taken, the kidney function improves.

Richard Bright's disease was characterized by albumin in the urine, which was a mark of general kidney failure. By 1914 kidney disorders were classified into three categories:
- Glomerulonephritis– inflammatory glomerular destruction.
- Nephrosclerosis– thickening of the small renal arteries.
- Nephrosis– degenerative process affecting the tubules.

Over a period of 30 years, several teams of doctors developed the artificial kidney. By 1970, most hospitals had them and this aroused an intense debate over people with kidney failure. It was difficult to say 'who should live,' and 'who should die.' On September 30, 1972 the U.S. Congress passed a law that extended medical coverage to all victims of 'end stage renal disease.'

In the next seven years, the kidney program increased in cost by more than a one billion dollars. This wasn't the only cost, because many of those needing dialysis were collecting federal disability payments. Government planners worried about the program, because 0.2% of the Medicare patients were using 5% of the funds, and the total was rising rapidly.

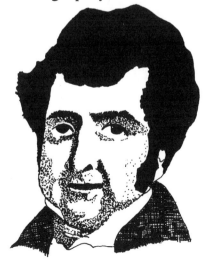

Richard Bright

The original intent of Congress was to help people whose lives could be made to function normally. The study groups that led to the recommendation were composed of young healthy people, with a strong will to live. Medical doctors began to place terminally ill patients and senile persons on dialysis to extend their lives. There were court cases in which families of patients requested that dialysis be terminated and the patient be allowed to die in peace.

Dialysis patients are often uncomfortable with cramps, nausea and weakness. They often have anemia, the bones degenerate and the men are usually impotent. The use of dialysis has resulted in a lot of unhappy patients, with a suicide rate seven times above average. Some patients simply kill themselves by missing dialysis appointments.

The National Institute of Health put hundreds of millions of dollars into research on artificial kidney machines. Then billions of dollars were put into the program to make the patients dependent on machines. Almost no money was spent on the possibility that the kidneys might be able to rejuvenate themselves given the proper herbs, diet and nutrients. Dialysis makes millions in profits for medical companies, but it makes slaves out of patients who feel powerless to control their lives.

In 1850 the French government issued a decree that all folk remedies were to be turned in for testing. The government promised to reward people with successful remedies. This resulted in many remedies being turned in, although I know of no tests and rewards.

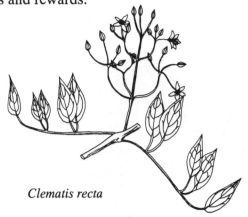

Clematis recta

One remedy that was turned in was the seed of ***Clematis recta*** for treating Bright's disease. A 38 year-old man had edema and albumin in the urine. He was given digitalis to remove the water, but it didn't work. Then Professor Suveur gave an infusion of clematis seeds. The results were remarkable: The excess water was eliminated, the albumin in the urine disappeared.

Several days later the professor had another chance to try the seeds. Once again they produced copious urination, and in a few days the problem seemed to be completely cured. Nothing more is heard of this remedy in the literature.

One of the first herbs used for dropsy and Bright's disease in the United States was reported in 1869. A woman suffered from chronic Bright's disease. The doctors finally told her that she was incurable. A neighbor visited the woman and told her that the condition could be cured by the inner bark of the common elder ***Sambucus canadensis*** mixed with hard cider. This is a 6-8% alcohol solution. The woman got the cider and scraped off the elder bark. She took ounce doses 3-4 times a day. In a few days improvement was quite marked, and soon she was well.

A Missouri doctor was called to see a seven year-old girl. Her limbs continued to swell, the face was puffy, and she had pain in her joints. There was a large amount of albumin in the urine. The doctors tried digitalis, squills, gamboge, Lugol's solution, ipecac, ***Veratrum viride*** and tartar emetic. The girl began to have violent spasms, and her pupils couldn't be seen. It became apparent that she was dying and had a short time to live.

A doctor who heard about the woman with Bright's disease came over, and told the attending doctor about hard cider and elder bark. He got the remedy, and in two days the girl began to look better. After three weeks of hard cider and elder bark, the little girl had fully recovered.

Mexico is the home of ***Agave*** plants. There are more than 250 species divided into the magueys and the amoles. The amoles contain saponins, which are soaplike chemicals. The leaves and roots of the amole plant ***Chlorogalum pomeridianum*** were sold in the markets as a substitute for soap. In the early days of California, the laundries grew this plant for soap.

The magueys have big fleshy leaves and are economically important. The pita magueys have thin leaves and they were used to produce fiber for twine and rope. The mescal magueys have thick stems and rootstocks, which ferment when made into a mash. This is the basis of the popular Mexican alcoholic drink known as mescal or tequila.

The pulque maguey *Agave atrovirens* is used in medicine as a laxative, diuretic, emmenagogue and galactogogue. The fresh sap is of special value for kidney problems. Mexican doctors found they could cure most patients with Bright's disease by having them drink the fresh sap. People affected with kidney disorders used to travel south of the Mexican border to take the treatments.

Here is an 1881 advertisement for the Mexican Pulque Company of Apam, Mexico: "I will state I rely upon its efficiency [*Agave atrovirens*], to cure Bright's disease of the kidneys, depending upon the presence of albumen in the urine, in all cases where the disease has not resulted in the final prostration and absolute debility. I can further prove the complete cure of several American and English residents here [in Mexico City], where in some cases the amount of albumen in the urine exceeded 2½%, the only remedy prescribed being pulque ad libitum." Signed Dr. A.W. Parsons, Harvard graduate.

The only thing occurring in literature in the way of a scientific test on this plant was done with rabbits. The kidneys were damaged with tartaric acid so that only 12% of the rabbits used as a control survived. A similar group of rabbits was given *Agave atrovirens*, and 73% survived, although it took some time for the injured kidneys to regain their function.

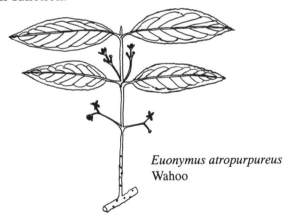

Euonymus atropurpureus
Wahoo

In 1898 Francis Hanson wrote how he used the green root bark of wahoo *Euonymus atropurpureus* in kidney disorders. He used ten drops of the tincture three times a day. By the second day the albumen was clearing in the urine and was usually gone in about a week. Hanson wrote:

"I believe wahoo is able to give every case of Bright's disease, that is not totally moribund a mighty hard tussle for existence. All the cases that I have had since I took up this plant have been 'nipped in the bud,' in very short order."

Another interesting case of kidney regeneration occurred when a woman at Fort Pierce, Florida, was dying of kidney failure. The doctors gave up hope and left the woman to die. A family servant asked permission to try a remedy, which her grandmother had used in the Bahamas. She sent her grandson up a coconut tree to pick some young green coconuts. They were hacked open and the soft coconut jelly was fed to the dying woman. An hour later her condition began to improve, and in a few days the woman was completely recovered.

Coconuts have a remarkable array of growth stimulants. Coconut milk causes cell division of single carrot cells, and of other plants. It is used in plant laboratories. The active substances are auxins, sugar alcohols, and several forms of inositols. The soft spongy green coconut was known as 'vara' in the South Pacific. High amounts of auxins can also be extracted with alcohol from immature corn kernels. Nobody has tried to use these substances to cure failing kidneys. The natural remedies have never been the subject of medical testing.

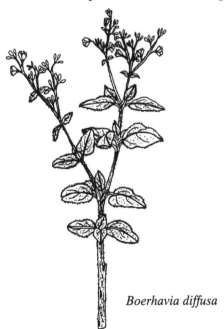

Boerhavia diffusa

Two plants have caught the attention of researchers in India as possible kidney rejuvenants. *Boerhavia diffusa* is used as a kidney sedative and diuretic. When ten grams a day of the crude herb powder was given to a group of kidney patients, four were healed, seven were greatly improved, and one found no relief.

Six patients with uremia were given 300 mgs. extract of *Tinospora cordifolia* at each meal. In five of the six patients clinical signs of the disease disappeared by the sixth day. The herb induced extensive urination and the amount of urea in the blood returned to normal levels. A month later the kidneys were checked and were still functioning normally.

Kidney failure may mean that urea is broken down into ammonia, which results in an ammonia smell on the breath. A century ago doctors discovered that *Arenaria rubra* removed the smell of ammonia from the urine. The smell of ammonia is generally a mark of liver damage, and this herb may have benefits for both the liver and the kidneys.

The European fava bean *Vicia faba* contains a powerful kidney stimulant. Rabbits were fed a standard ration of hay, bran and water, which resulted in 0.44 grams of urea and 0.07 grams of chlorides in the urine. When they were given an injection of a water extract of fava bean hulls, the excretion changed to 1.2 grams of urea and 0.5 grams of chlorides. The active substance in the bean hulls was isolated and found to be calcium glycerate. It promoted urogenesis, oxidation and deanimation of waste products. It could possibly help to aid kidney victims in regenerating their kidneys.

The famous Lloyd brothers of a century ago ground white kidney beans to a fine powder and soaked them in alcohol for about three weeks. Ten drops of the bean extract were taken every four hours for albumen in the urine. In a case where a coma was nearing, and the urine contained 10% albumin, the bean extract cleared up the urine in ten days.

Sarsaparilla is an old traditional blood and kidney herb. The first scientific work was done on it in 1931 in Germany. The kidneys of animals were damaged with uranium, and the animals were given a preparation of the herb. It had a distinct therapeutic action, and prevented the death of some of the animals. If the animals were too far gone, the herb had no value.

Researchers in the Philippines tested the value of the different species of sarsaparilla by remov-

ing most the kidneys of dogs, and placing them on a high protein diet. This resulted in high levels of urea in the blood. In the damaged dogs the urea levels shot up from 30 mgs. to 260 mgs. in six days. When the dogs received two grams of *Smilax* roots over a two-day period the urea level dropped to 120 mgs. Nine species of *Smilax* were tested and the most effective were *S. anceps, S. macrocarpa, S. ceylanica,* and *S. macrophylla.*

Another herb which attracted a lot of attention around 1925, was a Southeast Asian mint *Orthosiphon stamineus.* Doctors stressed that it was not a cure for failing kidneys. "Indian kidney tea," was successful in treating some cases of kidney failure. The tea is a strong gall stimulant, and has good results in kidney and liver illness. It is not a sure cure, but it is a valuable herb.

The Russian army medical journal printed an article on a doctor's experiences in using Icelandic moss *Cetraria islandica.* A patient had poor appetite, constipation, weakness and dropsy. He took a tablespoonful of a decoction of Icelandic moss every two hours. After four weeks of treatment the watery swelling disappeared. Other cases that the doctor treated got well with the remedy.

There are other kidney herbs which have no record of testing. Kidney disease in Russia was treated with birch tree buds. The kidney tea of the Seminole Indians was the flower of *Asimina reticulata.* A case of Bright's disease in West Virginia was reported cured by a tea of the roots of Queen of the Meadow *Eupatorium purpureum.* Some of the diuretic and liver regeneration herbs may be of value in the kidneys.

In Japan there has been an active look at some of the old kidney herbs. Rats were fed a diet of casein and adenine, which produced kidney failure. When a water extract of the roots of *Salvia miltiorhiza* was given to the rats it increased the flow of blood to the kidneys, and apparently resulted in partial repair. It decreased the urea and waste products in the blood. The active ingredient was isolated and found to be magnesium and ammonium-potassium lithospermates. When given to rats, it produced remarkable kidney improvement.

Japanese scientists found another herb that could be used to repair damaged kidneys. An extract of the roots of rhubarb improved kidney function, and decreased the level of urea and creatinine in the blood. It increased the calcium levels in the blood serum.

Many cases of kidney damage are known to be due to autoimmune disorders. The immune system becomes primed by disease agents, and attacks the kidneys as foreign tissue. A water extract of **Cinnamomum cassia** proved to be a strong immunosuppressant. Japanese scientists found that it was similar in strength to the drugs now used.

In the nineteenth century, if you went to a doctor complaining of kidney problems, the chances were good that he would have you take a solution of sodium citrate. This salt is part of the citrates in citrus fruits. When a bone is broken, the citrates in the fluids around the break increase rapidly as the repair process takes place. Citrates were a common medication of the last century, but they have been largely forgotten.

Thirteen dogs were given an injection of uranium nitrate. This damaged the kidneys and twelve of the dogs died in the following days. The next group of dogs received an injection of sodium citrate five days before the uranium nitrate and five days afterwards. The kidneys were badly damaged, but in twelve days they were almost totally repaired. This experiment is an indication that kidney regeneration can be helped with electronegative salts.

The pioneer of Vitamin E was Wilfred Shute of Guelph, Ontario. He noted that Bright's disease often followed severe throat infections. A four-year-old boy developed tonsillitis with a high fever, which was treated with sulfamerazine. In two days his urine was bright red with blood passing through the damaged kidneys. He was given 150 units of Vitamin E and the blood cleared from the urine the next day. The following day the albumin cleared up.

A 16 year-old boy developed a sore throat. In two days his face, ankles and fingers began to swell. The urine showed large number of red and white blood cells.He was given 300 units of Vitamin E. In four days all traces of blood and albumin disappeared from the urine. After recovering his friends noted that his face wasn't as fat as it was normally.

When rats are deprived of Vitamin E, the tubules of the kidneys degenerate. A trial was made of 13 women with poor kidney function and 25 mgs. a day of Vitamin E benefited ten cases. The improvement was quick, but it was transient unless the therapy was continued.

I would like to think that at least half of those needing dialysis could benefit from the herbs mentioned here. It is unlikely that those who have spent years on dialysis would benefit greatly, but it certainly would be worth trying. The human machine was made to regenerate itself, but all we have been able to do is think of mechanical support! A small amount of money spent on honest research could pay back many fold in productive working people.

KIDNEY STONES

November 4, 1660
"Hence to my father's where I found my mother in greater and greater pain of the stone."

March 26, 1662
"Up early. This being by God's great blessing the fourth same day of my cutting for stone this day four years ago, and am by God's mercy in very good health, and like to do well, the Lord's name be praised for it."

Diary of Samuel Pepys

"Rocks of lava, which neither iron nor fire can alone dissolve, split into pieces and dissolve when heated with fire and sprinkled with vinegar. Since we see these things taking place before our eyes, we might infer that the same principle is of use. Patients with the stone may in the nature of things, be cured with acid water on account of the sharpness of the solution."

Vitruvius -100

The Hippocratic School of medicine was located on the little island of Cos off of the present day Turkish coast. The treatment of stones was considered so special, that it was written into the doctor's oath. "I will not cut persons laboring under the stone, but will leave this to be done by men who are practitioners of this work." The lack of knowledge of anatomy and a high death rate for surgery made this important.

The first operation for stones was done at Meudon, France, in 1574. A thief sold valuables from a church and was condemned to death. Since the thief was troubled with stones, the doctors of Paris petitioned the king: "It would be useful to see the places where these maladies are concreted, and this could best be done by vivisecting a human being." The doctors got their wish, and remarkably enough, the man survived and was given a pardon after recovering.

Martin Luther developed kidney and bladder stones and said, "I am pregnant again and lie in the pains of childbed. I cry out on account of the pain caused by the stone, which is a disease of Germans, just as they say that in England gout is very widespread." A letter to his wife says: "Your art with the use of dung did not help." He tried pigeon dung, which Pliny recommended over the bladder area.

One of his doctor's remedies survives in an old manuscript: "For the stone of Dr. Martin Luther. Take a new vessel, fill it half-full with juniper berries, fill it up with wine and water, and let one-third boil off, and drink of it." Unfortunately, it didn't work.

In 1537 the attacks were so severe that his friends feared for his life. He vomited repeatedly and said: "Bless it for me, dear God, whether it be for death or for life! For if the disease lasts longer with me, I shall certainly become insane. But even should I perish, yet do I know that God is ever wise."

He was taken on a wagon through a bumpy road through the Thuringen Forest. A spring in the woods that seemed to help him is still called "Lutherbrunn." At Tambach, Germany, he was put up in an inn. He drank some red wine and was able to urinate, which he hadn't been able to do for days. The worst was over and he was able to go on with his religious work.

Samuel Pepys, the famous London diary writer of the seventeenth century, was troubled with stones and suffered greatly from the pain. While he was a student at Cambridge the suffering was too much and an operation was performed. He was given a mixture of licorice, marshmallow, cinnamon and rose water to soothe him, but no narcotics to kill the pain. The doctors removed a stone the size of a tennis ball, and Pepys was so relieved that every year on March 26th, he had a feast at his home in memory of the suffering. He kept his stone in an expensive box made for the purpose.

Paracelsus (1490 – 1541) explained the cause of stones and gout with the doctrine of 'tartsus.' He got the idea from wine barrels; if the barrel sat for a long period of time and allowed the wine to evaporate, the remainder formed concretions of minerals, in the dregs of the wine. This is the central idea behind what chemists call solubility. It is the amount of substance which will remain in a fluid without forming crystals.

Stones were found in an ancient Egyptian burial ground that dates back 7,000 years. The frequency with which people have this condition may depend on the water, although there is little difference between people in areas where there is soft or hard water. Stones are related to diet, and people in areas where there are oxalate containing foods have a higher rate of stones. The hot areas of the world are the 'stone districts.' In these areas people sweat a lot and water is lost through the skin. This concentrates the urine, and the minerals began to precipitate out as stones.

Urinary stones are related to some types of arthritis, but are not necessarily synonymous. About one person in a thousand in the US has urinary stones. Residents in Wyoming and Missouri have half the average, and people in South Carolina and Georgia have double the number. Farmers have a low rate of stones, and health workers suffer at higher than average rates.

The main symptom of stones is pain, although there are quiet stones, which may remain for years without pain. The pain generally begins in the kidney area and radiates downward towards the bladder. Often there is nausea and vomiting, and blood is present in the urine. Sometimes these symptoms are absent, and the only real detection of the problem is by x-ray.

Many stones have organic glue binding them together. This glue appears to be a result of a reaction between the endotoxins of gram negative bacteria and antibodies from the immune system. The kidneys remove the endotoxin, and they bind to antibodies and in turn bind to minerals. If the gut flora can be shifted towards gram-positive bacteria, these individuals are less likely to form stones.

Stones can vary in size from a pinhead to a coconut. If drugs that act as dyes are taken, these leave a daily growth ring. If we reduce the mineral content of the urine, the stones will slowly disappear. Calcium oxalate stones are the most common form in the US and England. When higher amounts of magnesium are added to the diet, oxalates won't form. These stones were treated by giving tablets of 420 mgs. of magnesium to two men. As long as they continued to take the magnesium, they remained free of stones. When they stopped taking them, the stones began forming in three to four weeks. Vitamin B6 is a stimulant of oxalate excretion. It increases the amount of citric acid in the body, which helps to remove stone forming minerals.

The first persons to suggest that stones were a deficiency disease were Thomas Osborne and Lafayette Mendel in 1917. The rats in the experiment had not been provided with Vitamin A, and 10% of them developed stones. Yoshitomo Fujimaki in Japan followed up this lead in 1926. He found that rats deficient in B and C vitamins didn't develop stones. A diet deficient in Vitamin A and calcium formed phosphate stones; first in the bladder, then in the kidneys. Each type of mineral deficiency, along with Vitamin A deficiency, produced a different type of stone formation. He x-rayed rats and then added a large amount of Vitamin A to the diet. When they were checked again, the stones disappeared. Supplements of Vitamin A in people should do the same thing for mineral stones. Gallstones are lumps of cholesterol, and do not respond to this treatment.

When rats are put on Vitamin B6 deficient diets, there is increased kidney damage and higher amounts of stone forming oxalates. Oxalate deposits scar the kidneys and create painful stones. An increase in this vitamin reduces the amounts of oxalates.

The first ideas on stone treatment were taking vinegar, because people knew that vinegar dissolved many minerals by forming soluble acetates. The stones that trouble the body are not usually formed of the minerals that respond to dissolution by vinegar.

The next idea for treating stones came from the observation that carbon dioxide dissolved calcium and magnesium minerals in water. This gas forms bicarbonates in minerals making them more soluble in water. In 1777 William Saunders put out a paper *Observations and experiments on the power of mephic acid in dissolving stones of the bladder.*

The famous English scientist Stephen Hales demonstrated that water mixed with carbonic acid could dissolve urinary calculus. He made stone dissolving water by mixing 1.9 grams of potassium carbonate and 1.2 grams of citric acid in separate cups of water. They were then poured together and drunk, which caused fizzing from the release of carbon dioxide. Hales showed that carbonic acid quickly made its appearance in the urine. It wouldn't dissolve uric acid stones, but it would dissolve mineral stones.

Polygonum aviculare is a low plant that grows in damp soils. A man from Kew, England, was noted for seeking out people suffering from stones and giving them the herb as a tea. In one case, two glasses of the tea reportedly caused pain, as a stone broke up and passed into the urine. Dozens of bad cases were said to have been cured by drinking the tea.

Verbesina heliantho-ides was known as gravel weed to the settlers of the Southeastern U.S. It is related to the sunflower and has four welt-like edges that

Polygonum aviculare
Smartweed

make the stem appear to be square. The first settlers learned about it from the Cherokee Indians. A tincture of the roots was said to be a sure cure for gravel. It was also used in kidney and bladder problems and was called 'diabetes weed.' In 1845 Dr. Turk wrote: "I have

Verbesina helianthoides
Gravelweed

never failed to cure gravel even of long standing, in four of five days with this root in alcohol and until I do fail I will continue to believe in its efficacy."

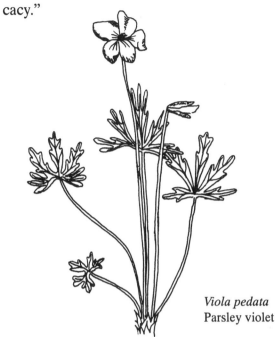

Viola pedata
Parsley violet

In 1696 a woman at Medford, Massachusetts, just outside of Boston, was worried about her son's life. An Indian came by and asked about her problem. He told her to get some parsley violet roots ***Viola pedata***, pulverize them and make a tea with hot water. Her son voided urinary stones and recovered.

In 1739 a nephew of the family suffered from stones. Violets were gathered and they cured the trouble. Thirty years later the same family had a friend, who was in great pain in the urinary tract. He drank violet tea, and was cured.

When a baby girl in a nearby farm reached the age of six weeks, she began to have attacks of pain. The girl would shriek with pain, and began to jerk. The family doctor tried everything but nothing worked, and he finally gave up. A friend recommended trying the parsley violet tea every hour. The baby had one more attack, and the problem was over. It is unlikely that the problem was stones, and the account suggests that the herb may have a wider use.

Dr. Samuel Butler was the first to write about using seven barks ***Hydrangea arborescens*** for stones. This is a shrub growing up to five feet tall. The bark layers are each a different color giving it the names nine barks, or seven barks. As a missionary to the Cherokees, Butler used the herb to cure Rattling Gourd and several other persons that he ministered to. It worked in about half of the cases, and it cured dribbling of urine.

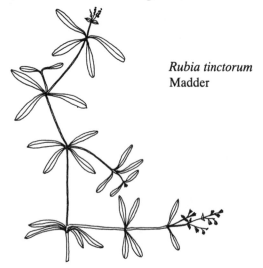

Rubia tinctorum
Madder

A Lady Elizabeth had suffered long from stones. She wrote: "I have been under the care of several physicians belonging to the army and taken many kinds of medicine for my complaint. I have found nothing to relieve me as the decoction of this plant has done."

German doctors found that madder **Rubia tinctorum** would dissolve many bladder stones. It was especially effective on stones composed of sodium and ammonium salts. Madder stimulated the muscular action and helped to expel the stones.

In India **Celosia argentea** grows as a weed with the crops. It is considered a specific in Ayurvedic medicine for dissolving stones. Glass beads were inserted into the bladders of rats and the irritation began forming stones. In ten days an 8 mg. glass bead had an average weight of 100 mgs. as urinary minerals formed around it. A tincture of *Celosia* was given to another group of rats. After being in the rat for ten days the usual glass bead weighed about 10 mgs.

In Southern China **Desmodium styracifolium** is used to treat urinary stones. Stone formation was encouraged in laboratory rats by giving them ethylene glycol. This caused 81% of them to have urinary stones, but only 19% in the group getting

the herbal extract had stones. The herb appeared to block the excretion of calcium and it increased the excretion of citrate. The citrate ion dissolves calcium and keeps it in solution.

Ordinary pumpkin seeds were tested in the stone forming districts of Asia. This probably doesn't indicate any special quality of the seeds, except they have a balance of calcium and phosphorus. In these areas the nutritional balance was so poor, that the addition of the seeds lower the risk of bladder stone formation.

In Egypt and the Sudan kidney stones are common. A long thick grass known as hamreb **Stipa tenacissima** is made into a tea. In 1962 Geoffrey Dale was traveling through and suffering from kidney stones. He tried antibiotics, antispasmodics and painkillers without results. Then he drank the tea three times a day and passed a large stone and was cured.

In Taiwan a variety of Chinese herbs were used to treat stones. Scientists recently found that **Uncaria kawakamii = U. hirsuta** was far stronger than any of the other herbs used in treating stones. The herb could act by making soluble minerals into bicarbonates, or by interfering with the protein binding glue of the stones.

Quercus stenophylla extracts have been studied in Japan with rats and implanted glass beads. The herb increases the urinary excretion of calcium and magnesium and decreases the phosphorus. Rats given a tincture of the leaves showed a marked reduction of stone formation on glass beads.

In Roman times Pliny recommended teas of **Paeonia officinalis, Cicer arietinum** and mints for dissolving stones. On the island of Cyprus the plant **Plantago coronopus** is called "lithospaston," meaning 'stone-dissolver.' It is a strong diuretic, and a tea is drunk until the pain of stones is relieved. It has never been clinically tested. The literature of the world contains a rich assortment of lithotropic plants. However, none of them have received any real attention. A study of these herbs might be able to eliminate many operations.

✿ ✿ ✿

HYPOGLYCEMIA

"All the healing of their diseases we told to Noah, together with the means of administration thereof; so that he might cure through the trees of the earth. Noah wrote everything as we taught him, in a book concerning all kinds of healing. The evil spirits were fended off from the children of Noah. He gave everything he had written to Shem, his oldest son, for he loved him more than all his sons."

The Book of Jubilees *(one of the once lost books of the Bible)*

A woman once came to Mahatma Gandhi and said to him, "Please tell my son to give up sugar." He replied, "Come back in three days, and I'll do that." The woman returned three days later and her request was granted. She then asked, "Why didn't you do this three days ago?" "Because I hadn't given up sugar myself!"

Searl Harris first described the problem of low blood sugar in an article in 1924. He recognized that it was just the opposite of diabetes in which the blood sugar is too high. The case that brought the disorder to his attention was a doctor who remarked that about an hour before lunch, he felt so weak and nervous and hungry that he could not work. He got relief from eating candy or fruit. With a good balanced diet he improved.

Harris noted a number of similar cases. Low blood sugar resulted in weakness and hunger, which was cured by eating. In many cases the diet was poor, and smoking, drinking black coffee and alcohol were additional factors.

When insulin came into use after 1925, doctors found that patients sometimes reacted with strange symptoms. They even went into comas, because the blood sugar dropped so much. By 1935 doctors solved the problem of insulin-induced low blood sugar. They found that a combination of calcium and insulin decreased the effectiveness, although potassium and iron increased the effectiveness of insulin. When a combination of zinc and insulin was made, the blood sugar levels lowered gradually. They did not drop to dangerous levels, and the combination lasted much longer. Zinc may also keep blood sugar constant in nondiabetic cases

Doctors called the problem of low blood sugar, 'hyperinsulinism' and 'glycopenia'. They found that some cases of epilepsy were cured after the blood sugar was raised to normal levels. Children who were considered to be 'dull' or 'slow learners' often had low blood sugar. Thyroid problems were found to be linked to the storage of sugar in the liver.

Writers project their own feelings, or the feelings of friends into the material they write. It has been theorized that 'Winnie the Pooh' suffered from hypoglycemia. He ate breakfast of "marmalade spread lightly over a honeycomb or two" and then set out for a walk in the woods. At 11 A.M., he suffered from peculiar cravings and "a sort of funny feeling began to creep over him. It began at the tip of his nose and trickled all through him, and out at the soles of his feet. It was just as somebody inside him were saying, "Now then, Pooh, time for a little something."

When Winnie the Pooh was at Owl's house, he hinted to Owl about "a small something about now, about this time in the morning, just a spoonful of condensed milk or whatnot, with perhaps a lick of honey." Owl wouldn't give him anything, and he tried to listen to what Owl was saying, but all he could do was shut his eyes and say "yes" or "no." The lovable children's storybook bear seems to have suffered from low blood sugar.

The *Minnesota Multiphasic Personality Inventory* is one of the best-known tests of how people feel and react. It is a multiple-choice test with questions like: "Do you think people are talking about you?" Neurotics and people with hypoglycemia tend to give deviant answers to 21 questions. Low blood sugar makes us more fearful and anxious, and our answers become abnormal.

Many American breakfasts invite problems. Coffee with sugar, doughnuts or toast with jam is high in sugar, but low in nutrition. The blood sugar level rises rapidly and the insulin level rises rapidly to control it. Then the blood sugar falls rapidly, and if the body's controlling mechanism isn't working well, it falls too low. High sugars and high carbohydrates cause low levels of blood sugar, and invite hunger and tired feelings. High protein breakfasts cause little hunger, and the sugar level stays constant. Alanine, one of the amino acids in meat proteins, is believed to keep the blood sugar at a constant level.

There are a number of plants which contain liver toxins, and liver damage almost invariably causes hypoglycemia. One of the worst offenders is the African tree **Blighia sapida** that is planted extensively in the Caribbean. It was named **Blighia** in honor of Captain William Bligh, who is forever immortalized in *Mutiny on the Bounty*. Eating the unripe fruits results in 'vomiting sickness,' which is a result of a liver toxin which causes severe hypoglycemia. The akee tree was been banned on some islands, and warnings are issued on others. It is grown in southern Florida as a curiosity.

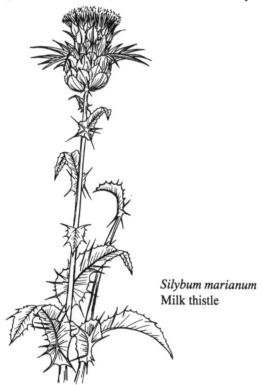

Silybum marianum
Milk thistle

Liver toxins are known to cause hypoglycemia. Would liver healing agents like the purple milk thistle **Silybum marianum** and artichoke leaves **Cynara scolymus** keep blood sugar levels normal? Evidence suggests that this is part of their function, but nobody has studied these plants.

When the liver is damaged by chloroform or carbon tetrachloride, it results in severe hypoglycemia. A chemical known as guanidine accumulates as a result of injury. Additional calcium seems to prevent further injury, and keeps blood sugar at normal levels.

In liver disease the blood sugar is low due to the liver injury. I have listed the herbs known to cure liver problems. It is likely that many of them would act to normalize the blood sugar levels.

Sugar must be stored in the liver so it can be released when we haven't eaten for awhile. The chemically bound sugar in the liver is known as glycogen, and the sugar in sweet corn is almost identical. Vitamin B2 (riboflavin) is believed to increase sugar storage. Orange juice is known to increase the storage of liver sugar in rats. The increased storage means that more sugar is available for release when needed.

Biotin is a B vitamin which acts with the enzyme pyruvate carboxylase to release stored sugar. In time of stress more biotin is needed to release the sugar for use in the body. There is a theory that 'crib death' is due to lack to biotin, so that not enough blood sugar is available to keep the brain and nervous system operating.

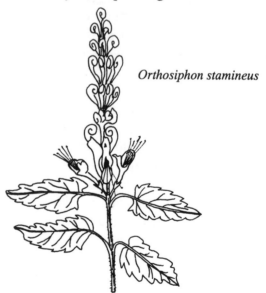

Orthosiphon stamineus

When rats were fed the roots of burdock **Arctium**, the sugar content of their livers rose by five times. In 1887 **Orthosiphon stamineus** was brought to England to be tested for gout and renal disorders. It is a mint with purple veins, which is used as a houseplant. Experiments showed that the plant stimulated the liver to store sugar.

Rutin is a bioflavanoid, commercially extracted from the buds of the Japanese pagoda tree *Sophora japonica*, which contains up to 22%. Buckwheat straw contains about 7% rutin, and it is commercially extracted with alcohol. When a group of rabbits was given 10 mgs. of rutin, blood sugar levels rose by 35%. The levels peaked in four to eight hours, but occasionally they continued rising for the next ten or more hours. When rabbits were given 20 mgs. of rutin the average blood sugar rise was 47%. Many hypoglycemia problems could be due to a low intake of bioflavanoids.

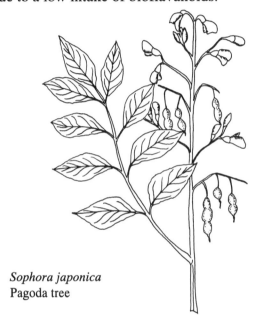

Sophora japonica
Pagoda tree

Apple tree leaves contain up to 2.3% phloridzin, which is extracted by strong alcohol. This chemical inhibits the process that generates high-energy phosphate bonds for energy. As a result of blocking the enzymes, the blood sugar rises rapidly. The bark of apple, cherry, plum and pear trees contain phloridzin. In 1835 experiments were done with these barks in the treatment of malaria. They showed that it produced high blood sugar. Unfortunately, it probably isn't good for you.

There are many plants which lower blood sugar but relatively few, which raise blood sugar levels. Some plants that raise blood sugar levels have an adrenaline-like effect, which depletes the glycogen in the liver. Both *Morinda citrifolia* and black cohosh *Cimicifuga racemosa* are known to produce feelings of happiness and well being. Could the improved feelings be due to higher blood sugar levels?

The crucial factor in hypoglycemia is a good diet. When the sugar and carbohydrates are eliminated in favor of more protein, the blood sugar does not rise and fall rapidly. The pancreas produces a steady amount of insulin, especially if our emotions and feelings remain balanced. These simple measures could benefit some people, now classified as neurotic or mildly mentally unbalanced.

✩ ✩ ✩

DIABETES DIETS

"It is a disease of the rich, and one that is brought about by gluttonous overindulgence in rice, flour and sugar. The order of disease is ushered in by the appearance of morbid secretions about the teeth, ears, nose and eyes. The hands and feet are very hot and burning, and the surface of the skin is shining as if oil had been applied to it. This is accompanied by thirst, and a sweet taste in the mouth. The different varieties of the disease are distinguished from each other by the symptoms of deranged humors, and by the color of the urine.

Charaka, the famous Ayurvedic healer of India c. -600

The distinguishing mark of diabetes was sweet urine, and a desire to drink large quantities of water. In -229, the Chinese writer Chang-Ke mentions a disorder that produced sweet urine. The medical books of ancient India called diabetes 'madhumea,' meaning 'honey urine.' In medieval times doctors studied the urine, and urine that attracted flies was a mark of diabetes. Before 1925 diabetes was a sentence of misery and death, for most doctors had no answers.

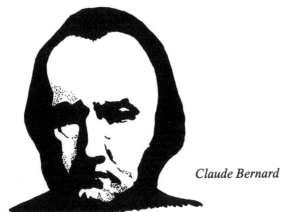

Claude Bernard

In 1857 Claude Bernard established that the liver was the organ where sugar was stored in the body and released. In 1869 a German medical student named Paul Langerhans found what is now called the Islands of Langerhans. At the time, it wasn't known what the islands of Langerhans did in the pancreas. In 1889 the German physiologists Joseph von Mering and Oscar Minkowski showed that the removal of the pancreas led to diabetes. In 1922 physiologists added another piece to the puzzle, by showing that removal of the liver led to a rapid drop in blood sugar.

In 1916 Edward Schaefer suggested the name insulin for the hypothetical hormone of the Islands of Langerhans. This suggestion was published in his Stanford lectures, which were published as *An Introduction to the Study of Endocrine Glands*. In 1921 Frederick Banting brought both pieces of the puzzle together by isolating insulin. The liver stored sugar; and an enzyme released it from the glycogen, as the blood sugar levels fell. The pancreas secreted more insulin, which acted as a sugar-burning catalyst, when the blood sugar levels become too high.

We treat diabetes with insulin, but there are cases of 'insulin resistant diabetes.' Insulin doesn't do any good in the condition. Another form is known as 'diabetes insipidus,' in which large amounts of urine free from sugar are passed. The disorder is in the posterior part of the pituitary gland. A true cure for most diabetes would be regeneration of the insulin-producing cells of the pancreas. It may not always be possible to regenerate the pancreas, but in some cases, the pancreas can be stimulated to produce extra insulin.

Israeli scientists studied the sand rat, which is common in the desert areas of the Middle East. When they changed its diet from green forage to laboratory pellets, the rats developed diabetes and died. Rats normally thrive on this mixture, but these developed hyperglycemia and cataracts. Autopsies showed that the beta cells of the pancreas degenerated. The normal food of the sand rat is the shrubby saltbush *Atriplex halimus*. Experiments showed that the plant's chromium kept the sand rats from becoming diabetic.

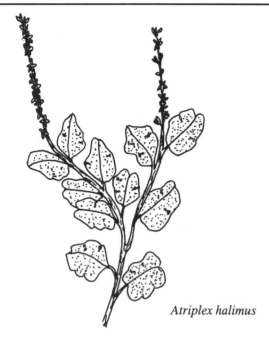

Atriplex halimus

The same thing apparently happens in people. Around 1940 the Pima Indians of southern Arizona changed their diet to a more European oriented diet. Their old foods were mesquite pods, acorns, Indian corn, lima beans, and tepiary beans. Tests show that mesquite pods and acorns were quite effective in controlling blood sugar. When these people switched to processed food, their genes reacted, with high rates of diabetes. About half of the Tohono O'odham (Pima) people over 35 years of age have diabetes.

In 1955 two researchers suspected that a particular factor in brewers yeast could prevent diabetes. They found that certain diets made rats mildly diabetic, and they could prevent this with portions of yeast. They suspected that it was a metal, and they tested 40 different metals. Manganese had some effect on blood sugar, but the only thing that kept the blood sugar level normal was chromium.

Chromium is the sixth most abundant element in the earth's crust and 15th most abundant in the ocean. It does not have insulin activity, and it acts as a co-hormone with insulin. Curiously enough, it is quite active in hypoglycemia. It keeps the blood sugar level stable, not too high or too low. When six diabetic patients were given chromium supplements of a milligram before meals, three of them had blood sugar levels return to near normal. About a third of diabetics have marked benefit. Supplements of 150 micrograms were successful in restoring the blood glucose levels of older people.

British doctors studied the curious case of a man who had high blood sugar levels. When he took alfalfa they plummeted and he became hypoglycemic. The high content of manganese in the alfalfa lowered the blood sugar levels. Alfalfa contains about 45 mgs. of manganese per kilogram. When diabetics were given manganese chloride, it caused a significant reduction in blood sugar level, but, typically, it did not bring them to normal levels.

The pancreas is rich in insulin, and the metal acts as a catalyst in the critical biochemical reactions. In India, a preparation of 'Jasad bhasma' (an Ayurvedic zinc compound), cured many mild cases of diabetes and helped diabetics to reduce their insulin needs.

Vanadium is a little known metal which is used in specialty alloys, but its function and need are unknown in humans. There is a marine tunicate **Ascidia nigra**, which has a bright yellow blood pigment, made of vanadium, instead of iron. When low levels of sodium vanadate was given to diabetic rats, it acted like insulin. Vanadium can be given by mouth, and it quickly lowers blood sugar levels.

Insulin acts as a catalyst for burning sugar. There is a popular high school chemistry demonstration of this action. When a match is applied to a sugar cube, it won't burn. Cigarette ash is sprinkled on the cube, and then the sugar burns. The minerals function as aids in allowing sugar to burn, just as insulin does in the body.

High levels of blood sugar is not necessarily the result of diabetes. It may be due to emotional stress. A group of Harvard medical students were tested before and after a tough examination. Three percent of the students had urinary sugar before the test, and 18% had extra sugar after it.

There are numerous cases in medical literature of people with traumas developing diabetes, or having their blood sugar go out of control. When a policeman was told his 18 year-old daughter had leukemia, his insulin requirement went out of control. When he learned it was not leukemia, it became normal. There are many cases where a narrow escape from death led to the person becoming diabetic.

Banting's co-worker James Collip predicted that plants could have insulin-like substances, since they had sugars. He was able to demonstrate that onions, lettuce, green beans and wheat leaves had weak insulin-like effects. His observations aroused the curiosity of doctors, and two studies were done in treating diabetics with plant extracts by 1928. A mixture of alfalfa, sweet clover, corn silk, onions, carrots, bran and rice polish were extracted with 40% alcohol and used in Beijing, China. Most of the diabetics in the study were able to control blood sugar by taking ten to 15 grams by mouth each day.

In 1796 Dr. John Rollo reported that he had good results treating a soldier with diabetes. The soldier was given a sparse diet of eggs and meat with a little bread and butter. He might have had a mild case of diabetes associated with obesity, which is common. By losing weight, many of these cases cure themselves.

In 1853 Dr. Bird Herepath successfully treated a case of diabetes with brewer's yeast. A tablespoonful three times a day cut the sugar in the urine by a third in two days. In six weeks the problem was cured and the patient regained his original weight. The doctors thought that the yeast fermented the sugar in the stomach and left nothing for the urine. The yeast is rich in B vitamins and nutritional factors, which was almost certainly the real cure.

A diet rich in vitamins may prevent or even cure diabetes. Vitamin E reduced the requirements of insulin in diabetics. It protects rats when alloxan, a chemical that destroys the insulin producing cells is added. Estrogen, Vitamin E and Vitamin K are known to help rats. Tests were made on groups of rats made diabetic with alloxin. Four milligrams of Vitamin E restored 3 out of 12 rats. Estrogen helped 4 of 15 rats return to normal in eight weeks. When estrogen was combined with Vitamin K, 7 of 11 rats returned to normal.

Thiamin does not directly help diabetes, but it can correct problems caused by diabetic acidosis. The acid condition can cause vomiting and lethargy. In once case a woman suffered severely, and when she was given 50 mg. of thiamin, the shortness of breath and other problems quickly disappeared.

The Egyptian Medical Society ran a study of Vitamin B3 nicotinamide. Diabetics received 400 mgs. of nicotinamide twice a day, which was reduced to 250 mgs. twice daily. In new diabetic cases the symptoms went away in three to four weeks, and most patients could return to a normal diet in six to eight weeks. In severe diabetes and older cases, the amount of insulin could be greatly reduced.

A study published in 1990 showed that nicotinamide was of benefit in both type I and type II diabetes. Type I diabetes is a result of immune system or oxidant injury to the insulin producing cells. It often cures early cases and reduces the amount of insulin needed in older cases.

A middle-aged man was taking four different drugs to control high blood pressure, arthritis, and gout. Elevated blood sugar pointed to diabetes, and he decided that five drugs was simply too much for one person. He began taking 500 mgs. of nicotinamide, a gram of Vitamin C and 50 mgs. of zinc. In four weeks nearly all of his problems disappeared. He felt more energetic and slept better.

A 64 year-old man suffered from diabetes, cough, shortness of breath and a pre-gangrene condition on his toes. His enlarged heart was now failing and he had severe insomnia. He began taking three tablespoonfuls of flax oil, two grams of Vitamin C and 500 mgs. of nicotinamide. In six weeks all of his conditions had significantly improved.

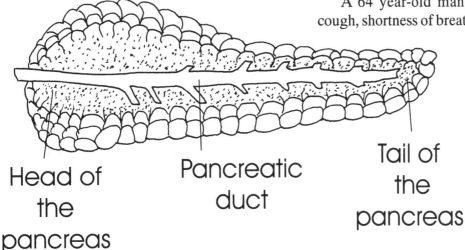

Head of the pancreas

Pancreatic duct

Tail of the pancreas

Diabetes often results in symptoms similar to pernicious anemia, which is due to a lack of Vitamin B12. A test was made of this vitamin as a therapy. An older woman suffered from leg pains and cold feet for five years. After the first B12 injection, the shooting pains dramatically decreased. Another woman suffered from diabetes for three years. Because of severe hand and feet cramps she couldn't lace her shoes. Several injections of Vitamin B12 brought the problem under control.

The amino acid choline is known to be of help in diabetes. Some patients could eliminate insulin completely by taking four grams per day. A combination of the different vitamins known to help might be of great benefit in diabetes.

Most of the old diabetic diets were bland and sugarless. In 1874 the roots of artichokes were proposed for diabetics. The roots contain inulin, which is not converted into sugar, like the starch of plants. Another diet, which became quite common, was nothing but oatmeal.

Oats have mild insulinlike properties, and although they do not completely substitute for insulin, an oat diet can be quite useful. Oatmeal diets were the subject of several medical reports around 1915. Patients ate oatmeal for three days and then followed it with two days of vegetables. After a few weeks small amounts of fish and meat were added. A diet of oatmeal didn't cure diabetes, but it did a good job of controlling it in 28% of diabetics.

Rice diets, potato diets and cereal combination diets were proposed. Combination diets of fast days, fat days, vegetable days and oatmeal days were tried. All of these diets had a little value in cases of mild diabetes, but they were ineffective, when the pancreas secreted little or no insulin.

The Arabs called diabetes "Donarah" or "Zalc el goliah," which referred to the greater amount of urine. Avicenna, the prince of physicians, treated diabetes with a mixture of *Artemisia pauciflora*, fenugreek seeds and hops. A trial was made of this formula in Tunisia by giving diabetics 2.5 grams of the powdered herbs, and increasing this to five grams over several days. If the sugar doesn't disappear from the urine, the dose is increased by five grams a day, until it reaches 45 grams.

A trial on 39 diabetics showed that nearly all people had a major reduction of sugar in the urine. In three weeks, an 87-year-old man went from 133 grams of sugar to 16 grams. A 62-year-old man went from 180 grams of sugar in the urine a day to 10 grams in a month. Five people had no sugar at all in the urine. It is known that fenugreek inhibits the transport of glucose and keeps the blood sugar relatively level. Treatment with ground seeds improves severe diabetes and decreases sugared urine in mild diabetes. Generally an initial level of two grams per kilogram of body weight will provide a significant blood sugar reduction.

The value of the foods for stabilizing blood sugar was studied in England by having groups of volunteers eat a portion of food, and then measure the blood sugar rise over a period of time. The foods which kept the blood sugar stable were kidney beans, black-eyed peas and lentils. The worst items were whole wheat bread, potatoes and brown rice. Oatmeal was the best cereal, with a modest blood sugar rise over a shorter period of time. Diet in diabetes is no longer as important as it once was, but it is still vital to good health. Good diet aids the general aspects of health, not just the problem of diabetes. James Dickey put the feeling of the experience in his powerful poem *Diabetes*: "One night I thirsted like a prince, then like a king, then like an empire, like a world on fire. I rose and flowed away and fell, once more to sleep."

✽ ✽ ✽

DIABETIC TEAS

"The nature of the disease is chronic and it takes a long period to form. The patient is short-lived if the constitution of the disease becomes completely established; for the weight loss is rapid and the death speedy. Moreover, life is disgusting and painful. The thirst is unquenchable with excessive drinking, which moreover is disproportionate to the large quantity of fluid excreted. More fluid is excreted, but one cannot stop either from drinking or excreting fluid. If they abstain from drinking for a while, their mouth becomes parched and their body dry. The organs seem as if they were scorched. They are affected with nausea, restlessness, and a burning thirst; and at no distant term they expire."

Arataeus +300

The word diabetes has its roots in the Greek word 'diabaino' meaning 'to run through.' In diabetes, people are always thirsty, and need to urinate frequently. The Persian water wheel was called a 'ziabethus,' because the main current of water was sent to the fields for irrigation, and water poured out from a side spout for home use. A similar version known as a 'picottish' is still used to water the fields of southern India.

In +160 Galen borrowed the word 'diabetes,' and because of his enormous prestige, the term remains in medical use. He wrote, "I am of the opinion that the kidneys are affected in the rare disease, which some people call chamber-pot dropsy, and others call it diabetes from the violent thirst. For my part I have seen the disease only twice when patients suffered from an inextinguishable thirst. This forced them to drink enormous quantities, the fluid was urinated swiftly, with a urine resembling the drink."

The sweet taste of the urine was first mentioned in the Ayurvedic books of India 3,000 years ago. Sushruta's book says that when a man suffers from honey urine, he is incurable. Many tribes had noticed that when urine attracts flies, the person has diabetes. In 1674 Thomas Willis rediscovered the sweet urine of diabetes. A century later, it was proven that this was sugar.

There are several hundred plants with antidiabetic activity, although no plant is a complete substitute for insulin. It is curious to note that many of the plants which affect the pancreas, also affect the kidneys and the thyroid. The fresh pods of the kidney bean *Phaseolus vulgaris* and *P. multiflorum* are active in clearing up kidney disorders. A tea of the pods lowers blood sugar levels and increases the alkalinity of the blood. A study was done on bean pod tea in Germany in 1927. In less severe cases of diabetes, a cup of tea with meals often eliminated the need for insulin. In severe cases insulin was required.

Vaccinium angustifolium
Blueberry

German peasants used blueberry leaves *Vaccinium angustifolium* for the 'evil inflammation of the blood.' They were one of the first plants to be tested for antidiabetic effects. A tea of the leaves reduces or eliminates sugar in the urine, but unfortunately the tea doesn't reduce the blood sugar, so its effect is useless.

Quebec doctors did a study of the berries of the staghorn sumac *Rhus hirta* = *R.* typhina after a patient found he was able to control his diabetes with a tea of the berries. They found that many people were able to use the tea in place of insulin, if the insulin needs were small. When the pancreas didn't produce any insulin at all, the tea didn't work. The active substance is a tannin. Many tannins reduce blood glucose, and a tannin in a tropical American plant *Coutarea latiflora* reduces blood sugar concentrations only in diabetic individuals.

Doctors in British Columbia, Canada, told an Indian man that he would have to take insulin for his diabetes. They were surprised when he appeared healthy and perfectly normal without insulin. His secret was drinking a tea of the roots of devil's club *Oplopanax horridus*. The plant attracted medical investigators, but they were unable to isolate the active chemical and the project was dropped. *Oplopanax japonicus* was once used in Japan for diabetes. Neither tea cured the patient, but it eliminated the need to inject insulin.

When supplies of drugs were cut off during WWII in the Philippines, pharmaceutical researchers began taking a look at the native plants of the islands. They collected 35 plants used for diabetes and found that five lowered blood sugar. They selected the leaves of a small tree *Lagerstroemia speciosa* for further development. The leaves are not highly active, and a concentrated solution had to be prepared. The first patient to receive it had a blood sugar level of 310. In eleven days it dropped to 172, and five days later it was at 125. This was sold in the drugstores of the Philippines.

Japanese researchers studied 31 plants used for diabetes in that country. *Rehmannia lutea* was the only effective remedy. French researchers evaluated a number of Chinese herbs, and found two that really lowered blood sugar. When a solution of *Rehmannia glutinosa* was injected into rabbits the blood sugar was 52% of its beginning value five hours later. An injection of *Atractylis ovata* lowered the blood sugar by 65% five hours later. The bark of *Rehmannia* is believed to block the effects of the immune system. Diabetes is generally an immune disorder, in which the immune system shuts down the insulin producing cells.

The kitchen spice turmeric is known to be helpful in some cases of insulin-resistant diabetes. In one case, a man in India wasn't able to control his blood sugar with high levels of insulin. By taking spoonfuls of turmeric, his blood sugar returned to normal levels.

Mathew King, a Native American spiritual elder, related his experience with diabetes in *Wisdomkeepers*. "Once while I was up on the mountain, I prayed to God to give us a cure for diabetes. And while I was there somebody said, "turn around." So I turned around and there was the most beautiful Indian woman I'd ever seen. She had long black hair and the most wonderful face. She was holding something out to me in her hand. It was those little berries of cedar, the dark blue berries on cedar trees. She held them out, but before I could reach out my hand she disappeared."

King spent time in the hospital with his diabetes, and then he remembered the vision that White Buffalo Calf Woman had given to him. He picked the berries of *Juniperus communis* and made a tea of them. He believed that the bitter tea took the sugar right out of his body.

This was the remedy used by the herbalist Dr. John Christopher. He once had a diabetic tell him that after taking a tea of the berries, he didn't need so much insulin. Doctor Christopher tried out the remedy on other diabetics and made a mixture of herbs for all of his diabetic patients. Some scientific work has been done with the berries in Spain. They do not seem to be a cure, but they allow the body to use insulin more efficiently.

In Pakistan, doctors did a trial of *Momordica charantia* powder on people with maturity-onset diabetes at a dosage of 50 mg./kg. Eight people taking the powder found that it eliminated the sugar in the urine in a week. Their average blood glucose level dropped from 246 mgs. to 155 mgs. The results were promising enough to suggest that many diabetics would not have to depend on imported insulin for the control of their disease.

Coccinia indica is a vegetable growing in the Bengal area of India. The active principle is weak, and it takes about three weeks for it to have an effect. A group of diabetics were given either a placebo or tablets of the freeze-dried leaves of the plant. At the end of the six-week trial, people taking the placebo had an average fasting glucose level of 181. The people taking the herb had a glucose level of 122. Only three patients on the placebo showed any improvement, but 11 of the 16 taking the herb showed significant improvement.

The peasants of Egypt are known to drink a willow leaf tea *Salix* species when they have diabetes. When rats were made into diabetics with alloxin, their blood sugar returned to normal levels in about four weeks with the leaves. Some of the rats were apparently cured, but when they stopped using the leaves, the blood sugar began to rise again.

Another peasant diabetic remedy of Egypt is the fruit of **Balanites aegyptiaca**. When it is separated into individual saponins, there is no diabetic activity for each, but together they show significant activity.

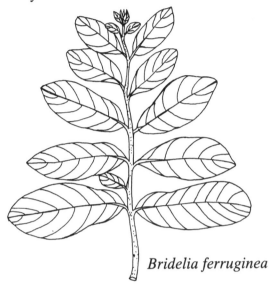

Bridelia ferruginea

The Institute for Traditional Medicine in Ghana, West Africa, reported on a woman who didn't like injecting insulin. She tried two local herbs known for diabetes. Each time her blood sugar went completely out of control she made a tea made of ten leaves of **Bridelia ferruginea** boiled in a pint of water. By drinking a cup of tea with each meal, it took 12 weeks to return her blood sugar level to normal.

In India the toadflax **Linaria muralis** was used in diabetes. It has a bitter unpleasant taste, and was also used in eye inflammation. Early in the twentieth century a Pennsylvania doctor reported that he discovered an excellent treatment for diabetes. This was the toadflax, also known as "butter and eggs" **Linaria vulgaris**. The folk name comes from the mixed yellow and white flowers. At the time of flowering, the upper parts of the plant are made into a tea. A half-cup of the tea is taken four times a day. The doctor never did make a complete report on his results.

Many of the old remedies are known, but remain untested. The Baja Peninsula of Mexico has a high incidence of diabetes. A survey of the local healers showed that the most common diabetic herbs are **Turnera diffusa, Hintonia latiflora** and **Bidens pilosa**.

It was once common for diabetics in the Eastern US to take a tea of **Chionanthus virginicus**. When taken with Epsom salts this was claimed to have excellent results.

In 1932 a major court case was fought over an herbal diabetic product. It was tested on 80 diabetics and the developers claimed that 60% of diabetics would not have to inject insulin, and the others who needed insulin could reduce the amount. The FDA's position was that only insulin cured diabetes, and that all plant preparations were quackery. Doctors testified on the witness stand that there was no historic evidence that diabetes was ever successfully controlled with herbs. They ignored at least a dozen articles in medical literature.

The winning of this case meant that all herbal preparations were taken off the market, and none were even tested for decades. Insulin is a highly profitable drug, and diabetes is a disorder that requires regular medical attention. Our medical system should be looking towards cures or controls, rather than promoting insulin along with the associated diabetic complications.

HERBAL DIABETIC CURES

"As to what belongs to the cure, it seems a most hard thing in this disease to draw propositions of curing, for that its cause lies so deeply hid, and its origin so deep and remote. For what is commonly thought, that the reins, and the other solid parts, containing or transmitting the serum and the blood are in the fault, because that they send away too hastily their contents. For that cause astringent medicines are chiefly and altogether to be insisted on. I say both reason and experience doth contradict both this hypothesis and practice. For that few or none are cured by this method; and it is highly improbable (if I may not say impossible) for that diuresis to proceed from such a cause."

Pharmaceutice Rationalis *Thomas Wills, +1617*

One of the important experiments on a recent space shuttle flight was the production of an ultrapure form of insulin in zero gravity. NASA officials told a group of gullible reporters that the new insulin might prove to be a cure for diabetes! Insulin is a medicine that replaces a deficiency, and it can never be a cure. The regeneration of the Islands of Langerhans of the pancreas, which produces insulin, would be a cure. Since it costs about $2,000 per pound to lift equipment and materials into orbit, an ultrapure form of insulin would be exceedingly expensive. Furthermore, nature usually does better with impure mixtures than pure substances.

The real answer to diabetes may lie in the genetic code, but answers appear to be in nutrition and herbs. Overweight people have a much higher rate of diabetes, so weight control is a key factor, as are the minerals zinc, chromium and manganese, which may be enzyme activators. Some vitamins are necessary to the health of the pancreas.

Doctor Aba de Hermany of Hungary believed that silicon was the secret of the diabetic plants used in folk remedies for diabetes. The most popular diabetic plants of Eastern Europe were nettles– *Urtica dioica,* yarrow— *Achillea millefolium, Galeopsis segetum* and *Polygonum aviculare.* The doctor produced a silicon water colloid of calcium silicate hydrate and a metasilicious hydrogel, which was widely used in Hungary and Yugoslavia. When given to a diabetic patient, the sugar in the urine decreased and the patient stopped craving water.

A 50 year-old woman was taking insulin and was put on a strict diet. Her condition steadily grew worse with much urination and fatigue. After taking three teaspoonfuls of the silicate, the sugar in the urine fell from 6% to 0.6% in two days. Her health returned, and there was no irritation or excess urination. In most cases the sugar disappeared from the urine with silicon; in others it reappeared after a few months, and then disappeared with a new dose of silica. Acetone is a mark of diabetes, and it disappears when silicon is taken. If insulin without silica is taken, the body continues to produce some acetone.

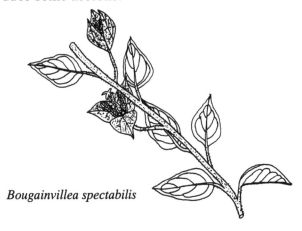

Bougainvillea spectabilis

Bougainvillea spectabilis is a plant from India, which is claimed to be a diabetic cure. An alcoholic extract of the leaves is very active and shows no toxicity. The agent is a form of the vitamin inositol known as pinitol. An oral dose of 10 mg./kg. is all that is necessary. Mice were given alloxin, which destroys the insulin-producing cells. The blood sugar rose to 270, but the mice given pinitol had a blood sugar level of 130 mg. Inositol has weak antidiabetic activity, but this form has potent activity, and may rejuvenate the pancreas, if the diabetes hasn't gone too far.

Scientists in India studied the antidiabetic action of the bark of ***Pterocarpus marsupium***, which was used in diabetes. Rats were given a chemical to destroy the insulin-producing cells, and then were given 1-epicatechin at a level of 30 mg./kg. The chemical regenerated the beta cells and produced a normal insulin level. The chemical is also present in the leaves of the hawthorn tree.

Some tribes of the Aligarh district of India use new leaves of the custard apple ***Annona squamosa*** and black pepper ***Piper nigrum*** against diabetes. Two to five leaves of the custard apple and five black peppers were mixed and taken every morning for three to eight weeks. Tests on diabetics showed that 80% benefited or were cured. It was adopted by some western-trained doctors in the areas.

A century ago James Dick was visiting a friend in New Zealand. His friend caught the flu, and a neighboring lady informed them that drinking a tea of eucalyptus leaves several times a day would cure the flu. It did go away, but at the same time his diabetes vanished. Dick took the remedy back to Edinburgh, Scotland, and gave it to a doctor for testing. He found that tablets of the pulverized leaves cured 15 out of 41 diabetic patients. It helped five others, and did nothing for the rest.

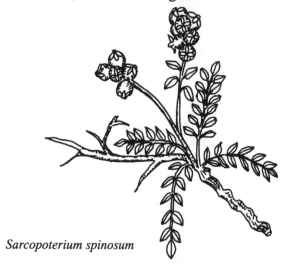

Sarcopoterium spinosum

The Bedouins of the Middle East had a thorny shrub ***Sarcopoterium spinosum = Poterium spinosum***, which they used to cure diabetes. The shrub does not decrease the blood sugar of normal people, but it acts in diabetes. A joint Syrian-German expedition was exploring the Syrian hills for new medical plants. They found that Bedouins with clinically diagnosed diabetes would boil the plant for about four hours to remove the extremely bitter taste, and then they would drink it for 30 to 40 days as a cure.

Doctor Stenmetz believed that the active principle stimulated the Islands of Langerhans in the pancreas and restored the insulin making function. The roots were only active during April through August, and most active in May and June. Different plants varied widely in their diabetic activity. The discovery was not commercialized.

Barbara Woodhouse, the famous British animal trainer, related an experience with diabetes in her book *Talking to Animals*. When she was training horses in Argentina she developed a severe case of diabetes and had to inject insulin twice a day. The condition grew worse until she was going into a diabetic coma. She lost so much weight that she looked like a skeleton, and was going blind. Her condition was deteriorating so rapidly, that she was considering suicide.

One weekend her ranch cook returned with fresh young leaves from the tree ***Phyllanthus sellowianus***. She was told that the natives used them as a diabetic cure, but the older branches were inactive. One the second day after taking the leaves as a tea, she stopped taking insulin. In six weeks she stopped drinking the tea, and the diabetes did not return. When she returned to England she brought along bundles of the leaves. She gave them to a friend who had taken insulin for 47 years. He was able to stop injecting insulin after drinking the tea for three days, but he had to continue drinking the tea to be free of diabetic symptoms.

One of the curious remedies of India is the use of ***Gymnema sylvestre*** leaves as a tea. The use is quite rational, for the tea abolishes the sweet taste of sugar. Its use as a diabetic remedy was believed to be mere superstition, since it didn't change the high levels of blood sugar or the sugar in the urine.

A recent study shows that the early researchers didn't wait long enough. Chemicals in the leaves slowly regenerate the isles of Langerhans. Studies with rats showed that the leaf extract doubled the number of beta cells in about a month. A 50% alcohol extract of the crushed dry leaves was given to 27 diabetics. All of them were able to slowly reduce the need for insulin. The extract offers hope as a cure when used long enough.

In Central America the Mayan healers used Billy Web bark *Acosmium panamense = Sweetia panamensis* to treat diabetes. The bitter bark was said to cure diabetes in about three months. It was also used for internal cleansing, dry coughs and uterine congestion.

In 1878 a Vermont doctor put down his herbal cure for diabetes in a medical journal. He was riding on a train, and opposite him were a man and his wife. The woman was so thirsty that she was drinking at least ten quarts of water a day. They had visited a number of doctors, and so far the woman was getting steadily worse, without a sign of a cure. After talking to him for a few minutes, Doctor Gerald wrote on a piece of paper: "Rx: *Lycopus virginicus* one ounce of the fresh plant to one pint of hot water. Take four to five tablespoonfuls per day."

The doctor didn't leave his address. A year later he was surprised to receive an enthusiastic letter from the traveler, who had gone to great lengths to track him down. The man wrote: "We tried your remedy and it proved just the thing. She is completely recovered, and is in good health and spirits. I have mentioned the matter to others having this affliction, and in each case it has worked wonders." He mentioned that he was sending a bushel of apples in gratitude for saving his wife's life, and that now he had located him, he wanted to pay the bill and give him a generous reward.

It is now known that many cases of diabetes are an immune disorder. The immune system recognizes the insulin secreting beta cells as foreign and destroys them. Both *Lycopus virginicus* and *L. europaeus* block the action of the immune system and keep the cells healthy. The Chinese diabetic herb *Rehmannia glutinosa* acts in the same way. Nigerian herbalists have claimed to cure a high percentage of diabetes with the roots of *Anthocleista vogelii* and *A. djalonensis*.

We often think of the wonder cures of the Amazon basin, and the remote areas of the world, but we have at least one interesting cure in the forests of the U.S. Around 1910 a Canadian doctor developed diabetes, and he began a series of experiments on himself. Red pepper reduced the excess blood sugar by half, and the effect lasted several weeks. *Grindelia robusta* also reduced the level of blood sugar. His surprise was finding that

an alcoholic extract of pipsissewa *Chimaphila umbellata* brought the blood sugar to normal in 23 days. It rose ten days later when he ate a great deal of starch, and then disappeared with more pipsessewa the next day. "Pipsissewa" is a Cree Indian word meaning "Its-juice-breaks-it." The idea refers to kidney stones.

It was tried on several people and these people were cured of their diabetes. Small doses didn't cure it, but larger amounts did. The results were printed in a medical journal, but doctors simply ignored it.

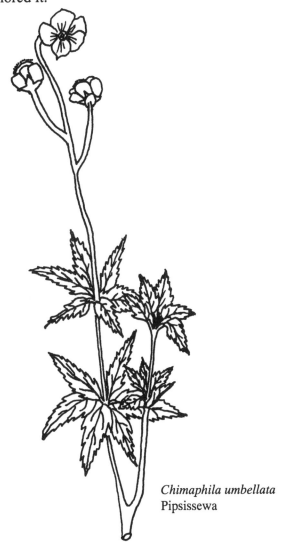

Chimaphila umbellata
Pipsissewa

The second part of the story happened around 1940. A geological engineer in Portland, Oregon, developed diabetes. His work demanded long stays in the wilderness, and he had difficulty controlling his diet and the amount of insulin. Then his marriage broke up, and he lost his job. Without money for medical care, he drove to a hunter's cabin in northeastern Oregon expecting to die. His condition deteriorated, and one-day an Indian woman who lived nearby stopped to talk. She remarked how bad he looked, and he told her that he had diabetes and no money for insulin.

The woman returned a little later with some fresh green leaves and told him to drink it as a tea either cold or warm, but he was not to heat it or it would be inactive. He drank the tea several times a day and recovered. Weeks later he stopped by to talk with his doctor in Portland. The doctor was interested and had the plant identified as ***Chimaphila umbellata***.

These observations were brought to Dr. Robin Williams, the head of the medical school at the University of Washington. He found that the enzyme arbutinase was the active material that controlled or cured diabetes. Tests of the enzyme were very encouraging, but no paper was put out. They found that the plants varied widely in activity, and experiments were carried out at two universities. At the time they were working with the plant, the first orally active form of insulin came out. The herbal extract was quietly shelved and remains almost unknown to this day. So we continue to take insulin, without realizing that the medical profession shelved an important cure.

PANCREATIC ENZYMES

"It is agni [fire] alone, that is located in the pitta, and gives rise to good and evil consequences, according as it is in a normal or an abnormal condition. These consequences are digestion and indigestion, vision and loss of vision, the normality and abnormality of temperature, the healthy and disease complexion, intrepidity and fear, anger and delight, confusion and lucidity and such other pairs of opposite qualities."

Charaka -600

A Japanese story tells about a farmer who was walking home through the woods when he saw a giant snake swallowing a man. Then the snake crawled up to a tree and finished up with some leaves. The farmer realized that the leaves were a digestive agent for the snake. Weeks later, he entered a village rice cake-eating contest. After eating a large stack, he finished up with some tree leaves. In a few minutes there was only a gelatinous pool on the floor with a mound of half-chewed rice cakes. The tree leaves contained a powerful digestive agent, but it was only good for digesting men!

This story isn't true, but it does illustrate the specificity of enzymes. Each enzyme does one thing, and it doesn't function outside of its job. The enzymes are the machines of the cells. Everything that is burned, built up, or broken down in the body is done with the aid of enzymes. When we have indigestion or allergies, our enzymes aren't functioning.

Life could not function without enzymes, and they are present in bacteria, fungi and higher forms of life. They are part of nature's recycling process in which matter decays, returns to the soil, and is in turn converted to new forms of life.

Perhaps the most powerful enzyme is found in the "nuytsia" ***Nuytsia floribunda,*** also known as the "West Australia Christmas tree." The US government tracking station near Perth, Australia had troubles with its underground communication lines. The roots of the nuytsia were dissolving the polyethylene cables. No known chemicals or enzymes can dissolve this plastic.

In 1833 two scientists published a report that an extract from malt changed starch into sugar.

They called the extract "diastase," from the Greek words meaning, "separating." In 1834, it was found that gastric juice could digest food in a test tube. The digestive substance was isolated and given the name of pepsin.

Our knowledge of the pancreas is largely related to the insulin, which it produces. Each of the million Islands of Langerhans has 3,000 insulin-producing cells scattered across the pancreas. This accounts for 1% of the cells of the pancreas. What does the other 99% of the pancreas do?

The pancreas is really two organs. The second function of the pancreas is the production of digestive enzymes, which act in the digestive tract. The acinus glands of the pancreas produce essen-

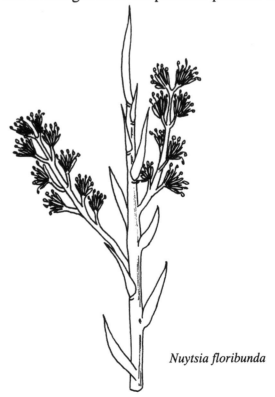

Nuytsia floribunda

tial digestive enzymes. Trypsin converts meat into amino acids. Chymotrypsin reduces milk into simpler molecules. Amylase breaks down complex sugars into simple sugars. Lipase changes fats into glycerin and fatty acids.

Food that has begun the digestive process in the stomach carries the hormone secretin and pancreozymin with it. When secretin reaches the pancreas, it triggers the flow of bicarbonates, which neutralizes the stomach acid. Pancreozymin stimulates enzyme secretion from the pancreas.

Just as a bad diet can contribute to diabetes, poor nutrition can contribute to poor secretion of digestive enzymes. It is known that some varieties of the avocado *Persea americana* have d-mannoheptulose, a substance that inhibits insulin secretion in animals and produces diabetes in some.

Cystic fibrosis is a disease that results from lack of pancreatic enzymes. Enzymes would normally break down the mucus-like material. With the material remaining unbroken, it clogs the lungs and causes severe breathing difficulties.

It is believed that food allergies result when not enough pancreatic enzymes react with the food in the stomach. The partially broken down foods trigger an immune response when they get into the blood. The herbs mentioned here may solve many problems with food allergies.

The liver and the pancreas have just as much to do with good digestion as the stomach or the intestinal tract. If their secretions are absent, we have dyspepsia or colic after eating. Hepatic (liver) colic makes eating so unpleasant that people develop anorexia, because the effects of eating are so disagreeable. It is not always clear where the disorder known as colic in babies originates. It may be 'pancreatic colic,' because a lack of pancreatic enzymes cause gas and digestive problems.

When rats were given supplements of amino acids, it was found that methionine increased the levels of the enzymes lipase and protase. Phenylalanine and isoleucine increased the levels of protase.

'Jureba,' the root of *Solanum paniculatum*, is an old remedy for improving digestion. Sufferers were once given one to three grams of the roots three times a day. The discomfort after meals improves rapidly and soon disappears. Although known as a 'hepatic herb,' it probably works on the pancreas.

Jureba is used in South America for gall bladder attacks. The appetite returns and there is no discomfort after meals. This indicates that it stimulates the pancreatic food-digesting enzymes.

The mint *Lycopus europaeus* was once used as a cure for diabetes, for it has something that blocks the immune system attack on the insulin-producing cells of the pancreas. It was once considered to be a valuable cure for digestive colic. The immune system may attack both the insulin-producing cells and the enzyme-producing cells.

A medical journal noted that around 1860 an Ohio root doctor was able to cure a case of flatulent colic after everything else had failed. His secret was *Lycopus europaeus*. The colic and digestive disturbances may have been due to lack of digestive enzymes from the pancreas. The herb restored them and brought the digestion back to normal.

Catharanthus roseus is an herb with hypoglycaemic activity, because it stimulates the insulin-secreting cells of the pancreas. Catharanthine is made from the alkaloids of this plant. Small amounts of this chemical triple the amounts of enzymes, and it is being actively researched for pancreatic disorders.

German researchers tested four herbs known to stimulate digestion to see if they stimulated either the liver or the pancreas. *Chelidonium majus*, *Artemisia absinthium* and *Curcuma longa* were

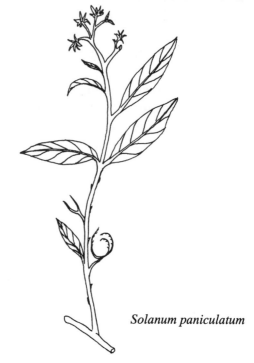

Solanum paniculatum

all strong cholagogues. ***Silybum marianum*** was a weak stimulant of lipase, the fat-splitting enzyme. Twenty minutes after being taken, turmeric (***Curcuma***) produced a modest increase in lipase and increased the starch-splitting enzyme by four times. A tincture of ***Chelidonium*** must have two active agents in it. Twenty minutes after being taken, it produced a rise in pancreas enzymes. This fell off to normal levels after an hour. Then it rose to a higher level after another 40 minutes. The lipase enzyme was increased by 17 times its normal values.

Inositol, the B Vitamin, is an active part of the starch-splitting enzyme alpha amylase. The leaves of the diabetic herb ***Bougainvillea spectabilis*** may be a powerful digestive tincture, for they are active in diabetes.

Lemon oil contains the terpenes limonin and limonene. These oils were enriched with zinc and copper and dissolved in alcohol. The mixture was called compound 561 and was tested in laboratory animals. An hour after taking the mixture, the level of pepsin in the stomach rose by five times and the level of hydrochloric acid was markedly increased. The compound doubled or tripled the production of the common pancreatic enzymes. Unlike substances that stimulate the release of pancreatic juices, this stimulated the production of enzymes in tests on dogs.

Perhaps the most powerful of all pancreatic stimulants is the sap of a small tree found in eastern Africa and Madagascar. A preparation based on ***Harungana madagascariensis*** has proven to be a miracle tonic for indigestion sufferers in Germany. It is a small tree with brilliant orange pigments in the sap. These contain anthroquinones, which are similar to those in rhubarb roots or cascara bark.

People who have suffered from indigestion and gas all their lives feel great after taking it. The problem with the herb is that after taking it regularly, the effect slowly wears off. In order to prolong the action, it is taken several times a week, with short rest periods, so that the stimulation doesn't wear off.

Since the extract of ***Harunga madagascariensis*** stimulates the digestive enzymes of the pancreas, would it also stimulate the insulin producing cells? It was tested on 22 diabetic patients and in seven cases the herb was able to control diabetes. That is a rather poor record for such an interesting herb.

In many cases, allergies are due to a lack of pancreatic enzymes to aid in the digestion of food. The stimulation of the enzyme-producing centers of the pancreas may greatly help people with allergies and cystic fibrosis. Little research has been done into this question.

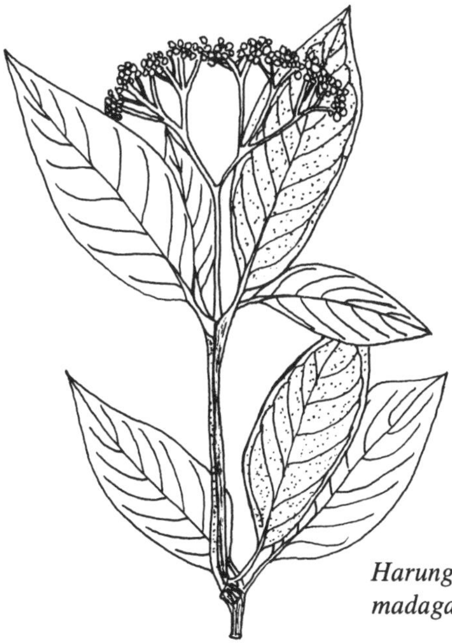

Harungana madagascariensis

☆☆☆

GOITER

"There were mountaineers,
Dew-lapp'd like bulls, whose throats had hanging at them,
Wallets of flesh."

Tempest *William Shakespeare*

"The inhabitants [of Yarcan] are also great craftsmen, but a large proportion of them have swollen legs and 'great crops' at the throat which arises from some quality in the drinking water."

Marco Polo

In previous centuries it was considered normal to have a bulging throat or a spare tire appearance about the neck. In the European Alps, people had such bulging protrusions about their necks that they became the basis for the misshapen figures that we find on old European buildings known as gargoyles. Paracelsus was the first to establish the relationship between cretinism and endemic goiter. Lack of iodine produced hunchback cretins, although nobody knew that it was due to the lack of a mineral. The German word 'kroph' meant goiter and in towns such as 'Krophsberg,' nearly everyone had goiter due to the lack of iodine.

In Tibet, medicine men developed theories to explain the different forms of throat swellings. There was the small 'lucky goiter,' which meant that you would become rich within a year. Then there was the 'unlucky goiter,' which meant that you would lose your job. Goiters were believed to be caused by bad karma, evil spirits, fatty meat and menstrual blockage. Doctors advised exercise and avoiding crayfish, oranges and peaches.

Around +1180, Roger of Palermo recommended the ashes of burned sponges and seaweed in treating goiter. In 1811 iodine was isolated from burnt seaweed. Five years later William Prout tried using it as a medicine. In 1820 Jean Coidet gave a tincture of iodine to 150 people with goiter, and an effective agent had finally been discovered.

The problem of goiter is paradoxical, because it normally results from the lack of iodine in food and drinking water. However, in places along the ocean, where people eat a lot of iodine-rich seaweed, goiters can result from too much iodine.

Robert McCarrison investigated the problems of health and nutrition in the villages along the Himalayas. He found that villages at the headwaters of streams had few goiters, but villages downstream had increasing numbers of goiters. He had a group of people drink boiled downstream water and another group drank the same unboiled water. The second group had signs of goiter in a few weeks. The communities upstream dumped their sewage into the water, and the bacteria in the water blocked iodine metabolism, and caused goiter.

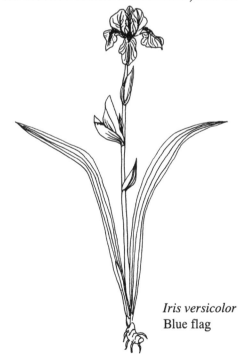

Iris versicolor
Blue flag

There are a number of poultice type remedies which might have reduced the swelling of the neck. A steamed leaf of **Cynoglossum macrostylum** was said to rapidly reduce goiters when used as a poultice. A water cream of **Iris versicolor** was said to take three days to reduce goiters when put over the throat. A few drops of iris tea several times a day was reported to have reduced large goiters down to normal in two or three months. In the US an ointment of **Phytolacca americana** was reported to reduce goiter. A poultice of cypress leaves **Cupressus** species was pulverized and mixed with wine and put on the goiter. Each day a new poultice was applied, and a cure for goiter was supposed to take about a week.

There are a number of plants taken as teas to aid in the reduction of goiter. Goiter was common among the Siberians because of their habit of eating fish and 'sea cabbage' (kelp). They drank a tea of 'goiter grass' **Phlomis tuberosa**. In Russia a tea of **Veronica officinalis** was also used for reducing goiters. Russian healers used a tea of **Genista tinctoria** for all thyroid disorders. In India the goiter herbs are **Eichhornia crassipes** and **Bauhinia variegata**. In Europe a tea of **Clematis graveolens** was reported to cure goiter.

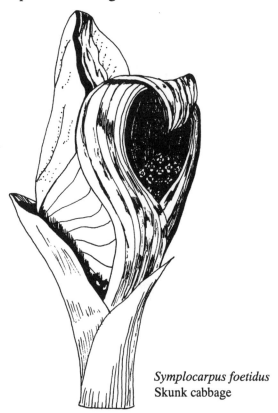

Symplocarpus foetidus
Skunk cabbage

The early settlers of the US found that skunk cabbage **Symplocarpus foetidus** contained something that reduced goiter. In early spring, the plant reduced goiters effectively, but it was ineffective in July. The plant has a high level of iodine, but it seems to contain both thyroid stimulants and inhibiting factors.

Just as there are plants which cure goiter, there are plants which cause goiters. Cabbage, rutabagas and onions are all goiter-causing plants. They contain chemicals that block the use of iodine by the thyroid. In 1943 Edwin Astwood isolated the thyroid blocking agents, and they were tried in overactive thyroids. When large amounts of English walnuts **Juglans regia** are eaten they will produce goiter. In countries where they are a common part of the diet, neck swelling is common.

There was an epidemic of goiter among school children in Australia caused by a free milk program in the public schools. The farmers found that they could raise large amounts of feed for their cattle by growing kale **Brassica oleracea acephala**. The goiter-causing chemicals got transferred into the milk and caused problems.

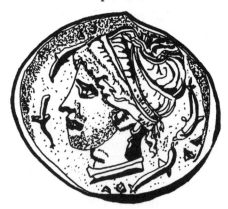

Greek coin with goiter

Aristotle was the first Greek writer to describe goiter. He thought that people with a thick neck were spirited and rash. On the Greek coins of this era, we find that the Greek gods Apollo and Athena suffered from goiter. Many other historic figures, including Cleopatra, are shown with a goiter.

The Chinese were believed to have discovered the first therapy for goiter in -1600 by giving patients burnt sponges and seaweed. Pliny mentions their medical use, but he does not specifically relate them to goiter in Roman times. The medical school of Salerno that dominated Europe during medieval times used seaweed and sponges to treat thyroid problems.

The link between iodine, goiter and seaweed was much slower to be established. The great geographer Alexander von Humboldt studied the frequency of goiter in the mountains of South America during his trips there from 1799 to 1804. He noted that goiter was present where there was great variation of day and night temperatures. It was also present where there was little variation, so that couldn't be the cause. He noted the legend that people from the mountain, who went down to the hot valley of Rio San Francisco, lost their goiters. When his donkey driver went down into the valley, his goiter became about a third smaller.

It surprised von Humboldt to find that goiter had appeared in Santa Fe de Bogota, only 30 years prior to his visit. The residents attributed this disease to the 'impurity' of the Zipaquira salts. Through the years they switched supplies of salts. The old salt had been 'contaminated' with iodine, and the new salt was free from it.

In 1811 Bernard Courtois was using kelp to manufacture saltpeter, which he obtained from the beaches of Normandy. He burned the seaweed and added sulfuric acid to it. Violet vapors rose from the reaction and condensed into glistening black crystals. He took the crystals to the leading chemists of the time, and they identified it as a new element. It was named 'iodine' from the Greek word 'violet'.

Iodine is soluble in water, and over the centuries the rivers carry it into the oceans. Ocean plants collect iodine, and the dry weight may contain up to 1% iodine. In 1825 a French chemist made the connection between iodine and seaweed observations. In 1895 Eugene Bauman discovered that iodine worked in the thyroid gland. This launched a new fad; people wore little bottles of iodine around the neck, as a charm to keep away goiter.

Iodine alone doesn't always stimulate thyroid activity. If the thyroid isn't producing enough thyroxin, we are always tired, fatigued, and possibly overweight. The thyroid controls the amount of energy and muscle strength. We need an active thyroid to function well. Pantothenic acid of the B vitamin group stimulates the activity of the thyroid. The triply unsaturated fat in flax oil is another thyroid stimulant. These work with iodine in keeping us healthy and energetic.

A young man developed a cyst on the thyroid, which had to be removed along with part of the thyroid gland. A week later he began to yawn frequently. As his pulse rate slowed, the yawning rate increased. This led to the idea that yawning was a mechanism which squeezes the thyroid gland when the body needs more thyroxin. Yawning compresses the gland, and thyroxin gets into the blood and contributes to the wake-up process. When he was given the thyroid hormone, he stopped yawning.

Although the cause of goiter was known, it took more than a hundred years to overcome the problem. A study was done of thousands of school children at Akron, Ohio, and nearly 50% of them had mild goiter, which was preventable by trace amounts of iodine. This stimulated a search of simple methods to prevent goiter. The addition of iodine to salt and the availability of ocean fish have made goiter uncommon.

GRAVES' DISEASE

"I met a gentleman in my village very frequently, but had no opportunity of examining him. He presented the hairless face and head, the heavy swollen features, the slow speech and movements characteristic of the disease. Meeting his medical man, who was also at this seaside village for a spell, I asked what was the matter with the patient. He told me that there was absolutely nothing amiss, that he had seen many consultants and all agreed that he was free from ailment. Three days later myxoedema was described; and on reading it I promptly wrote to my friend and colleague, but as up to that time no remedy had been found, the result was inevitable."

Alexander Campbell 1883

There are three common thyroid problems and many conditions requiring the expertise of a specialist. The most common is probably an underactive thyroid, which results in overweight, and general sluggishness. An overactive thyroid resulted in thin, active, nervous people. Graves' disease is caused by the immune system attacking the thyroid gland. Combinations of this disorder and a lack of iodine create a mixture of thyroid conditions that baffled early doctors.

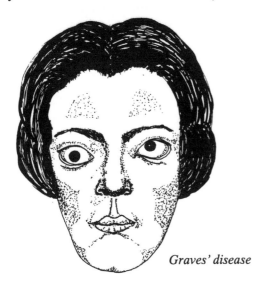

Graves' disease

In 1835 Robert Graves published this description of a disorder. "Lady aged twenty, became affected with some symptoms which were supposed to be hysterical. This occurred more than two years ago; her health previously had been good. After she had been in this nervous state about three months, it was observed that her pulse had become singularly rapid. This rapidity existed apparently without any cause and was constant, the pulse being never under 120, and often much higher. She next complained of weakness on exertion and began to look pale and thin. Thus she continued for a year, but during this time she manifestly lost ground on the whole, the rapidity of the heart's action having never ceased. It was now observed that the eyes assumed a singular appearance, for the eyeballs were apparently enlarged, so that when she slept or tried to shut her eyes, the eyes were incapable to closing. When the eyes were open the white sclerotic could be seen to a breadth of several lines all around the cornea."

Robert Graves got the credit for the first good English description. At about the same time other European doctors called it Parry's disease, Flajani's disease and Basedow's disease. The puzzled doctors described the swollen throat, the bulging eyes, the fast heartbeat and the tremor of the hands. It affects 19 out of a thousand women, but less than two of the same number of men.

It has been called hyperthyroidism, but the thyroid does not seem to be more active than normal. It is also called toxic goiter, hyperplastic goiter and dysthyroidism. These names are a cover-up for our ignorance. The skin yellows with the disorder because a functioning thyroid is needed to convert carotene into Vitamin A. When the thyroids of laboratory animals are removed, the carotene level in the blood rises, but the amount of Vitamin A falls. The ability of the eye to adapt to dark conditions is also reduced.

The Romans realized that slaves with bulging eyes fatigued rapidly, and they had low value.

Aristotle mentions the disorder and remarks that people suffering from it were stupid. Around the year +900, the Byzantine Emperor Leon VI issued the *Vasilika*, a legislative work, distinguishing between disease and health. People with goiter and bulging eyes were considered to be healthy. In his time people with thyroid disorders were social outcasts, because bulging eyes were considered to be a sign of demon possession. In many areas the 'evil eye' is still a stigma.

The abnormal thyroid condition is often accompanied by phobias. When a survey was made of people with Graves' disease, 22 of 115 had monophobia, the fear of being alone. Another 15 people had ochlophobia, the fear of crowds, and some went out only at night when there were only a few people. When the thyroid problem was treated, the phobias went away.

The thyroid was thought to be a gland that merely speeded the rate of metabolism. In 1915 it was discovered that feeding thyroid to tadpoles caused them to metamorphose into frogs. It was then realized that the thyroid has a complex action on the entire body.

Since the thyroid hormone controls the metabolism of the body, and is important to growth, an underactive thyroid will literally slow the body down and make a child appear sluggish. It slows down heat production and people with poor thyroid activity tend to have lower body temperatures. The problem appears more often in women and interferes with the menstrual cycle. It can be diagnosed by taking the body's temperature first thing in the morning, before exercise increases it. It is usually treated with thyroid extract.

Vitamin F, which is a mixture of unsaturated fatty acids, increases the activity of the thyroid. Flax oil is the richest source of the triple unsaturated fatty acids. When the oil was used in large quantities to reduce the swelling of the prostate in older men, the goiters of several men were reduced. The oil decreased the calcium in the blood by 11%, increased the phosphorus by 8% and increased the iodine by 307%.

Pantothenic acid is an essential vitamin which stimulates lactobacillus flora. It increases the activity of the thyroid, and protects the thyroid from toxic conditions. It is found in yeast and in tomato juice.

Thyrotoxicosis seems to be accompanied by low levels of Vitamin B12. This vitamin restores the ability of the cells to function normally. No tests have been done on humans, but the results on animals show definite benefit.

Vitamin E is useful in autoimmune disease. The vitamin repairs the membranes and this prevents the escape of enzymes that alter tissue proteins and cause the formation of autoimmune antibodies. Levels of a thousand units of Vitamin E have done wonders over a period of about six months in clearing up skin disorders caused by autoimmune diseases.

Many reports have appeared on the remarkable properties of a chemical found in *Coleus barbatus = C. forskolii*. Forskolin is a potent activator of the cyclic AMP generating system. This system activates and generates the muscular response of the body. It is a powerful stimulator of an underactive thyroid.

In Russia and Eastern Europe *Genista rumelica = G. lydia* var. *rumelica* is used to treat thyroid problems. It increases the heartbeat, breathing rate, and the general muscular tone. Ironically enough, it seems to decrease the action of the thyroid. Speedwell *Veronica officinalis* is another treatment for Graves' disease. Two cups of the tea are drunk daily.

In 1925 a British doctor claimed that manganese was an active nutrient for the thyroid. When people with Graves' disease were given additional manganese they needed less thyroid extract, the skin color improved, and the swelling on the neck decreased. He found that symptoms associated with heart failure improved, which didn't respond to digitalis. The dropsy disappeared with the manganese. He claimed to have cured five cases of angina pectoris (chest pain) with potassium permanganate.

The action of boron is little understood in the body, but it has cured some cases of Graves' disease. In one instance a patient was treated with x-rays, electrotherapy and quinine without improvement. Each day the patient took three grams of sodium borate. Soon the heartbeat fell to 90 and the tremor and insomnia disappeared. The patient gained weight, and the enlarged thyroid was reduced to half its volume.

A 50 year-old woman had persistent heart palpitation and an enlarged thyroid. She took two to four grams of sodium borate in a 5% water solution by mouth after meals. In three weeks her pulse fell from 120 to 80 and she began to gain weight.

Another method of treating the hyperactive thyroid is to give people massive doses of Vitamin A. Taking 200,000 to 400,000 units of Vitamin A reduces sweating, irritability, nervousness, and tremors of the hands. In one case taking 300,000 units of A for a week reduced the pulse from 120 to 109 and the feelings of nervousness left. After three more weeks the pulse fell to 88 beats per minute and all symptoms disappeared. Other reports indicate that it may take several months of high levels of Vitamin A to bring the thyroid activity back to normal.

The standard medical treatment for the disorder was to have the person take a solution of radioactive iodine. The radiation destroys the excess cells of the thyroid and the difficulty disappears. While taking high levels of Vitamin A for more than a few weeks has some risk, it is probably more effective and less dangerous than using radiation.

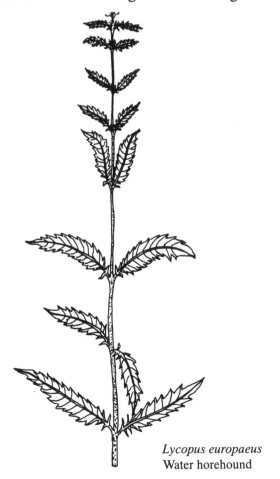

Lycopus europaeus
Water horehound

One person accidentally discovered help for his thyroid problem characterized by a rapid pounding heart and weakness. After taking four teaspoonfuls of lecithin granules per day, he no longer needed thyroid medication. When the lecithin was stopped, the heart began to pound again.

It now appears that the mysterious thyroid disorder is an autoimmune system disorder in which immunoglobins in the blood attack the thyroid, causing it to swell. They recognize the body's own tissues as being foreign. It is interesting to find that the same herb is listed in old medical accounts as a cure of Graves' disease and diabetes. This herb had substances which block the receptor-binding ability of immunoglobulins.

The inhibitors in *Lycopus europaeus* and *L. virginicus*, which bind the TSH (thyroid stimulating hormone) and prevent it from stimulating the adenylate cyclase in the thyroid membranes, are chiefly ellagic and caffeic acids. It was first reported as a cure for diabetes in 1856, and by 1911 it was found to be a cure for Graves' disease. The reports were forgotten and are virtually unknown today.

A woman had been a missionary to the slums, but she had to give it up, because of weakness, shortness of breath and rapid heartbeat. She went to Hahneman Medical College with the signs of Graves' disease, which were tremors of the hands and marked exophthalmos (bulging eyes). They told her that the problem was incurable. Fortunately she found a doctor who prescribed *Lycopus virginicus*. By drinking the tea there was a slow gradual improvement and she was normal in about a year.

A 41 year-old schoolteacher had a pulse of 116. He was unable to sleep, his hands trembled and with the slightest exertion, he was out of breath. He began by taking five drops of a *Lycopus* tincture. It took him two years to return to being completely normal.

There has been interest in Europe in using *Lycopus* to treat endocrine and autoimmune disorders. Water extracts of the leaves have weak activity, but alcoholic extracts have strong activity. Curiously enough, as the phenolic components in the leaves oxidize, they become more active.

In Ukrainian folk medicine *Potentilla alba* was used to treat headaches, palpitation, tachycardia and sleeplessness. The root tincture had high thera-peutic activity without adverse reactions. From 1-3 tablespoonfuls of the tincture were taken 2-3 times a day. This produced a decrease in the size of the thyroid. The tachycardia, tremor, blood pres-sure, and cholesterol levels returned to normal. In a test of 19 people, all received significant benefit, but not all were cured.

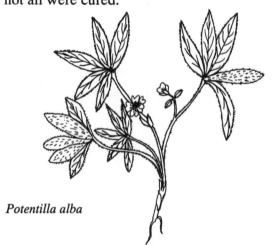

Potentilla alba

case a patient had been treated with iodine and thy-roid extract and was steadily getting worse. Tak-ing small amounts of goldenseal after meals for six weeks cured her.

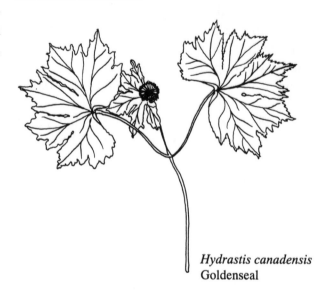

Hydrastis canadensis
Goldenseal

Goldenseal *Hydrastis canadensis* has an ef-fect on immune system disorders of the thyroid. During pregnancy the immune system is de-pressed, or is sensitive due to foreign proteins from the pregnancy, and goiter may appear at this time. A British doctor treated 25 cases of goiter and cured them in six weeks to three months. In one

These herbs may affect other immune system disorders. Multiple sclerosis, some allergies, neu-ralgias and palsies are disorders in which the im-mune system attacks the nerves or causes pain. The herbs may not be a cure, but they could be a help-ful therapy to problems which have no ready an-swers.

✿ ✿ ✿

BIBLIOGRAPHY

Note:All titles have been put into English for the sake of my readers. I have listed the titles in the way that a person would find them when going into a large university library. Books are listed by author first.

1 HEADACHE HERBS

Acta Medica Philippina 1:1, 199, 1964 "Effects of an Azasteroidal Alkaloid from *Kibatalia gitingenesis*" H.R. Estrada

Arzneimittelforschung 27:2039, 1977 "Anti-nociceptive Substances from the Roots of *Angelica acutiloba*" S. Tanaka et al.

Brain 20:194, 1897 "The Diet Treatment of Headache, Epilepsy and Mental Depression" A. Haig et al.

Clinical Journal of Pain 5:49, 1985 "Beneficial Effect of Capsaicin Application to the Nasal Mucosa in Cluster Headache" F. Sicuteri et al.

Curare 3:203, 1980 "Folk Phytotherapeutic Methods Used in Poland for the Relief of Headaches" A. Paluch

Drugs of the Future 4:216, 1981 "Butylidenephthalide" K. Hillier

Giornale Medico di Roma 1:601, 1865 "*Verbena officinalis* in Certain Headaches" A. Gavini

Headache 1:Jan/21, 1962 "Clinical Study of Headache Relief with a Niacin Containing Compound" H.D. Ogden et al.

Journal of Ethnopharmacology 36:193, 1992 "Headache Treatments by Native Peoples of the Ecuadorian Amazon" E.B. Russo

Lancet 1:143, 1906 "On the Relief of Certain Headaches by the Administration of One of the Salts of Calcium" G.W. Ross

Laryngoscope 61:138, 1951 "Headaches and Vertigo Associated with Hypoglycemic Tendency" J.A. Harrill

Medical and Physical Journal 1:286, 1799 "Dissertation on the Sick Headache" N. Dwight

Medical Record 153:404, 1941 "A Clinical Study of the Effect of Desiccated Garlic on Intestinal Flora" E. Weiss

Medical Standard 6:171, 1889 "Potassium Iodide for Headache" J.H. Bertrand

New England Journal of Medicine 235:541, 1946 "The Cause, Relief and Prevention of Headaches Arising from Contact with Dynamite" A.M. Schwartz

New York Academy of Medicine; Bulletin 48:661, 1972 "Headaches in History and Literature" A.P. Friedman

Planta Medica 50:331, 1984 "2-Acylindole Alkaloids from the Leaves of *Pterotaberna inconspicua*" P. Bakana

Plantes Medicinales et Phytotherapie 21:47, 1987 "Contribution to the Pharmaceutical Study of *Scabiosa atropurpura*" E.M. Requena et al.

Plantes Medicinales et Phytotherapie 21:285, 1987 "Study of an Active Analgesic and Antipyretic from *Dittrichia viscosa*" W. Greuter

Practitioner 42:337, 1889 "The Diagnosis and Treatment of Headaches Accompanied by Diminished or Increased Blood Pressure" E.L. Jones

Prevention 19:May/28, 1967 "Herb for Headache" C.T. Grant

Prevention 23:Oct/232, 1971 "Headaches Relieved with Vitamin E" F. Roberts

Prevention 23:Nov/40, 1971 "Eyesight and B_{12}" M. Burke

St. Louis Eclectic Medical Journal 7:292, 1880 "Remedies for Headache" L.H. Washington

2. MIGRAINE HEADACHES

American Journal of Clinical Nutrition 41:774, 1985 "Amelioration of Severe Migraine by Fish Oil (W-3) Fatty Acids" T. McCarren

British Medical Journal 2:1133, 1923 "Treatment of Migraine by Calcium Lactate" A.D. Bigland

British Medical Journal 291:569, 1985 "Efficacy of Feverfew as a Prophylactic Treatment of Migraine" E.S. Johnson et al.

Chinese Medical Journal 92:260, 1979 "Radix Puerariae in Migraine" G. Xiuxian et al.

International Archives of Allergy 7:205, 1955 "Historical Development of the Ergot Therapy of Migraine" E. Rothlin

Journal of Ethnopharmacology 29:267, 1990 "Ginger (*Zingiber officinale*) in Migraine Headache" T. Mustafa et al.

Journal of the American Osteopathic Association 49:502, 1950 "The Effects of dl-Methionine and Some Members of the B Complex on Migraine" A.P. Cline et al.

Lancet 2:412, 1959 "Mechanism of Migraine" J. Hamilton

Lancet 2:446, 1966 "A New Remedy for Migraine" E. Ask-Upmark

Medical Age 7:392, 1889 "Cascara Sagrada in Migraine" S.E. Morgan

Minnesota Medicine 9:87, 1926 "Calcium Lactate as a Preventive in Migraine" C.E. Riggs

Quarterly Journal of Crude Drug Research 1:104, 1961 "Tonga" E.F. Steinmetz

Semaine Therapie 43:307, 1967 "Migraine and *Fumaria officinalis*" Y. Barre

Therapeutic Gazette 5:77,187,437, 1881 & 7:260, 1883 & 10:424, 1886 (Articles on Tonga)

Therapeutische Monatschefte 1:138, 1887 "Treatment of Migraine with a Home Remedy (Salt)" S. Rabow

Union Pharmaceutique 64:323, 1923 "Analgesic Action of Camomile" H. Leclerc

Berzelius, Jons *Jons Jacob Berzelius; Autobiographical Notes* Royal Swedish Academy of Sciences, 1934

3. ORIGINS OF MENTAL PROBLEMS

Arzneimittelforschung 11:49, 1967 "Phytogenic Drugs as Remedies Against Central Nervous and Mental Disorders" V.H. Haas

Canadian Psychiatric Association Journal 18:41, 1973 "Lactate Infusion in the Treatment of Free-floating Anxiety" J.A. Bonn et al.

Diseases of the Nervous System 9:231, 1948 "Thyroid Therapy in Some Mental Disorders" L. Danziger et al.

Journal of the Arkansas Medical Society 14:75, 1917 (Discussion) C.S. Peltus

Journal of the American Medical Association 90:880, 1929 "Cerebral Stimulation" A. Loven et al.

Journal of the Formosa Medical Medical Association 78:61, 1979 "A Study on the Antihypertensive Action of Uncarine" C.C. Chang et al.

Journal of the National Medical Association 58:12, 1966 "Relative Hypoglycemia as a Cause of Neuropsychiatric Illness" H.M. Salvzer

Lancet 1:70, 1976 "Does Phenylethylamine Cause Schizophrenia?" M. Sandler et al.

Medical Hypothesis 34:131, 1991 "Subtle Vitamin B_{12} Deficiency and Psychiatry: A largely Unnoticed but Devastating Relationship?" J. Dommisse

Medical Record 150:303, 1939 "Vitamin B Therapy in Inflammatory and Degenerative Diseases of the Nervous System" W.J. McCormick

Military Medicine 140:101, 1975 "Significance of Abnormal Liver Function" R.L. Farrel et al.

New Scientist 100:46, 1983 "Eat Your Way to Mental Health" G. Fery

New Scientist 148:Oct 7/50, 1995 "Which Doctor?" P. Aldhous

New York State Journal of Medicine 30:1430, 1930 "The Cure of Suicidal Ideas by Lowering of the Diastolic Pressure" J. Benjour

Post-Graduate 21:810, 1906 "Isotonic Sea Water in the Treatment of Mental Diseases" Dr. Marie et al.

Scientific American 220:Feb/69, 1969 "The Biochemistry of Anxiety" F.N. Pitts Jr.

South Dakota Journal of Medicine and Pharmacy 5:243, 1952 "Bacteriological Studies in Idiopathic Epilepsy and Schizophrenia" E.C. Rosenow

Southwestern Journal of Anthropology 27:259, 1971 "A Traditional African Psychiatrist" R.B. Edgerton

Levinson, Harold N. *Phobia Free* New York: N. Evans and Company, Inc, 1986

4 MENTAL ILLNESS HERBS

Annales Medico-Psychologiques 95:452, 1937 "Using *Orthosiphon stamineus* to Treat Psychosis Due to Liver-Kidney Insufficiency" J. Trillot et al.

Arogya – Journal of Health Science 2:136, 1976 "Action of *Luffa tuberosa* on Septal Rats" K.S. Karanth et al.

Fate 27:Jan/49, 1974 "Can Fasting Cure Mental Illness?" S. Drippner

Indian Journal of Psychiatry 4:8, 1962 "Preliminary Report of an Indigenous Drug *Acorus calamus* in Psychiatric Disorders" N.G. Fozedar et. al.

Indian Journal of Psychiatry 6:131, 1964 "Clinical Observations of *Paspalum scrobiculatum*" L.P. Shala et al.

Journal de Practischen Arzneykunde und Wundarzneykurst 71, 1795 "The Workings of Gratiola in Insanity" L.F. B. Lentin

Journal of Research in Ayurveda and Siddha 1:333, 1980 "Studies on the Anti-Anxiety Effect of the Medhya Rasayana Drug Brahma (*Bacopa monniera*)" R.H. Singh et al.

Lancet 1:1030, 1889 "Pilocarpine in Threatening Mania" E.F. Willoughby

Lancet 1:1236, 1972 "Cholinergic Reversal of Manic Symptoms" D.S. Janowsky et al.

London Medical and Physical Journal 42:197, 1819 "*Hedera sylvestris* in Treating Mania" E. Sutliffe

London Medical Journal 6:120, 1785 "Account of the Effects of Camphor in a Case of Insanity" W. Oliver

Menninger Clinic Bulletin 29:256, 1965 "Ancient Psychopharmacotherapy" P.E. Feldman

Nagarjuin 8:426, 1965 "Certain Herbal Remedies for the Treatment of Mental Illness in Indian Medicine" R.H. Singh

Philosophical Transactions of the Royal Society 35:347, 1727 "Touching the Efficacy of Camphor in Manical Disorders" D. Kinneir

Pisani 84:327, 1960 "Sialic Acid in Neuropsychiatry" A. Scoppa

Practitioner 17:7, 1875 "A Contribution to the Investigation of the Therapeutic Action of Hyoscyamine" R. Lawson

Publication of the University of Ibadan #25:1, 1971 "The Traditional Background of Medical Practice in Nigeria"

W.H.O. Chronicle 3:436, 1977 "Traditional Healing Methods for Mental Disorders" T.W. Harding

5. SCHIZOPHRENIA

American Journal of Psychiatry 92:201, 1935 "The Aschner Treatment of Schizophrenia" K.E. Appel et al.

American Journal of Psychiatry 141:1034, 1984 "Ladislas Meduna and the Origins of Convulsive Therapy" M. Fink

British Journal of Psychiatry 122:240, 1973 "Pyridoxine and Schizophrenia" L. Bucci

International Journal of Addiction 13:375, 1978 "Apomorphine Revived; Fortified, Prolonged and Improved Therapeutic Effect" S.A.L. Halvorsen et. al.

Journal of Applied Nutrition 27:#2/9, 1975 "Copper, Zinc, Manganese, Niacin and Pyridoxine in the Schizophrenic" C.C. Pfeiffer et al.

Journal of Orthomolecular Psychiatry 3:301, 1974 "Controlled Fasting Treatment for Schizophrenia" A. Cott

New Scientist 85:642, 1980 "A Singular Solution for Schizophrenia" D. Horrobin

Pharmaceutical Journal 51:618, 1882 "The Hellebores of the Ancients" C.W. Dod

Psychiatrisch-Neurologische Wochenschrift 36:73,1934 & 36:79, 1934 "The Aschner Method of Treating Schizophrenia in Women" R. Carriere

Psychopharmacologia 2:295, 1961 "Effect of *Paspalum scrobiculatum* Extract on Acutely Disturbed Schizophrenia Patients" U.R. Deo et al.

Rivista di Patologia Nervosa e Mentale 43:424, 1934 "Action of Lobelin Injected Into Catatonic Patients" I. Rizzatti et al.

Science 191:401, 1976 "Wheat Gluten as a Pathogenic Factor in Schizophrenia" M.M. Singh et al.

Science 200:567, 1978 "Schizophrenic Symptoms Improve with Apomorphine" C.A. Tamminga et al.

Aschner, Bernhard *The Art of the Healer* New York: Dial Press, 1942

6. THE TRANQUILIZER STORY

Academie Royale de Medicine de Belgique Brusselles 1:567, 1967 "A Study of the Hypotensive, Diuretic and Tranquilization of Purified *Morinda* Extracts" J. La Barre et al.

Annales Pharmaceutiques Francaises 21:289, 1963 "On the Tranquilizing Action of Some Medical Herbs" R. Paris et al.

Antiseptic 39:197, 1942 "Insanity Herb *Rauwolfia serpentina* Benth." J.S. Chowhan

Archives Internationales Pharmacodynamie 143:41, 1963 "Pharmacodynamical Effect of a Volatile Fraction Isolated from *Seseli sibiricum*" K.S. Jamual et al.

Arzneimittelforschung 41:584, 1991 "Clinical Efficacy of a Kava Extract in Patients with Anxiety Syndrome" E.Kinzler et al.

Arzneimittelforschung 45:124, 1995 "Sedative Action of Extract Combinations of *Eschscholtzia californica* and *Corydalis cava*" H.L. Schafer et al.

Biochemical and Biophysical Research Communications 165:547, 1989 "Benzodiazepine-Like Molecules as Well as Other Ligands for the Brain Benzodiazepine Receptors, are Relatively Common Constituents of Plants" J.H. Medine et al.

British Medical Journal 2:789, 1928 "The Therapeutic Value of Valerian" Dr. Manson

C.R. Bulgare Academie des Sciences 30:1657, 1977 "Studies on the Central Depressive Action of Methanol Extract from *Geranium macrorhizum*" P.N. Manolov et al.

Current Therapeutic Research 16:621, 1974 "Glazlovine Versus Diazepam: A Double-blind Clinical Trial" B. Buffa et al.

Fracastoro 46:347, 1947 "A New Pharmaceutical with Neurosedative Action, An Extract of Coltsfoot *Petasites officinalis*" C.E. Baccaglini

Indian Journal of Medical Research 58:103, 1970 "A Pharmacological Study of *Cyperus rotundus*" N. Singh et al.

Journal of Ethnopharmacology 33:73, 1991 "Neuropsychopharmacologic Properties of a *Schumanniophyton problematicum* Root Extract" E. Amadi et al.

Journal of Pharmacology and Pharmacotherapy 19:170, 1967 "The Mechanism of the Tranquilizing Action of Asarone from *Acorus calamus*" M.K. Menon et al.

Life Sciences 1:225, 1962 "Tranquilizing Activity of Jatamansone- A sesquiterpene from *Nardostachys jatamansi*" R.B. Arora et al.

Medical History 2:87, 1958 "Notes on *Rauwolfia* and Ancient Medical Writings of India" K. Somers

Naturwissenschaften 51:411, 1964 "Pharmacological Screening of *Valeriana wallichi, Lallemntia royleana* etc." C. Chatterjee et al.

Presse Medicale 60:658, 1940 "Hypotensive Action of Somborg- *Blumea balsamifera*" H. Leclerc

Presse Medicale 70:2809, 1972 "The Tranquilizer of Helen of Troy" A. & P. Plichet

Recherche #295:84, 1997 "Is Peppery Kava, A Cure for Stress" V. Lebot

7   EPILEPTIC HERBS

Annales Pharmaceutiques Francaises 42:35, 1984 "Anticonvulsant Activity of *Onestis ferruginea*" C. Declume et al.

Brain 80:251, 1957 "The Conditioned Inhibition of Uncinate Fits" R. Efron

British Medical Journal 2:789, 1882 "Treatment of Epilepsy by Borax" S. Lockie

British Medical Journal 2:258, 1974 "Anticonvulsant Action of Vitamin D in Epileptic Patients" C. Christiansen et al.

Chicago Medical Journal 24:299, 1867 "Epilepsy Treated by Lactate of Zinc" C.F. Hart

Dublin Journal of Medical Science 22:327, 1856 "A Comparative View of the Effect of Some Remedies Used in Epilepsy" J. Osborne

Fitoterapie 53:147, 1982 "Studies on Some Plants Used as Anticonvulsants in Amerindian and African Traditional Medicine" S.K. Adesina

Indian Journal of Experimental Biology 4:99, 1966 "Effect of Marsiline on the Behavioral and Other Changes in the Central Nervous System Induced by Psychotropic Drugs" P.K. Day et al.

Indian Journal of Physiology and Allied Science 22:75, 1968 "The Anti-epileptic Potency of Some Phyto-Products With Special reference of EEG Changes" D.C. Dey

International Medical Digest 1:701, 1920 "Boron Salts in the Treatment of Epilepsy" P. Marie et al.

IRCS Medical Science 10:88, 1982 "Treatment of Epileptic Patients with the Chinese Herbal Medicine 'Saiko-seishi-to'" Y. Narita et al.

Journal of the American Medical Association 238:1805, 1977 "Low Manganese Level May Trigger Epilepsy" P. Sampson

Journal of Traditional Chinese Medicine 5:267, 1985 "Studies of Qingyangshen – root of *Cynanchum otophyllum*" K. Peigen et al.

Lancet 1:482,510, 1862 "On a Proposed Remedy for Epilepsy and Other Spasmodic Affections" J.W. Ogle

Massachusetts Magazine 3:157, 1791 "Experiments Made with the Common Cow Parsnip in the Relief of Epilepsy" J. Orne

Medical Age 4:153, 1886 "Peach-root Tea in Epilepsy" J.L. Dorset

Medical and Physical Journal 1:182, 1799 "Medicines Successfully Employed in Epilepsy"

Medical Life 37:167, 1930 "The Folklore and Cultural History of Epilepsy" L. Kanner

Ohio Medical and Surgical Journal 9:528, 1857 "*Paeonia officinalis* in the Convulsions of Children" Dr. Livezey

Pediatrics 20:33, 1957 "Intake of Vitamin B_6 and Infantile Convulsions" O.A. Bessy

Pharmaceutical Journal 177:274, 1956 "Studies on *Leontice Leontopetalum Linn.*" J. McSheffety et al.

Prevention 22:April/31, 1970 "B_6 Controls Convulsions" J. Nightingale

Southern Clinic 1:248, 1879 "A Case of Epilepsy – New Remedy, Apparent Cure" C.M. Shields

Therapeutic Gazette 8:108, 1884 "Burdock Seed in Epilepsy" W.H. Bentley

West Indian Medical Journal 35:121, 1986 "Demonstration of Anticonvulsant Properties of an Aqueous Extract of Spirit Weed *Eryngium foetidum*" O.R. Simon

8   PARKINSON'S DISEASE

Annals of Neurology 16:723, 1984 "Octacosanol in Parkinsonism" S.R. Snider

Archives of Neurology 24:869, 1930 "The Effect of Stramonium in Parkinsonism" E.D. Hoedimaker et al.

Bulletin de l'Academie de Medicine 100:801, 1929 "The Biological Action of Magnesium Salts" P. Delbert

Canadian Journal of Physiology and Pharmacology 49:1106, 1971 "Blockade of the Antiadrenergic Action of Bretylium of an Aqueous Extract of the Leaves of *Rhoeo spathacea*" M. Garcia et al.

Journal of Medicinal Chemistry 14: 463, 1971 "Seeds as Sources of L-Dopa" M.E. Daxenbichler et al.

Journal of the Royal Society of Medicine 84:491, 1991 "Treatment of Parkinson's Disease in Ayurveda" M. Gourie-Devi et al.

Journal of the Society of Oriental Medicine 7:49, 1956 "Treatment of Tremor and Muscular Rigidity with *Magnolia obovata*" K. Ogawa et al.

Lancet 2:640, 1969 "Beans- A Source of L-Dopa" B.H. Natelson

Medical Herald 9:348, 1887 "On the Treatment of Shaking-Palsy" J.C. McCartney

Medical Record 153:409, 1941 "Some Side-Effects in Vitamin B Therapy" W.J. McCormick

Planta Medica 48:43, 1983 "Neuromuscular Blocking Actions of Alkaloids from a Japanese Crude Drug (Flos Magnoliae) in Frog Skeletal Muscle" I. Kimura

Prevention 10:Oct/33, 1958 "A Treatment of Parkinson's Disease"

Southern Medical Journal 77:1577, 1984 "Treatment of Parkinson's Disease with L-Methionine" J.R. Smythies et al.

9 NERVE DISORDERS

Acta Pharmaceutica Sinica 9:486,566, 1984 "The Anticonvulsive Action of 3-N-butylphthalide and 3-N-Butyl-4, 5 Dihydrophthalide" Y. Shu-Ren et al.

American Journal of Medical Science 9:310, 1831 "Observations on the Remedial Powers of the *Cimicifuga racemosa* in the Treatment of Chorea" J. Young

Annals of Neurology 20:165, 1986 "Preliminary Trial of Colchicine in Chronic Progressive Multiple Sclerosis" H.J. Weinreb et al.

Archives of Dermatology 70:181, 1954 "Lupus Erythematosus" A.L. Welsh

British Medical Journal 1:600, 1975 "Myasthenia Gravis Associated with Penicillamine Treatment for Rheumatoid Arthritis" R.C. Bucknall et al.

Canadian Medical Association Journal 108:1356, 1973 "Multiple Sclerosis and Other Demyelinating Diseases" H.T. Mount

Chemical Abstracts 93:179,561, 1980 "Effect of Ganoderms on Elevated Serum Aldolase Levels in Experimental Muscular Dystrophy" G. Liu et al.

Chemical Abstracts 117:220,065, 1992 "Acetylcholine Esterase Inhibitors Containing Alkaloids [*Aristolochia fangchi*]" T. Yamaguchi et al.

Chemical Abstracts 121:73,903, 1994 "Treatment of Muscular Dystrophy with Glycyrhizine" Y. Antoku et al.

Diseases of the Nervous System 11:131, 1950 "Pyridoxine and Thiamin Therapy in Disorders of the Nervous System" S. Stone

Eyes, Ears, Nose and Throat Monthly 22:227, 1943 "Manganese Therapy of Myasthenia Gravis" E.M. Josephson

Garden 10:Nov/16, 1986 "New Use for a Time Tested Botanical [Colchicine]" H.J. Weinreb

Indian Journal of Experimental Biology 13:369, 1975 "Spasmolytic Constituents of *Cedrus deodare*" V.N. Puri et al.

Journal of Animal Science 17:1183, 1958 "Selenium, Vitamin E and Linseed Oil as a Preventive of Muscular Dystrophy in Lambs" J.F. Proctor et al.

Journal of the Geological Society of London 137:559, 1980 "Geomedicine in Norway [Selenium]" J. Lag

Journal of the Indian Medical Association 33:129, 1959 "Cyanocobalamin in Chronic Bell's Palsy" M. Mitra et al.

Medical Hypothesis 5:365, 1979 "Multiple Sclerosis: the Rational Basis for Treatment with Colchicine and Evening Primrose Oil" D.F. Horrobin

New England Journal of Medicine 293:152, 1975 "Choline for Tardive Dyskinesia" K.L. Davis et al.

New Zealand Medical Journal 99:639, 1986 "Bee Venom and Chronic Inflammatory Disease" R.B. Fisher

Presse Medicale 38:244, 1930 "The *Lotus corniculatus*" H. Leclerc

Revista Brasileira de Medicina e Farmacia 1:37, 1925 "Botanical and Pharmacognostic Studies of Muria Purama" R.A. Dias da Silva

Revue Neurologie 4:299, 1992 "A Pilot Study in Ginkgolide B, A Specific Inhibitor of PAF-Factor, in the Treatment of Acute Episodes of Multiple Sclerosis" B. Brochet et al.

10 PARALYSIS

Archives of Pediatrics 68:309, 1951 "Iodine in the Treatment of Poliomyelitis and Other Paralytic Diseases" R.R. Scobey

Brain 54:247, 1931 "Experimental Production and Degeneration in the Spinal Cord" E. Mellan

Fortscher der Therapy 15:333, 1939 "Treatment of Postdiphtheric Paralysis with Vitamin B_1" P. Feige

Free Radical Biology and Medicine 6:599, 1988 "Protective Effect of Vitamin E on Spinal Cord Injury By Compression and Concurrent Lipid Peroxidation" K. Iwasa

Indian Journal of Physiology and Pharmacy 5:174, 1961 "The Influence of Some Amino Acids on Neuromuscular Transmission" M. Sirsi

Journal of Research and Education in Indian Medicine 8:23, 1989 "Medicinal Plants and Plant Products Used by the Street Herbal Vendors in the Treatment of Poliomyelitis in Children" K.H. Sinha et al.

Journal of the American Institute of Homeopathy 49:145, 1956 "*Karwinskia humboldtiana*" E.G. Trevino

Journal of the American Medical Association 96:1858, 1931 "Treatment of Dementia Paralytica" C.A. Neymann

Medical Gazette 9:186, 1882 "The Opium Habit, Its Successful Treatment with *Avena sativa*" Dr. Sell

Medical Record 154:389, 1941 "The Nutritional Aspect of Bedsores" W.J. McCormick

Medical Record 155:45, 1942 "Indian Treatment of Paralysis" H. Jones

Minerva Medica 44:1193, 1953 "Observations on the Action of *Betula alba* in Polio Paralysis" D. Dadone

Muchener Medizinische Wochenschrift 78:1697, 1931 "The Treatment of Polio Myelitis with Veratrin" H.A. Stappert

Nature 255:166, 1975 "Domic and Quisqualic Acids As Potent Amino Acid Excitants of Frog and Rat Spinal Neurons" T.J. Biscoe et al.

New York State Journal of Medicine 45:1673, 1945 "Dermatologic Aspects of Poliomyelitis" J.G. Reyes

Presse Medicale 69:182, 1961 "Nivalin: A New Medication of Myasthenia and Neuro-muscular Dystrophies" M. Pestel

Prevention 16:May/17, 1964 "Magnesium, the Miracle Mineral" J.I. Rodale

South African Medical Journal 1:53, 1979 "The Effect of Allantoin in Cellular Multiplication and Degenerating and Regenerating Nerves" J.M. Loots et al.

Neveu, Auguste *La Polio Guerie* Montreuil, France: Vie Claire, 1963

11 THE MYSTERY OF PAIN

Acta Rheumatologica Scandinavica 8:161, 1962 "Pain: A Chemical Explanation" O. Lindahl

Advances in Pain Research and Therapy 5:305, 1983 "Use of D-Phenylalanine, an Enkephaline Inhibitor in the Treatment of Intractable Pain" K. Budd

Agriculture Research Reviews 9:#2/40, 1971 "Pain: Cultural Contexts in Research and Application" V.A. Christopherson

American Journal of Medical Science 197:766, 1939 "The Use of Vitamin B_1 in Rest Pain of Ischemic Origin" M. Naide

American Journal of Psychology 52:331, 1939 "Pain: History and Present Status" K.M. Dallenbach

Annals of Surgery 123:96, 1946 "Pain in Men Wounded in Battle" H.K. Beecher

Arzneimittelforschung 38:892, 1988 "Pharmacological Studies of Lappaconitine" M. One

Bulletin of the History of Medicine 48:540, 1974 "A Historical Phenomenological Study of Bodily Pain in Western Man" D. De Moulin

Journal of Pharmacy and Pharmacology 45:1046, 1993 "Potent Antinoceptive Activity of a Hydroalcoholic Extract of *Phyllanthus corcovadensis*: F. Gorski et al.

Nature 287:185, 1980 "What We Don't Know About Pain" P.D. Wall et al.

Nature 379:29, 1996 "Analgesic Effects of Myrrh" P. Dolara et al.

Obstetrics and Gynecology 29:275, 1967 "Bromelain Therapy for the Prevention of Episotomy Pain" G.I. Zatuchni et al.

Practitioner 26:132, 1881 Rapid Breathing as a Pain-Obtunder" W.G. Bonwill

Scientific American 204:Feb/41, 1961 "The Perception of Pain" R. Melzack

12 NEURALGIA

American Journal of Medical Science 73:304, 1877 "The Relationship of Pain to the Weather" S.W. Mitchell

American Journal of Surgery 59:83, 1943 "Control of Somatic Pain" W. Bates

British Journal of Hospital Medicine 1:46, 1968 "The Neurology of Facial Pain" B. Wyke

British Medical Journal 1:576, 1874 *"Gelseminum sempervirens* (Yellow Jasmine) in Facial Neuralgia" E. Mackey

Dental Headlight 22:17, 1901 "Castor Oil as a Remedy for Neuralgia" H.N. Moyer

Journal of the American Academy of Dermatology 17:93, 1987 "Treatment of Chronic Post Herpetic Neuralgia with Topical Capsaicin" J.E. Bernstein et al.

Lancet 1:426, 1832-3 "Cases of Neuralgia Successfully Treated with *Colchicum autumnale*" W. Goss

Lancet 1:360,835, 1880 "On Tonga: A Remedy for Neuralgia Used by the Natives of the Fiji Islands" S. Ringer et al.

Lancet 1:1175, 1885 "A Cuban Cure for Neuralgia" A.L. Esperon

Lancet 2:556, 1943 "Anodyne Power of the Cynara" J.C. Badeley

Medical Review 19:176, 1916 "The Elderberry in Neuralgia" H.J. Vetleson

Royal Society of Tropical Medicine and Hygiene, Transactions 19:492, 1926 "Colchicum in the Treatment of After-pains of Dengue Fever" J.W. Tomb

Harris, Wilfred *Neuritis and Neuralgia* London: H. Milford, 1926

13 TRIGEMINAL NEURALGIA

Acta Psychiatrica et Neurologica 24:403, 1949 "Ferrous Carbonate in the Treatment of Tic Douloureux" L.M. Davidoff et al.

L'Art Medicale #114:187, 1912 *"Chelidonium majus* in Right Facial Neuralgia" A. Noack

Bulletin de Therapeutique 47:556, 1854 "High Doses of Roman Chamomile in Facial Neurolgies" Dr. Lecointe

Cincinnati Lancet and Clinic 11:345, 1883 "Ice in Tic Douleureux" R.G. Simpson

Dental Digest 59:214, 1953 "Vitamin B_{12} in Tic Douloureau" L.P. Strean

Edinburgh Medical Journal 35:614,762, 1890 "On the Cure of Facial Neuralgia, Odontalgia and Allied Neurosis" G. Leslie

General Dentistry 32:441, 1984 "Tic Douloureux: Report of Successful Treatment" S.M. Hayes

Journal of the American Medical Association 65:895, 1915 "Pilocarpine in Trifacial Neuralgia" J.L. Tracy

Journal of the Neurological Sciences 2:105, 1965 "Avicenna and Trigeminal Neuralgia" N.O. Ameti

Lancet 1:62, 1834 "Employment of Laurel Leaves in Tic Douloureux" C. Loudon

Lancet 1:439, 1954 "Treatment of Trigeminal Neuralgia with Vitamin B_{12}" S.J. Surtees et al.

Mayo Clinic Proceedings 41:453, 1966 "History of the Numbering of the Cranial Nerves" C.W. Rucker

Neurology 2:131, 1952 "Relief of Pain in Trigeminal Neuralgia by Crystalline Vitamin B_{12}" W.S. Fields

Science 89:439, 1939 "The Relief of Symptoms in Major Trigeminal Neuralgia with Vitamin B_1" H. Borsook et al.

Townsend Letter #23:3, 12985 "Tic Douloureux: Its nature, Causes, Control and Its Implications" D.E. Babcock

Transactions of the American Neurological Association 70:176, 1944 "The Relief of Tic Douloureux Using Large Doses of Ferrous Carbonate" L.M. Davidoson

U.S. Army Medical Department Bulletin 8:535, 1948 "Trigeminal Neuralgia" L. Davidoff

Wiener Medizenische Blatter 9:972, 1886 "The Treatment of Trigeminal Neuralgia with Castor Oil" C. Gussenbauer

Stooken, Bryon *Trigeminal Neuralgia, Its History and Treatment* Springfield, Illinois: C.C. Thomas, 1959

14 SCIATICA

Antiseptic 62:735, 1965 "Role of *Semecarpus anacardium* in the Management of Sciatica" S.N. Tripathi et al.

British Medical Journal 2:1550, 1898 "The Application of Hydrochloric Acid in Sciatica" R.A. Bayliss

John Hopkins Hospital Bulletin 38:159, 1917 "Sarco-Iliac Strain" W.S. Baer

Journal de la Societe de Medicine et de Pharmacie de l'Isere 12:65, 1888 "Treatment of Sciatica by the External Application of Flowers of Sulfur" L. Duchesne

Journal of the American Medical Association 30:95, 1898 "The Alleged Accidental Discovery of the Value of Hydrochloric Acid in Sciatica"

Nature 60:125,150, 1889 "Strawberry for Gout" D. Ferguson

New York State Journal of Medicine 51:1171, 1951 "The Treatment of Sciatica with Glucurone" J.H. Hodas et al.

New York State Journal of Medicine 59:154, 1959 "The Buckling Sign- A Determinative in Sciatic Nerve Tension" A.A. Michele

St. Lewis Courier of Medicine 20:154, 1888 "Flowers of Sulfur in Sciatica"

Therapeutic Gazette 5:401, 1881 "The Seeds of *Persea gratissima* as a New Therapeutic Agent in the Treatment of Intercostal Neuralgia" H. Froehling

15 LOCAL ANESTHESIA

Chemical Abstracts 40:7411, 1946 "Some Pharmacological Properties of the Alkaloid of *Fritillaria sewerzowii*" E.S. Zolotakchina

Edinburgh Medical Journal 33:564, 1887 "Drumine: A New Local Anesthetic" I.C. Geddes

Indian Journal of Pharmacy 34:10, 1972 "Local Anesthetic Activity of *Plumeria rubra*" I.M. Chak et al.

Indian Veterinary Journal 49:503, 1972 "*Lycopersicon esculentum* as a Local Anesthetic Agent" N.C. Banerjee et al.

Journal of Materia Medica 14:17, 1875 "Aconite as a Local Anesthetic in Tetanus and in Filling Teeth" P.W. Allen

Journal of Research in Indian Medicine 10:#1/29, 1975 "Local Anesthetic Effect of the Leaves of *Ziziphus jujuba*" N.C. Sahu et al.

Journal of the American Chemical Society 70:4234, 1948 "Herculin, an Insecticidal Component of the Prickly Ash Bark" M. Jacobson

Journal of the American Medical Association 53:1393, 1909 "Quinine and Urea Hydrochloride as a Local Anesthetic" A.E. Hertzler et. al.

Lancet 2:98,287, 1848 "On Cold as a Means of Producing Local Insensibility" J. Arnott

Lancet 1:990, 1884 "On the Use of Cocaine for Producing Anesthesia in the Eye" C. Koller

Laryngoscope 1:117, 1896 "Guiacol as a Local Anesthetic in Diseases of the Ear, Nose and Throat" G. Laurens

Lloydia 33:393, 1971 "The Isolation and Identification of the Numbing Principle in *Chrysanthemum anethifolium*" R.W. Doskotch et al.

Medical Review 18:148, 1915 "Anesthesia of the Trigeminal Nerve by Inhalation of Oleum Sinapis" L. Flodquist

Medical Times and Gazette 2:517, 1855 "Local Anesthesia by Means of Cold" J. Arnott

National Medical Journal 3:Sept/47, 1961 "Devadali- *Luffa echinata*, a Promising Local Anesthetic" B.R. Shamachar

Phytochemistry 23:1173, 1984 "On the Pungent Principle of *Matricaria pubescens*" H. Greger

Revista Universidad Nacionalde Cordoba 35:211, 1948 "Etiopina, A Nitrogenous Organic Base Extracted from *Zantedeschia aethiopica*" J. Carlomago

Science 51:497, 1920 "Local Anesthetics" H.G. Barbour

16 GENERAL ANESTHESIA

Association Medical Journal 1:479, 1853 "On the Anesthetic Properties of the *Lycoperdon proteus* or Common Puffball" B.W. Richardson

Bulletin of the Torrey Botanical Club 64:401, 1937 "Notes on the Botanical Components of Curare" B.A. Krukoff et al.

Contact Point 24:69, 1954 "Anesthesia and Analgesia Before Horace Wells" W.F. Fenke et al.

Janus 31:24, 1927 "Research in the History of Anesthesia Before 1846" M.L. Baur

Journal of Ethnopharmacology 11:309, 1984 "Non-narcotic Orally Effective, Centrally Acting Analgesic from an Ayurvedic Drug" C.K. Atal et al.

Journal of Pharmacy and Experimental Therapy 60:69, 1937 "Action of *Erythrina americana*, a Possible Curare Substitute" A.J. Lehman

Journal of the History of Medicine 1:573, 1946 "Historic Notes on the Pharmacology of Anesthesia" C.E. Heaton

Pharmaceutical Journal 7:519, 1847 "On the Use of Mandrake as an Anesthetic in Former Times" T.H. Silvester

Presse Medicale 45:1430, 1937 "The Pharmacology of *Piscidia erythrina*" H. Leclerc

Proceedings of the American Academy of Arts and Science 40:487, 1904 "The Mandragora of the Ancients in Folklore and Medicine" C. Randolph

Therapeutic Gazette 5:183, 1881 *"Gelsemium sempervirens"*

Ellis, Edgar S. *Ancient Anodynes, Primitive Anesthesia and Allied Conditions* London: W. Heinemann, 1946

17 THE HERBS OF SLEEP

Alkaloid Clinic 5:532, 1882 *"Avena sativa"*

Biochemical Pharmacology 23:2807, 1974 "Protective Effect of Adenosine and Nicotinamide Against Audiogenic Seizure" M. Maitre et al.

Bollettino Societa Italiana di Biologia Sperimentale 28:113, 1952 "Genesis of Sleep (Magnesium and Vitamin B_{12})" V.M. Bucaino

Chemical and Pharmaceutical Bulletin 34:1672, 1986 "Isolation of Sedative Principles from *Perilla frutescens*" G. Honda et al.

Economic Botany 16:288, 1962 "The Drug Aspects of the White Sapotes" J.F. Morton

Experientia 20:390, 1964 "The Hypnotic Constituents of *Stipa vaseyi*, Sleepy Grass" W. Epstein et al.

Herbal Gram #26:34, 1992 "Traditional Chinese Medicine" A. Leung

Japanese Journal of Psychiatry and Neurology 45:167, 1991 "Treatment of Persistent Sleep-Wake Schedule Disorders in Adolescents and Vitamin B_{12}" T. Ohta et al.

Journal of Clinical Pharmacology 13:475, 1973 "Cardiac Effects of Chamomile Tea" L. Gould et al.

Journal of Experimental Medical Science 7:53, 1963 "The Chemistry and Pharmacy of Marsiline, A Sedative and Anticonvulsive Principle Isolated from *Marsilia minuta* and *M. rajasthensis*"A Chatterjee et al.

Medical Press and Circular 34:230, 1882 "The Odor of heliotrope as a Narcotic" M.D.

Medicinsk Forum 19:116, 1966 "A Soporific Agent in Clams" T. Johnesson

Merck's Report 20:173,271, 1911 "The Sleepy Grass of New Mexico" O. Farwell

Practitioner 176:122, 1956 "Hops for the Sleepless"

Science and Culture 29:619, 1963 "The Chemistry and Pharmacology of Marsiline" A Chatterjee et al.

Sleep 6:257, 1983 "Successful Treatment of Human Non-24 Hour Sleep Wake Syndrome" B. Kamgar-Parsi et al.

18 SENILITY

Arzneimittelforschung 17:1541, 1961 "On the Cerebral Effect of a Plant Preparation From *Ginkgo biloba*" R. Henner

Brain 99:67, 1976 "Aluminum, Neurofibrillary Degeneration and Alzheimer's Disease" D.R. Crapper et al.

British Journal of Psychiatry 121:207, 1972 "Senile Dementia: A Changing Perspective" D.A. Alexander

Clinical Trials Journal 22:149, 1985 *"Ginkgo biloba* Extract" G. Vorberg

Journal of Ethnopharmacology 28:349, 1990 "Effects of Shosaikoto, An Oriental Herbal Medicinal Mixture on Age Induced Amnesia in Rats" S. Amagaya et al.

Journal of Ethnopharmacology 38:129, 1993 "Plants in Treating Senile Dementia in Northwest Amazon" R.E. Schultes

Journal of Gerontology 14:344, 1959 "Air Ionization and Maze Learning in Rats" J. Jordan et al.

Journal of the American Geriatrics Society 17:477, 1969 "Prevention of Senile and Presenile Dementia by Dihydroxy-coumarin (Dicumarol) Therapy" A.C. Walsh

Landarzt 44: Aug 20/iv, 1968 "Treatment of Cerebro-organic Changes Due to Age with Kavaform" J.F. Kurz

Nature 209:109, 1966 "Correlation of Dementia and Counts of 'Senile Plaques' in Cerebral Gray Matter of Elderly Subjects" M. Roth et al.

New Scientist 148:Oct 14/10, 1995 "When Sage May be the Wisest Remedy" J. Itzhaki

Quarterly Journal of Crude Drug Research 9:1373, 1969 "Dioscorea (Yams) – The Food of the Slaves with Potentials for Newer Drugs" C.R. Karncik

Quarterly Journal of Medicine 36:189, 1967 "Dementia and Foliate Deficiency" R.M. Strachan

Nagatsu, T .*Basic Clinical and Therapeutic Aspects of Alzheimer's and Parkinson's Disease* New York: Plenus Press, 1990

19 MEMORY HERBS

American Journal of Mental Deficiency 59:235, 1954 "The Experimental Administration of *Celastrus paniculata* in Mental Deficiency" J.V. Morris et al.

American Journal of Psychiatry 120:320, 1963 "Effects of Ribonucleic Acid on Memory Defect in the Aged" D.E. Cameron et al.

Archives of Neurology 26:25, 1972 "Ancient Art of Memory" B.M. Patten

British Medical Journal 2:852, 1951 "Indian Remedies for Poor Memory" S. Hakim

Clinical Trials Journal 22:149, 1985 "*Ginkgo biloba* Extract: A Long-term Study of Chronic Cerebral Insufficiency in Geriatric Patients" G. Vorgberg

Dental Abstracts 13:387, 1968 "Foresee New Drug Supply from Plants"

Economic Botany 11:263, 1957 "A Unique Reported Use for the Fruit of *Semecarpus anacardium* in Ancient Arabian and Indian Medicine" J. King

Journal of Research in Indian Medicine 12:#1/18, 1977 "Studies on the Psychiatropic Effect of *Convolvulus pluricaulis*" R.H. Singh et al.

Kango 20:Aug/104, 1968 "Brain Metabolism Improving Agents" M. Shimizu

Medizinische Monattschrift 10:112, 1956 "The Old Time German Art of Memorizing" G. Eis

Pharmazeutische Monatschrift 16:353, 1936 "Sinicuichi, the Magic Drink Causing Oblivion" V.A. Reko

Presse Medicale 15:1592, 1986 "Activity of *Ginkgo biloba* Extract on Short Term Memory" I. Hindmarch

Prevention 35:Feb/152, 1983 "Memory Aided by B_6" A. Allen

Science 201:274, 1978 "Human Serial Learning: Enhancement with Arecholine and Choline and Impairment with Scopolamine" N. Sitaram et al.

Yates, Frances *The Art of Memory* London: Routledge and K. Paul, 1966

20 DEAFNESS

American Bee Journal 114:68, 1974 "Treatment of Deafness with Propolis" R. Pershakov

American Journal of Cancer 17:971, 1933 "Effect of Bone Marrow from Young Animals" H. Rosenstein et al.

British Medical Journal 1:621, 1931 "Bath Treatment for Deafness" J. Adam

Bulletin de l'Academie Naturale de Medicine 145:16, 1961 "Fifteen Years Experience in the Treatment of Deafness with Amino Acids and Vitamins" G. de la Farge

California Medical Journal 17:174, 1896 "Tincture of Mullein Flowers" O.S. Laws

Eye, Ear, Nose and Throat Medicine 92:75, 1950 "Observation on the Treatment of Deafness and Tinnitus with Parenteral Vitamin A in Massive Doses (Lobel)" J.R. Anderson et al.

Geriatrics 38:17, 1983 "Hearing Loss May be Linked to Zinc Deficiency" G.E. Shambaugh Jr.

Lancet 2:93, 1849 "Glycerin, A Remedy in Deafness" J. Brown

Lancet 1:64, 1851 "Glycerin in the Treatment of Certain Forms of Deafness" T.H. Wakely

Massachusetts Medical Journal 20:241, 1900 "The Good Effects of Pilocarpine in Certain Forms of Deafness" J.C. Emery

Medical and Surgical Reporter 39:401, 1876 "The Aboriginal Method of Treating Diseases of the Ear" A.L. Turnbull

Nature Medicine 2:1060, 1996 "Stimulating Hair Cell Regeneration: On A Wing and a Prayer" E.W. Rubel et al.

Society of Experimental Biology and Medicine, Proceedings 72:172, 1949 "Hearing in Guinea Pigs Deficient in the Anti-stiffness Factor" R. Wulzen et al.

Wakely, Thomas *Clinical Reports on the Use of Glycerin in the Treatment of Certain Forms of Deafness* London: S. Highly, 1851

21 MENIERE'S DISEASE

American Journal of Otolaryngology 14:94, 1993 "Vitamin B_{12} Deficiency in Patients with Chronic Tinnitus and Noise-Induced Hearing Loss" Z. Shemesh et al.

Annals of Otology, Rhinology and Laryngology 52:45, 1943 "The Treatment of Meniere's Syndrome with Magnesium Salts" A. Schick

Annals of Otology, Rhinology and Laryngology 70:836, 1961 "Placebos, Anti-Sludging Drugs and Disorders of the Ear" E.P. Fowler

Annals of the New York Academy of Science 243:468, 1975 "Dimethyl Sulfoxide Therapy in Subjective Tinnitus of Unknown Origin" A.Z. Caro

Archives of Otolaryngology 46:681, 1947 "Pyridoxine (B$_6$) Used in the Treatment of Vertigo" A. Lewy et al.

Australassian Journal of Pharmacy 30:1255,1348, 1949 "Meniere's Disease or Labyrinth Vertigo" E. Colman

Chinese Medical Journal 1:343, 1975 "Treatment of Sudden Deafness with Radix *Puerariae*" Beijing Research Institute

Exerpta Medica: Oto-Rhino-Laryngology 3:#1393 & #1709, 1950 "Theory of Dissolution of Otoliths by Intravenous Injection of Sodium Bicarbonate" S. Fujisaki

Laryngoscope 75:1491, 1965 "Historic Aspects of Meniere's Disease" T.G. Wilson

Mayo Clinic Proceedings 37:474, 1962 "Citrus Bioflavanoids, Ascorbic Acid and the B Vitamins in the Treatment of Certain Types of Neurosensory Deafness: Preliminary report" H.L. Williams et al.

Memorabilien-Zeitschrift fur Rationelli Praktische Aerzte 16:388, 1897-8 "Hearing and Meniere's Disease Treated with *Cimicifuga racemosa*" A. Robin

Presse Medicale 45:364, 1937 *"Cimicifuga racemosa-* Its Use in Treating Ear Noises" H. Leclerc

Prevention 35:Jan/144, 1983 "Bioflavanoids Stopped the Spinning" S. Verriere

22 ANEMIA

Agriculture Research 33:Jan/4, 1985 "Sickle Cell Cramps Relieved" V. Mazzola

American Journal of Physiology 80:400, 1927 "Anemia- Influence of Fresh and Dried Fruits" F.S. Robscheit-Robbins et al.

Blood 77:1334, 1991 "Vanillin, A Potential Agent for the Treatment of Sickle Cell Anemia" D.J. Abraham et al.

Clinical Pharmacology and Therapeutics 7:147, 1966 "Treatment of Pernicious Anemia: Historical Aspects" W.B. Castel

C.R. Societe de Biologie 108:79, 1931 "Action of Extracts of *Sophora japonica* on Red Blood Cells" King Li Pin et al.

C.R. Societe de Biologie 115:1132, 1934 "Action of *Codonopsis tangshen* on the Blood Count and Blood Pressure" King Li Pin et al.

Johns Hopkins Hospital Bulletin 35:180, 1924 "A Comparison of the Effects of Germanium Dioxide and of Sodium Germanate on the Blood of the Albino Rat" J.E. Nowrey

Journal of the American Medical Association 215:762, 1971 "Sodium Citrate Orally for Painful Sickle Cell Crises" L. Barreras et al.

Lloydia 34:383, 1971 "Reversal of Sickling and Crenation in Erythrocytes by the Root Extract of *Fagara zanthoxyloides*" E.A. Sofowora et al.

Medical Librarian and Historical Journal 1:176, 1903 "A Sketch of the Treatment of Chlorosis with Iron" H.A. Christian

Orvosi Helilap 89:317, 1948 "The Effect of Spinach Extract on Experimental Anemia" J. Uri

Pennsylvania Medical Journal 26:86, 1922 "Pernicious and Secondary Anemias Treated with Geranium Dioxide" J.L. Lenker

Planta Medica 56:41, 1990 "Phenylalanine is the Predominant Antisickling Agent in *Cajanus cajan* Seed Extract" G.I. Ekeke et al.

Presse Medicale 63:887, 1949 "A Serious Case of Anemia Treated with Methionine" H. Bernard et al.

Proceedings of the Society for Experimental Biology and Medicine 26:835, 1929 "Inorganic Elements of Spinach in Treatment of Nutritional Anemia" H.S. Mitchell et al.

Public Health Reports 45:1175, 1930 "An Anemia of Dogs Produced by Feeding Onions" W.H. Sebrell

Transactions of the Royal Society of Tropical Medicine and Hygiene 81:510, 1987 "Antisickeling Agent in an Extract of Unripe Papaw Fruit (*Carica papaya*)" K.D. Thomas

23 SALTS AND THE BLOOD

American Heart Journal 108:188, 1984"Magnesium: Nature's Physiologic Calcium Blocker" L.T. Iseri

American Journal of Cardiology 12:6551, 1963 "Electrolytes and the Electrocardiogram" B. Surawicz

Archiv fuer Experimentelle Pathologie und Pharmakologie 178:109, 1935 "The Form of Calcium Which Acts on the Heart" K. Pohle

Arzneimittelforschung 16:1488, 1966 "Effect of Magnesium Asparaginate on the Coronary Circulation" P. Gorog et al.

British Medical Journal 1:616, 1907 "On the Use of Calcium Salts as Cardiac Tonics in Pneumonia and Heart Disease" L. Brunton

Canadian Medical Association Journal 15:913, 1925 "Calcium and Potassium Chlorides in the Treatment of Arterial Hypertension" W. Addison et al.

Circulation 69:849, 1984 "Sydney Ringer, Calcium and Cardiac Function " W.B. Fye

Comparative Biochemistry and Physiology 2:241, 1961 "Ringer Solutions and Some Notes on the Physiological Basis of Their Ionic Compositions" A. Lockwood

Journal of Physiology 4:29, 1883 "A Further Contribution to the Problem" S. Ringer

Journal of the American Medical Association 206:2515, 1968 "Sydney Ringer (1835-1910) Clinician and Pharmacologist"

Journal of the American Medical Association 230:130, 1974 "Soft Water, Heart Attacks and Stroke" A.G. Shaper

Medical Proceedings 5:487, 1959 "The Treatment of Coronary Artery Disease with Parenterol Magnesium Sulfate" R.S. Parsons et al.

Medical Record 143:208, 1936 "The Cardiotherapeutics of the Alkaline Earth Salts, Calcium, Potassium and Barium" E. Podolsky

Therapeutische Haltmonatsch 35:758, 1921 "Calcium in Cardiac Therapy" G. Singer

Selye, Hans *The Prevention of Cardiac Necrosis* New York: Ronald Press Co., 1958

24 THE ELECTRIC CHARGE MYSTERY

British Medical Journal 1:727,1192, 1932 "Aluminium and Health" A. Francis

Lancet 2:301, 1920 "Coagulation of the Blood" M. Bloch

New York Medicine 5:35, 1949 "Hemoglobin Research and Coronary Thrombosis" E. Klein

Science 218:145, 1982 "Coagulation as a Common Thread in Disease" J.L. Marx

Society for Experimental Biology and Medicine, Proceedings 46:476, 1941 "Treatment of Lead Poisoning with Sodium Citrate" S.S. Kety et al.

Transactions of the American Therapeutic Society 95,1948 "Sludged Blood" M.H. Knisely et al.

Bajusz, Eors *Electrolytes and Cardiovascular Diseases* [pages 260-76] New York: S. Karger, 1966

Clement, Mark *Aluminum, A Menace to Health* London: True Health Publishing Co.

Riddick, Thomas *Control of Colloid Stability Through Zeta Potential* Waynewood, Pennsylvania: Livingstone Publishing Co., 1968

25 PREVENTING BLOOD CLOTTING

American Journal of Clinical Nutrition 35:1452, 1982 "The Relationship Between High Fibrinolytic Activity and Daily Capsicum Ingestion in Thai's" S. Visudhiphan et al.

Archives Internationales de Pharmacodynamie 139:75, 1962 "Anticoagulant and Cardiovascular Actions of Callophylloide" R.B. Arora et al.

Arzneimittelforschung 20:1629, 1970 "The Therapeutic Effect of Rutin and Coumarin in Experimental Thrombophlebitis" V.M. Foldi et al.

British Medical Journal 3:351, 1968 & 1:845, 1969 "Effect of Onions on Blood Fibrinolytic Activity" I.S. Menon et al.

Canadian Journal of Biochemistry and Physiology 41:1325, 1963 "The Antithrombic Activity of Carrageenin in Human Blood" W.W. Hawkins

Chemical and Pharmacological Bulletin 35:1275, 1987 "Anti-Thrombic Actions of 70% Methanol Extract and Cinnamic Aldehyde from Cinnamic Cortex" H. Matsuda et al.

International Journal of Vitamin Research 43:494, 1973 "Effect of Methoxylated Flavones on Erythrocyte Aggregation and Sedimentation" R.C. Robbins

Journal of Laboratory and Clinical Medicine 60:641, 1962 "Antipeptic and Antithrombic Properties of Carrageenin" W.W. Hawkins et al.

Journal of the American Chemical Society 106:8295, 1984 "(E,2)-Ajoene: A Potent Antithrombic Agent from Garlic" E. Block et al.

New England Journal of Medicine 303:756, 1980 "Chinese Food and Platelets" T.O. Cheng

New England Journal of Medicine 302:1191, 1980 "Szechwan Purpura" D.E. Hammerschmidt

26 AIDING BLOOD CLOTTING

American Journal of Botany 29:353, 1942 "Presence of Anti-Hemorrhagic Material in Roots of the European Bindweed" A. Bakke et al.

American Journal of Medical Science 204:665, 1942 "The Influence of Blood Transfusion and Injections of Bursa Pastoris (Shepherd's Purse) Extract on Clot Resistance in Two Hemophiliacs" A.D. Copley et al.

American Medicine 3:729, 1902 "On the Effect of the Digestion of Gelatin; Its Styptic Properties" H.C. Wood

Dublin Hospital Gazette 6:19, 1859 "On the Treatment of Purpura Hemorrhagica by the Administration of Tincture of Larch Bark" S.L. Hardy

Edinburgh Medical Journal 38:639, 1893 "Hemorrhage from the Aveoli Checked by Puff-ball (*Lycoperdon giganteum*)" W.R. Smith

Journal-Lancet 60:422, 1940 "*Capsella bursa-pastoris* as a Hemostatic after Prostatectomy" A.E. Greenberger et al.

Journal of Laboratory and Clinical Medicine 63:359, 1964 "Activation of Hageman Factor by Solutions of Ellagic Acid" O.D. Ratnoff et al.

Journal of the American Chemical Society 63:929, 1941 "Hemorrhagic Degeneration and the Labile Methyl Supply" W. Griffith et al.

Journal of Materia Medica 9:238, 1870 "On the Use of the Nettle in Uterine Hemorrhage" E.A. Anderson

Medical Record 44:143, 1893 "The Hemostatic Properties of Puffball" A.L. Hall

New Remedies 1:207, 1872 "On the Hemostatic Properties of *Alnus incana*" T.R. Dupins

Ohio State Journal of Dental Science 5:479, 1885 "The Hemostatic Properties of *Ambrosia artemisiaefolia* Ragweed" J.H. Hall

Pharmazeutische Zentralhalle 63:437,465, 1922 "Hemostatic Action of Common Plants" L. Kroeber

Retrospect of Practical Medicine 42:77, 1861 "On the Use of Larch Bark in Hemorrhages" J.M. O'Ferral

Therapeutic Gazette 4:64, 1880 "*Asclepias curassavica* – Blood Flower" C.W. Hansen

Therapeutic Gazette 21:655, 1897 "*Senecio aureus* as a Hemostat in Capillary Hemorrhage" F. Gundrum

27 THE ACID-BASE BALANCE

American Journal of Nursing 75:980, 1975 "Reviewing Acid-Base Balance" J.E. Sharer

American Journal of Physiology 62:459, 12922 "The Effect of Intravenous Sodium Bicarbonate on Intestinal Movements" C.E. King et al.

American Journal of Physiology 130:9, 1940 "Variability of Blood pH and Its Association with Meteorological Factors" M. Berg et al.

American Medicine 22:385, 1916 "Pregnancy Toxemia, A Study of Acidosis in Pregnancy" W. Williamson

Annals of Internal Medicine 14:409, 1914 "Specific Role of Foods in Relation of the Urine" N.R. Blatherwick

Annals of Otology, Rhinology and Laryngology 39:584, 1920 & 41:1124, 1932 "The Upper Respiratory Tract as Guide to Nutritional Disasters" D.C. Jarvis

British Medical Journal 1:195, 1903 "On the Use of Alkalies for the Relief of Pain" H.C. Thomson

Bulletin de la Societe de Chemie et Biologique 31:325, 1945 "Effects of Vitamins on the Alkaline Reserve" R. Lecoq

Canadian Journal of Surgery 15:37, 1972 "Acid-Base Changes in Patients with Intractable Pain and Malignancy" R.J. Evans

Hospital Medicine 4:May/61, 1968 "Metabolic Alkalosis" F.J. Takacs

Journal of Clinical Pathology 12:195, 1959 "Acidosis and Alkalosis; A Modern View" S.C. Frazer et al.

Journal of the American Medical Association 70:531,611, 1918 "Acidosis in Cases of Shock, Hemorrhage and Gas Infection" W.B. Cannon

Medical Life 30:343, 1923 & 32:189, 1925 "History of Acidosis" M. Kahn

Respiration 25:201, 1968 "Indications for the Use of Sodium Bicarbonate in The Treatment of Intractable Asthma" J.C. Mithoeffer et al.

Society for Experimental Biology and Medicine, Proceedings 26:182, 1928 "Effect of Intravenous Injections of Alkali on Physiological Action of Curare" W.F. Wenner et al.

Society for Experimental Biology and Medicine, Proceedings 162:38, 1979 "Influence of Environmental pH on the Preservation and Inactivation of Herpes Simplex" G. Lancz

Transactions of the American Therapy Society59,1941 "The Importance of the Acid-Alkali Balance of the Blood" C.E. Wooding

Zentralblatt fur Bakteriologie 21:134,186, 1897 "Newer Tests on the Alkalization of Blood" J.V. Fodor

28 ARTERIOSCLEROSIS

Acta Medica Scandinavica 101:83, 1939 "Iodine Therapy in High Blood Pressure and Arteriosclerosis" N. Alwall

American Journal of Cardiology 11:283, 1963 "Diet and Arteriosclerosis: Truth and Fiction" I. Snapper

American Journal of Clinical Nutrition 34:824, 19981 "Oat Bran Intake Selectively Lowers Serum Low Density Lipoprotein Cholesterol Concentrations of Hypercholesterolemic Men" R.W. Kirby et al.

American Journal of Digestive Disease 19:381, 1952 "Results of Betaine Treatment of Arteriosclerosis" L.M. Morrison

American Journal of Pathology 25:481, 1948 "Arteriosclerotic Lesions in Pyridoxine-Deficient Monkeys" J.F. Rinehart

Annals of the Indian Academy of Medical Sciences 5:1, 1969 "Bengal Gram- An Effective Hypocholesterolemic Substance" K.S. Mathur

Artery 4:487, 1978 "Studies of the Antiarterosclerotic Action of *Nepeta hindostana* in Pigs" O.P. Agarwal et al.

Atherosclerosis 33:397, 1979 "The Antiatheromatous Action of Silicon" J. Loeper et al.

Dia Medicine 16:151, 1944 "Decholesterolization by Means of Artichoke *Cynara scolymus*" A.H. Roffo

Experimental Pathology 10:180, 1975 "Influence of Eggplant *Solanum melongena* Preparation on Cholesterol Metabolism in Rats" D. Dritchevsky et al.

Experientia 28:254, 1972 "Anti-hypocholesterolenic Effect of a Sulfur Containing Amino Acid Isolated from Cabbage" M. Fujiwara et al.

Experientia 31:549, 1975 "The Use of Crocetin in Experimental Atherosclerosis" J.L. Gainer et al.

Giornale Clinical Medicine 47:595, 1966 "A Study of Silicon for Treating Human Arteriosclerosis" J. Loeper et al.

Historie Medicine 3:Oct/81, 1953 "Phytotherapy of Hypercholesterol" F. Decaux et al.

Journal of Chronic Diseases 4:461, 1956 "A Practical Method for the Reduction of Serum Cholesterol in Man" H.A. Schroeder

Journal of Nutrition 100:1307, 1970 "Effect of Curcumin on Serum and Liver Cholesterol Levels in the Rat" D.S. Rao

Lancet 2:303, 1963 "Cholesterol Lowering Effect of Rolled Oats" A.P. de Groot

Lancet 1:454, 1977 "Silicon, Fiber and Arteriosclerosis" K. Schwarz

Medical History 17:304, 1973 "Leonardo da Vinci's Views on Arteriosclerosis" K.D. Keele

Panminerva Medica 3:74, 1961 "1-4-Dicaffeyl-quinic Acid, the Active Principle of the Artichoke" M. Mancini

Presse Medicale 19:1005, 1911 "Experimental Arteriosclerosis and Sodium Silicate" M. Gouget

Proceedings of the Society for Experimental Biology and Medicine 69:283, 1948 "Absorption of Aortic Arteriosclerosis by Choline Feeding" L.M. Morrison et al.

Prevention 39:Jan/24, 1987 "A Real Fish Story" C.D. Neal

Progress Medicale 36:189, 1921 "Silica in the Treatment of Arteriosclerosis" L. Scheffler et al.

Schweizer Medizinische Wochenschrift 54:455, 1924 "Action of Potassium Iodine on Circulation" D. Bloom

29 BLOOD PURIFIERS

Chemical and Pharmacological Bulletin 27:1464, 1979 "Effects of Crude Drugs on Congestive Edema" Y. Yamahara et al.

Journal of the American Institute of Homeopathy 32:681, 1939 "Sassafras in High Blood Pressure" H.E. Vander Bogert

Perfumery and Essential Oils Record 54:581, 1963 "Sanguinaria" E.S. Maurer

Proceedings of the Pennsylvania German Society 45:#2/1, 1935 "Folk Medicine of the Pennsylvania Germans" T. Brendle

Petulengro, Leon *Romanie Remedies and Recipes* New York: E.P. Dutton, 1936

Scully, Virginia *A Treasury of American Indian Herbs* New York: Crown Publishers

Nameless *Secret Remedies* London: British Medical Association, 1909

30 LOW BLOOD PRESSURE

Annales de Medicine Interne 131:508, 1980 "Corrective Effects of Yohimbine in Orthostatic Hypotension Induced by Tricyclic Antidepressents" A. Laurier et al.

Archives of Internal Medicine 69:721, 1942 "Induced Thiamin (Vitamin B$_1$) Deficiency and the Thiamin Requirement of Man" R.D. Williams et al.

Biologie Medicine 43:464, 1954 "The 24 Hour Cycle of Blood Pressure" A.C. Guillaume

C.R. Societe de Biologie 113:97, 1933 "Preliminary Notes on the Pharmacobiodynamic Effects of a False Kinkelba, *Kindeliba dekita*" F. Mercier

Journal of Ethnopharmacology 15:261, 1986 "Acute Antihypertensive Effect in Conscious Rats Produced by Some Medical Plants Used in the State of Sao Paulo" R. De A. Ribeiro

Journal of Pharmacy and Experimental Therapy 47:79, 1933 "The Pressor Action of Yohimbine and Quebrachine" S.J. Weinberg

Journal of the American Geriatrics Society 39:601, 1991 "Orthostatic Hypotension Induced by Vitamin B$_{12}$ Deficiency" A. Lossos et al.

Journal of the American Medical Association 257:3231, 1987 "Orthostatic Hypotension and Pernicious Anemia" W.B. White

Lancet 337:557, 1991 "Licorice and Blood Pressure" S. Brandon

Medical Life 37:60, 1930 "The Story of Blood Pressure" C.J. Brim

Medical Officer 96:285, 1956 "The Assessment of Blood Pressure at Routine Medical Examination" H.T. Phillips

Medizinische Monatsschrift 7:375, 1953 "Therapeutic Experiences with Glutamic Acid with Special Reference to Hypotension" E. Acker

Northwest Medicine 34:325,380, 1935 "Hypotension" O. Pepper

Revue Generale de Clinique et de Therapeutique 53:30, 1939 "Use of *Silybum marianum* and *Carduus mariana* as a Vascular Tonic in Hypotension: Two Cases" H. Leclerc

Schweizerische Medizine Wochenschrift 73:746, 1946 "Symptomatic and Causal Therapy of Pollen and Hypotensive Allergy" J. Strebel

Science 212:559, 1981 "Tyrosine Increases Blood Pressure in Hypotensive Rats" L.A. Conlay et al.

Science and Culture 24:241, 1958 "Some Chemical, Pharmacological and Antibacterial Properties of *Coleus aromaticus*" A. Chatterjee

Science News 138:344, 1990 "High Pressure Hormone" K.A. Fackelmann

31 HIGH BLOOD PRESSURE

Acta Medica Scandinavica 101:83, 1939 "Iodine Therapy in Hypertension and Arteriosclerosis" N. Alwall

American Journal of Medical Sciences 178:470, 1929 "Watermelon Seed Extract in the Treatment of Hypertension" T.L. Althausen et al.

Boston Medical and Surgical Journal 56:509, 1859 "*Veratrum viride* as an Arterial Sedative" E. Cutter

British Medical Journal 2:951, 1935 "*Crataegus oxyacantha* in Hypertension" J. Graham

Canadian Medical Association Journal 15:913, 1925 "Calcium and Potassium Chlorides in the Treatment of Arterial Hypertension" W. Addison

C.R. Academie des Sciences 258:5760, 1964 "On Some Pharmacological Effects of a Rapid Strong and Prolonged Hypotensive Plant" M. Raymond-Hamet

Journal of Pharmaceutical Sciences 71:475, 1982 "Hypotensive Activity of *Cecropia obtusifolia*" H. Virio et al.

Journal of the Formosa Medical Association 78:61, 1979 "A Study of the Antihypertensive Action of Uncarine, an Alkaloid of *Uncaria formosana* Used in Chinese Herb Medicine" C. Chang et al.

Journal of Orthomolecular Medicine 7:221, 1992 "Nutritional treatments for Hypertension" E.R. Braveman et al.

Lancet 1:784, 1986 "History of Salt Supplies in West Africa and Blood Pressure Today" T. Wildon

Lancet 335:765, 1990 "Blood Pressure, Stroke and Coronary Heart Disease" S. MacMahon et al.

Medical Council 23:751, 1918 "Citric Acid Treatment of High Blood Pressure" H. Nemenway

Medical Record 144:373, 1936 "Treatment of Vascular Hypertension with Active Molecular Iodine" F. Damrau

Medical Record 156:485, 1943 "Vitamin A in the Treatment of Arterial Hypertension" M. Villaverde

Naturwissenschaften 70:95, 1983 "Effects on Rats of Aqueous Extracts of Plants Used as Hypotensive Agents" B Lasserre et al.

New York Medical Journal 100:918, 1914 "Pilocarpine in High Blood Pressure" W.D. Robinson

New York Medical Journal 115:752, 1922 "Weight Reduction and Its Remarkable Effect on High Blood Pressure" R.H. Rose

Philippine Journal of Science 71:361, 1940 "Pharmacological Study of Quaternary Alkaloids and Fluid Extract of *Phaeanthus ebracteolatus*" F. Garcia

Presse Medicale 68:1478, 1955 "Treatment and Prevention of Hypertension, the Roots of *Morinda citrifolia*" Dang Van Ho

Royal College of General Practitioners 18:207, 1969 "High Blood Pressure- Ancient, Modern and Natural" R.G. Sinclair

Science 96:161, 1942 "Treatment of Experimental Renal Hypertension with Vitamin A" G.E. Wakerlin et al.

Shikoku Acta Medica 22:518, 1966 "The Effect of Administration of Vegetable and Fruit Juices on Experimental Hypertension Due to Sodium Chloride" R. Nose

Tohoku Journal of Experimental Medicine 78:347, 1963 "The Effect of Water-washed Rice in the Diet on the Growth, Excretion of Sodium in Urine and Blood Pressure of Rats" T. Koyanagi et al.

Toulouse Medical 49:57, 1948 "The Hypotensive Action of Extracts of *Buxus balearica, Hedera helix* and *Galium aparine*" R. Delas et al.

Vrachebnoe Delo 10:1051, 1957 "*Lagochilus* Therapy for Hypertension" E. Kopin

32 SECRETS OF THE BLOOD

Anthropological Journal of Canada 11:#4/18, 1973 "The A, B, O Blood types: Their Bearing on Amerindian Origins and Britain's Neolithic" L.J. Salter

Antiseptic 56:449, 1959 "Ancient Concept of the Blood" B.S. Johri

Bioscience 26:557, 1976 "Blood Groups: Why do They Exist?" W.J. Miller

Chemtech 1:697, 1971 "Reducing Fluid Friction with Okra" W. Castro et al.

The East 24:Jan/50, 1989 "Questions of a Sojourner in Japan"

Endeavour 13:72, 1989 "The Evolution of Blood Cells; Facts and Enigmas" D.A. Millar et al.

Glasgow Medical Journal 12:53, 1938 "The History of the Circulation of the Blood" L. Aschoff

Journal of Social Psychology 1:494, 1930 "A Study of Temperament and Blood Groups" T. Furukawa

Journal of the Siam Society 30:29, 1937 "An Ancient Chinese Test for Proving Parentage" F.H. Giles

Marquette Medical Review 17:Nov/7, 1951 "The Use of Okra as a Plasma Replacement in Laboratory Animals" D. Roth

Nature 331:178, 1988 "Functioning Hemoglobin Genes in Non-Nodulating Plants" D. Bogusz

New York Medical Journal 108:93, 225, 1918 "The Blood and the Soul in Ancient Belief" J. Wright

Nursing Mirror 118:July 31/iii, 1964 "The Circulation of the Blood: Theories Since Galen" S. Stevenson

PHP Intersect 1:Sept/12, 1985 "Let Your Blood Groups Do the Talking" K. Suzuki

Psychiatry 6:175, 1943 "Bloody: The Natural History of a Word" A. Montagu

St. Bartholomew's Hospital Journal 40:149,166,211,238, 1933 "The History of the Hedgehog's Rosary"

Texas State Journal of Medicine 35:403, 1939 "Actions and Uses of Castilian Malva Solution in Infectious, Necrotic and Gangrenous Lesions" R.P. Thomas Jr.

Transactions of the Royal Society of Canada 18:#5/1, 1924 "The Miraculous Micro-organism" F.C. Harrison

33   SECRETS OF THE PULSE

Annals of the New York Academy of Sciences 61:665, 1955 "Anatomical and Functional Change in the Peripheral Vascular System During Certain Induced Increases in Vascular Fragility" R.E. Lee et al.

British Heart Journal 13:423, 1951 "The Ancient Art of Feeling the Pulse" D.E. Bedford

Bulletin of Historical Medicine 10:209, 1941 "An Epitome of Ancient Pulse Lore" E.F. Horine

China Medical Journal 42:884, 1928 "The Pulse Lore of Cathay" K.C. Wong

Edinburgh Medical Journal 14:33, 1868 & 15:47, 1869 "On the Aneurysm by Iodide of Potassium" G.W. Balfour

Federation Proceedings 11:738, 1952 "Factors Determining the Contour of the Pressure Pulse Recorded from the Aorta" R.S. Alexander

Indian Journal of the History of Medicine 12:11, 1967 "The Pulse in Indian Medicine" P. Kutumbiah

International Clinics 3:92, 1911 "Dynamic Diagrams of the Pulse" T.F. Christen

Journal of Biomechanical Engineering 107:268, 1985 & 111:88, 1989 "On the Detection of Messages Carried in Arterial Pulse Waves" K. Dai et al.

Journal of Chronic Diseases 3:618, 1956 "The Normal Pulse Wave and Its Modification" H. Lax

Journal of the American Medical Association 64:1380, 1915 "The Contour of the Normal Arterial Pulse" C.J. Wiggers

Journal of the American Medical Association 201:105, 1967 "Vascular Abnormalities in Children with Diabetes Mellitus" A.W. Feinberg

Milwaukee Medical Journal 6:393, 1898 "The Pulse: Its Diagnostic and Prognostic Value" T.S. Dabney

Amber, R.B. *The Pulse in the Occident and the Orient* New York: Dunshaw Press, 1966

Coca, Arthur *The Pulse Test* New York: Lyle Stewart, 1959

Ewart, William *How the Feel the Pulse and What to Feel In It* New York: William Wood and Company, 1892

Mackenzie, James *The Study of the Pulse, Arterial, Venous and Hepatic, and of the Movements of the Heart* Edinburgh: Y.J. Pentland, 1902

34 SECRETS OF THE HEART

American Heart Journal 2:188, 1926 "Voluntary Pulse Control" A. Hymars

Clio Medicine 9:51, 1954 "The Heart in the Bible and Talmud" F. Rosner

Journal of the American Medical Association 259: 2553, 1988 "Cardiovascular and Renal Effects of Long Term Antihypertensive Treatment" M. Hartford et al.

Journal of the American Veterinary Medical Association 185:1347, 1984 "Cardiomyopathy Associated with Vitamin E Deficiency in 7 Gelada Baboons" S.K. Liu et al.

Lancet 2:41, 1974 "Hypoxia, Saffron and Cardiovascular Disease" S. Grisola

Medical Record 160:19, 1947 "Vitamin E in Heart Disease" A. Vogelsang et al.

Quarterly Journal of Medicine 15:107, 1946 "The Heart in Anemia" A. Hunter

Science 220:81, 1983 "Normalization of Depressed Heart Function in Rats by Ribose" H.G. Zimmer

Scientific American 205:Oct/132, 1961 "The Electrocardiogram" A. Scher

Wall Street Journal June 18/1, 1959 "Experiments on Rats Indicate Sugar May Spur Heart Ailments" A.J. Large

35 A MEDICAL DETOUR

Alive: Canadian Journal of Health and Nutrition #112:Sept/20, 1991 "The Choice is Yours: Knife or Spoon" W. MacDonald

American Heart Journal 39:729, 1950 "Results of Treatment of Coronary Arteriosclerosis with Choline" L.M. Morrison

American Heart Journal 67:433, 1964 "Intractable Heart Failure- Management with 5 to 7 Days of Fasting" A.J. Merrill

International Journal of Cardiology 49:191, 1995 "Salutary Effect of *Terminalia arjuna* in Patients with Severe Refractory Heart Failure" A. Bharani et al.

Journal de Pharmacie et de Chimie 2:321, 1942 "A Coffee Substitute *Cassia occidentalis*" M.P. Bruere

Kardiologija 9:#2/130, 1969 "Calcium Pantothenate in the Treatment of Chronic Heart Failure" N.V. Klykov

Lancet 234:308, 1938 "Vitamin C in Heart Failure" W. Evans

Newsweek 105:Mar 4/ 72, 1985 "A Tale of Two Hearts" M. Clark et al.

Planta Medica 55:276, 1989 "New Antihepatotoxic Naptho-pyrone Glycosides from the Seeds of *Cassia tora*" S. Wong

Psychology Today 18:Oct/ 58, 1984 "Life on the Cutting Edge" J. Rogers

Science 211:42, 1981 "Consensus on Bypass Surgery" G.B. Kolata

Time 121:April 4/62, 1982 "Death of a Gallant Pioneer" C. Wallis

Time 128:Aug 18/58, 1986 "Stilling the Artificial Beat" A. Toufexis

36 HERBS OF THE HEART

Acta Physiologica Academiae Hungaricae 35:183,189, 1969 "Pharmacology of Cherry *Prunus avium* Stalk Extract" E. Hetenyi et al.

American Journal of Chinese Medicine 8:86, 1980 "Mexican Medical Plants Used in Treatment of Cardiovascular Diseases" X. Lozoga

Archives Internationales de Pharmacodynamie 280:241, 1986 "Effects of the Water Extract of *Chrysanthemum indicum* on Coronary and Systemic Hemodynamics in the Dog" T. Kato et al.

Archivos de la Sociedad de Biologia de Montevideo 12:261, 1945 "Evidence of a Heart Stimulating Substance in the Fungus *Agaricus campestris*" R. Caldieyro

Berichte Uber die Gesamte Physiologie 115:126,1939 "Cardiovascular Effects of the Leaves of *Asarum europaeum*" I.A. Lerma

British Medical Journal 2:768, 1874 "Rheumatic Fever by Cynara" E.Copeman

Chemical Abstracts 35:7035, 1941 "Pharmacological Investigation of the Effect of the Tincture of *Spigelia* on the Isolated Animal and Human Heart and Human Coronary Vessels" I. Sivertsev

C.R. Societe de Biologie 85:527, 1921 & 86:399, 1922 "Cardiotonic Action of Nettle Juice" H. Hermann et al.

Indian Journal of Experimental Biology 15:485, 1977 "Protective Effect of Fruit Extracts of *Emblica officinalis*" M. Tarique et al.

Journal of Cardiovascular Pharmacology 9:193, 1987 "Mode of Cardiotonic Action of Helenalin" M. Itoigawa

Journal of Pharmacy and Experimental Therapy 69:309, 1940 "The Action of a Flavone Glucoside on the Heart" R.A. Ward

Journal of Pharmacy and Pharmacology 33:317, 1981 "Calcium Antagonist Action of a Coumarin Isolated from Aian-Hu, A Chinese Traditional Medicine" T. Kozawa

Medical Abstracts, Korea 3:117, 1976 "Pharmacological Action of Extracts of *Scutellaria baicalensis* on Cardiovascular System" Y.Y. Ro et al.

Medical Anthropology 3:401, 1979 "Indigenous Medicine Among the Hausa of Northern Nigeria" N. Etkin

Medizinische 18:692, 1956 "Clincial and Laboratory Experiments on the Mode of Action of Hawthorn Extracts" H. Werner

Pharmazeutische Zentralhalle 68:425, 1927 "Seventeenth Century Heart Remedies" A. Martin

Philippine Journal of Science 115:317, 1986 "Pharmacological Studies on *Jatropha Curcas* as a Possible Source of Anti-arrhythmic (Beta-blocker) Agent" F.R. Fojas et al.

Planta Medica 32:133, 1977 "Beneficial Effect of *Taxus baccata* in Experimental Myocardial Necrosis" S.J. Hussain et al.

Science 220:81, 1983 "Normalization of Depressed Heart Function in Rats by Ribose" H.G. Zimmer

Therapie 6:113, 1951 "Cardiovascular Effects of a Cactus *Pereska grandifolia*" R. Legant et al.

37 THE IRREGULAR HEART

American Heart Journal 39:703, 1950 "The Effects of Magnesium Upon Cardiac Arrhythmias" C.D. Enselberg

American Journal of Chinese Medicine 14:119, 1986 "The Antiarrhythmic Effects of *Sophora flavescens* in Rats and Mice" S. Dai

American Journal of Medical Science 194:53, 1937 "Vagal Reflex, Irritability and the Treatment of Paroxysmal Auricular Tachycardia with Ipecac" S. Weiss et al.

American Journal of Medical Science 229:89, 1955 "The Basis of Quinidine Therapy" G.E. Burch et al.

British Heart Journal 8:115, 1946 "The Action of Magnesium on the Heart" P. Szekely

Bulletin de la Society des Sciences Medicale 8:389, 1927 "A New Cardiac Drug *Lycopus virginicus*" M. Page

Cardiology 74:124, 1987 "Antioxidants as Antiarrhythmic Drugs" V.V. Frolkis et al.

Clinical Journal 4:37, 1894 "A Lecture on the Therapeutics of Heart Disease" S. Taylor

Journal of Pharmaceutical Science 51:851, 1962 "Defibrillatory Substance from *Pteryxia terebinthina*" G.H. Bryan

Journal of Pharmaceutical Science 63:1936 1974 "Preliminary Study of Potential Antiarrhythmic Effects of *Crataegus monogyna*" E.B. Thompson et al.

Journal of Pharmacology and Experimental Therapeutics 117:62, 1956 "Ajmaline and Serpentine in Experimental Cardiac Arrhythmias" R.B. Arora et al.

Mayo Clinic Proceedings 17:294, 1944 "A Remarkably Early Reference to the Use of Cinchona in Cardiac Arrhythmia" R.A. Willius

Medical News 64:239, 1894 "A Case of Paroxysmal Tachycardia, of Long Standing Relieved by the Use of Beechwood Creosote" W. Cornett

Medical Times and Gazette 1:161,217, 1867 "Remedial Uses of the *Prunus virginiana*" C. Allbutt

Nutrition Today 16:Sept/31, 1981 "Selenium" A. Szent-Gyorgyi

Planta Medica 24:133, 1973 'Preliminary Phytochemical and Pharmacological Investigation of the Roots of Different Varieties of *Cichorium intybus*" S. I. Balda et al.

Prencia Medica Argentina 35:2317, 1948 "Pharmacological and Chemical Study of a New Active Substance from *Pogonopus tubulos*" M. Sato

Science 102:69, 1945 "Fagarine, A Possible Substitute for Quinidine" V. Deulofeu

St. Louis Medical Journal 3:242, 1876 *"Collinsonia canadensis"* I.J.M. Gross

Tohoku Journal of Experimental Medicine 141:Supp/453, 1983 "Antiarrhythmic Action of Coenzyme A10 in Diabetes" T. Fujioka

Shamberger, Raymond *Biochemistry of Selenium* New York: Plenum Press, 1983

38 ANGINA PECTORIS

American Medicine 22:623, 1916 'Angina Pectoris With Special Reference to the Use of *Crataegus oxyacantha* in its Treatment" J.A. Hofheimer

American Practitioner 2:275, 1870 "Use of Sulfur in Angina Pectoris" E. Richardson

Annual Review of Pharmacology 15:259, 1976 "Selenium in Biology" D.V. Frost et al.

Drugs of the Future 8:865, 1983 "Puerarin" J. Ru-yun

Heart 1:230, 1909 "Breast Pain" Dr. X

Journal of Historic Medicine 35:288, 1980 "Coronary Arterial Spasm: A Historical Perspective" R.N. MacAlpin

Journal of Traditional Chinese Medicine 4:293, 1984 "Therapeutic Effect of *Crataegus pinnatifida* on 46 Cases of Angina Pectoris – A Double Blind Study" W. Weiliang et al.

Medical Analectic 2:392, 1885 "Berries of the Snow-Ball Tree in Angina Pectoris" Dr. Manguby

Medical Proceedings 4:67, 1958 "Parential Magnesium Sulfate in the Treatment of Angina Pectoris" A.L. Agranet

Southern Medical Journal 77:896, 1984 "Angina: From Heberden to Prinzmetel" J.D. Cantwell

Therapeutic Gazette 49:313, 1925 "Castor Oil as a Remedy in Angina Pectoris" L.F. Bishop

39 THE DIGITALIS STORY

Acta Cardiologica 40:357, 1985 "The Foxglove 1785-1985" R.B. Singh

American Heart Journal 83:845, 1972 "Experiments of Nature: Whole Leaf and Purified Alkaloids" G.E. Burch

American Heart Journal 111:615, 1986 "Digitalis: 200 Years in Perspective" J. Somberg et al.

American Journal of Medical Science 170:647, 1925 "Clinical Observations on the Value of Calcium Chloride as a Diuretic and Its Influence on the Circulatory Mechanism" H.N. Segall et al.

American Journal of Physiology 249:Nov/C367, 1985 "200 Years of Digitalis.The Emerging Central Role of the Sodium Ion in the Control of Cardiac Force" C.O. Lee

Heart 2:273, 1910 "Digitalis" J. MacKenzie

Medical Record 151:131, 1940 "Digitalis in the Dietary Treatment of Obesity" I. Bran

Halluin, Maurice D' *Resurrection du Coeur: La Vie du Coeur Isole* Paris: Masson, 1904

40 DIGITALIS SUBSTITUTES

Canadian Medical Association Journal 31:310, 1934 "The Search for Heart Remedies" E. Podolsky

Canadian Medical Association Journal 73:295, 1955 "Clinical Trial of *Ornithogalum umbellatum* on the Human Heart" A. Vogelsang

Eclectic Medical Journal 14:184, 1855 "Decoction of Oats as a Diuretic"

Ellingwood's Therapist 2:295, 1908 *"Phaseolus vulgaris"* V. Ramm

Indian Journal of Medical Research 60:462, 1972 "Cardiac Stimulant Activity of the Saponin of *Achyranthes aspera*"S.S. Gupta

Journal of the American Medical Association 235:194, 1985 "Squill – Energetic Diuretic" W.E. Court

Midland Medical and Surgical Journal 2:80, 1830 *"Asperula odorata"* in Dropsy" J.K. Walker

Scientific American 254:Feb/76, 1986 "The Heart as an Endocrine Gland" M. Cantin et al.

Tohoku Journal of Experimental Medicine 4:149, 1923 "The Cardiotonic and Diuretic Action of Kobu *Laminaria japonica*" M. Watanabe

Zoologica 49:137, 1967 "Birds, Butterflies and Plant Poisons; A Study in Ecological Chemistry" L.P. Brower et.al.

Ramm, H. August *Bohnenhulsenthee Mittheilungen fur Aerzte und Kranke* Preez, 1898

41 BEYOND THE HEART ATTACK

Alkaloids 23:227, 1984 "Constituents of Red Pepper Species: Chemistry, Biochemistry, Pharmacology and Food Science" T. Suzuki et al.

American Journal of Clinical Nutrition 35:1452, 1982 "The Relationship Between High Fibrinolytic Activity and Daily Capsicum Ingestion in Thais" S. Visudhiphan et al.

Arzneimittelforschung 38:1583, 1988 "The Protective Effect of *Allium sativum* and *Crataegus* on Sioprenalin-Induced Tissue Necroses in Rats" A.G. Ciplea et al.

Canadian Medical Association Journal 44:174, 1940 "Some factors in the Causation of Internal Hemorrhage" J.C. Paterson

Chemical Abstracts 80:91250x, 1974 "Cardiovascular Action of Capsaicin in Anesthetized Dogs and Unanesthetized Dogs with Radioelements" A. Ueno

IRCS Medical Science 10:446, 1982 "Decreased Total Serum, Myocardial and Aortic Cholesterol Levels Following Capsicum Treatment" P. Ki et al.

Journal of Pharmaceutical Sciences 71:1174, 1982 "Cardiotonic Principles of Ginger *Zingiber officinale*" N. Shoji et al.

Journal of the International Academy of Preventive Medicine 6:139, 1980 "Bromelain: Its Use in Prevention and Treatment of Cardiovascular Disease – Present Status" S.J. Taussig et al.

Medical Hypothesis 20:271, 1986 "Ginger: Inhibition of Thromboxane Synthetase and Stimulation of Prostacyclin" J. Backon

New England Journal of Medicine 328:1444, 1993 "Vitamin E Consumption and the Risk of Coronary Disease in Women" M.J. Stampfer et al.

New Scientist 118:June 2/46, 1988 "Hidden Powers of the Pineapple" G. Bickerstaff

New York Medical Journal 92:850, 1910 "A Scientific Interpretation of Kusatsu on the Japanese Method of Restoring Life" A. Abrams

Prevention 5:June/36, 1953 "Vitamin E Used Internally for Heart Disease" J.I. Rodale

Prevention 31:Sept/138, 1976 "B$_6$ – Maybe the Answer to Heart Disease" J. Kinderlehrer

Surgery, Gynecology and Obstetrics 93:97, 1951 "The Use of Calcium Chloride in the Treatment of Cardiac Arrest in Patients" J.H. Kay et al.

Rath, Matthias *Eradicating Heart Disease* San Francisco: Health Now, 1993

Schulte, Wildred *Alpha Tocopherol in Cardiovascular Disease* Toronto: Tyerson Press, 1954

42 SECRETS OF THE LIVER

American Journal of Obstetrics and Gynecology 78:141, 1959 "Amenorrhea as a Manifestation of Chronic Liver Disease" P. Green et al.

Antiseptic 43:322, 1946 "Role of the Liver in Health and Disease" M. Hussain

Eyes, Ears, Nose and Throat Monthly 19:176, 1940 "Further Observations on Liver Extract in Ophthalmologic Conditions" R. Bernard

Journal of the Indian Medical Association 27:14, 1956 "A Short Note on Heptology from the Earliest Times to 1900" D.S. Reddy et al.

Lancet 2:1142, 1928 "The Liver in Primitive Medicine"

Life 59:Nov 26/97, 1965 "Happiness is a Bad Liver" P. Dragadze

Medical Record 78:940, 1910 "The Philosophical Anatomy of the Liver" E. Souchon

New York Medical Journal 63:347, 1896 "The Eyes and the Liver" H.H. Seabrook

Panminerva Medical 2:524, 1960 "The Liver and Eczema" F. Ottolenghi-Lodigiani

Saturday Evening Post 195:May 5/12, 1923 "Our Lordly Liver" W. Hutchinson

University of Pennsylvania Medical Bulletin 20:238, 1908 "The Liver in Antiquity and the Beginnings of Anatomy" M. Jastrow

Crille, George W. *Bipolar Theory of Living Processes* New York: Macmillan, 1926

43 LIVER REGENERATION

American Journal of Clinical Medicine 22:30, 1915 "Five Hepatic Remedies" F. Ellingwood

Antiseptic 66:615, 1970 "Therapy of Anorexia with Liv 52" K. Bai et al.

Arzneimittelforschung 16:127, 1966 "Effects of *Cynara scolymus* Extract on Hepatic Regeneration in the Rat" T. Maros et al.

Chinese Medical Journal 3:173, 1977 "Protective Action of Schizandrin B on Hepatic Injury in Mice" Pao Tien Tung et al.

Current Science 72:546, 1997 "Protective Role of Ashwagnadha [*Withania somnifera*] in Cadmium-Induced Hepatotoxicity and Nephrotoxity in Male Mouse" S. Panda

Fitoterapia 57:307, 1986 "Natural Products and Plants as Liver Protecting Drugs" S.S. Nanda et al.

Food and Cosmetics Toxicology 15:173, 1977 "Regeneration of Rat Liver in the Presence of Essential Oils and Their Components" L.L. Gerskbein

Gazette Medicale Italino 135:659, 1976 "Controlled and Open Clinical Trials of Various Amino Acids on Liver Diseases of Varying Severity" G.B. Cavassini

Indian Drugs 30:355, 1993 "Plants with Hepatoprotective Activity: A Review" S. De et al.

Journal of the American Chemical Society 79:32992, 1957 "Selenium as an Integral Part of Factor 3 Against Necrotic Liver Degeneration" K. Schwartz et al.

Medical Record 161:220, 1948 "Clinical Study of Methionine on Hepatic Impairment" A. Debraille et al.

Rastiteleresursy 22:#1/83, 1986 "Effect of an Extract from *Odontites vulgaris* on the Functional State of the Rat Liver in Acute Toxic Hepatitis" I.O. Ubasheer et al.

Rastitleresursy 25:575, 1989 "Hepato-protective Properties of the Extract from the Aerial Parts of *Salsola collina*" A.I. Vengerovskii

Rivista di Biologia 54:537, 1961 "Action of Some plant Auxins on Liver Regeneration in the Rat" R.D. Volpe et al.

Wall St. JournalApril 12/1, 1984 "Transplants Increase and So do Disputes Over Who Pays the Bills" D. Wessil

Bertelli, Aldo *New Trends in the Therapy of Liver Diseases* New York: Karger, 1975

44 CIRRHOSIS OF THE LIVER

American Journal of Chinese Medicine 16:127, 1988 "The Pharmacological and Pathological Studies on Several Hepatic Protective Crude Drugs from Taiwan" Huio Fen Chiu et al.

American Journal of Pathology 18:661, 1942 "Effects of Yeast and Food Intake on Experimental Carbon Tetrachloride Cirrhosis of the Liver in Rats" J. Post

Archiv fur Experimental Pathologie und Pharmacie 206:674, 1949 "Experimental Study of Protection Against Poison" O. Eicher

Clinica Chinica Acta 4:728, 1959 "Protective Effect of Ornithine and Aspartic Acid in Chronic Carbon Tetrachloride Intoxication" F. Salvadore et al.

Indian Drugs 30:355, 1993 "Plants with Hepatoprotective Activity – A Review" S. De et al.

IRCS Journal of Medical Science 14:439, 1986 "Antihepatotoxic Activity of *Salvia haematodes* and *Artemisia absinthium*" S. Akbar

Journal of Hepatology9:105, 1989 "Randomized Controlled Trial of Silymarin Treatment in Patients with Cirrhosis of the Liver" D. Ferenci et al.

Journal of Physiology 97:103, 1939 "The Effect of Choline on the Fatty Liver After Carbon Tetrachloride Poisoning" H. Barrett et al.

New England Journal of Medicine 318:1709, 1988 "Colchicine in The Treatment of Cirrhosis of the Liver" D. Kershenobich et al.

Quarterly Journal of Studies on Alcohol 1:517, 1940 "Vitamin Deficiencies and Liver Cirrhosis in Alcoholism" N. Jolliffe

Scientific American 232:June/22, 1975 "How the Liver Metabolizes Foreign Substances" A. Kappas et al.

Society of Experimental Biology and Medicine, Proceedings 113:203, 1963 "Prevention of Experimental Dietary Hepatic Injury by Extracts of Some Tropical Plants" P. Gyorgy

Southern Medical Journal 36:353, 1942 "Alcohol and Cirrhosis of the Liver" R.S. Boles

Toxicology and Applied Pharmacology 45:723, 1978 "The Protective Effect of *Eclipta alba* on Carbon Tetrachloride Induced Acute Liver Damage" K. Ma-Ma et al.

45 JAUNDICE

American Journal of Clinical Nutrition 25:626, 1972 "Yerakon in the Bible and Talmud: Jaundice or Anemia" F. Rosner

Antiseptic 66:353, 1968 "Liv 52 in Infectious Hepatitis" S. Ray

Current Medical Practice 9:451, 1965 "Treatment of Jaundice with an Indigenous Drug *Picrorhiza kurroa*" G.N. Chaturvedi et al.

Eastern Pharmacist 27:May/86, 1984 "Herbal Remedy for Jaundice"

Experientia 41:699, 1985 "Antihepatoxic Constituents of *Garcinia kola* Seeds" M.M. Iwu

Indian Medical Record 22:175, 1902 "*Moringa pterygosperma* in Jaundice with Cases" R.D. Sinta

Japanese Journal of Pharmacy 2:102,139, 1953 "Study on *Gardenia florida* as a Remedy for Icterus" T. Miwa

Journal of Ethnopharmacology 48:89, 1995 "...The Nigerian Plant *Cochlospermum planchonii* as a Zinc Salt" R. Aliyu et al.

Medical Brief 10:63, 1882 "*Chionanthus virginicus*- Old Man's Gray Beard- A New Remedy for Jaundice" I.J.M. Gross

Medicina et Pharmacologia Experimentalis 16:407, 1967 "Chemical Fractionation of Antiviral Plants" S.C. Chou et al.

Practitioner 15:104, 1880 "On the Treatment of Jaundice" H. Cook

Southern Surgeon 5:50, 1936 "Jaundice: Diagnosis, Treatment and Prognosis" R.L. Sanders

Texas State Journal of Medicine 29:39, 1933 "Cenzo in the Treatment of Catarrhal Jaundice" P.I. Nixon

Toxicology and Applied Pharmacology 46:353, 1978 "Action of *Carica papaya* Extracts on Jaundice Produced in Rats by Saponosides of *Brennania brieyi*" B. Boum et al.

Hill, John *A Method of Curing the Jaundice by the Herb Agrimony* London: R. Baldwin, 1768

46 THE FUNCTION OF BILE

American Journal of Medicine 39:98, 1965 "Physiochemical Characteristics of Bile and Their Relation to Gallstone Formation" K. Juniper Jr. et al.

American Journal of Roentgenology 19:341, 1928 "Cholecystographic Studies After the Administration of Some of the Popular Cholagogues" W.H. Stewart et al.

British Medical Journal 3:813, 1972 "Bile Acids: A pH Dependent Antibacterial System in the Gut" I.W. Percy-Robb et al.

C.R. Societe de Biologie 108:1100, 1932 "Choleretic Action of the Compositae" E. Chabral

C.R. Societe de Biologie 109:275, 1932 "Choleretic Action of the Labiates" E. Chabral et al.

Deutsche Medizinische Wochenschrift 57:1673, 1931 "Investigation Into the Action of Turmeric On Liver and Gall Bladder Function"

Helvetica Chirurgica Acta 15:75, 1978 "Gallbladder Surgery and Emetin" V.E. Melchior

International Clinics 34:#1/187, 1924 "The Gall-Bladder: Its Past, Present and Future" J.E. Sweet

Journal de Medecine et de Chirurgie Pratiques 108:141, 1937 "Using *Curcuma xanthorrhiza* in Hepatic and Bilary Therapy" H. Leclerc

Medical Journal and Record 135:440, 1932 "The Therapeutic Effect of Elegiac Acid and Bile Salts in Diseases of the Bilary Tract" R. Finkelstein et al.

Medical Record 142:261, 1935 "The Importance of Bile and Transient Occasional Hepatic Acholia" M. Einhorn

Mitteilungen aus der Medizinischen Akademia zu Kioto 13:676,710, 1935 "The Influence of Japanese and Chinese Drugs on Bile Secretion in Rabbits" I. Sato

Planta Medica 53:239, 1987 "A Comparative Study of the Efficacy of *Pavetta indica* and *Osbeckia octandra* in the Treatment of Liver Dysfunction" I. Thabrew et al.

Review of Gastroenterology 8:225, 1941 "The Biliary System" C.J. Brim

Society of Experimental Biology and Medicine, Proceedings 43:474, 1940 "Effect of Whole Bile and Bile Salt of Swine on Gastric Mobility of the Dog" J.M. Winfield

47 GALLSTONES

Acta Manilana 15A:25, 1976 "Chemical Factors Involved in Cholesterol Gallstone Formation – Possible Prevention and Medical Treatment" M.D. Navarro et al.

Alkaloidal Clinic 13:104, 1906 "Wild Yam in Bilious Colic" J.H. Hall

American Journal of Roentgenology 26:904, 1931 "An Effective Gall-Bladder Stimulant to Supplant the Fat Meal" L. Levyn

L'Art Medicale #111:368, 1910 "A New Treatment of Bile Stones *Triumfetta semitriloba*" M. Jousset

Boston Medical and Surgical Journal 98:133, 1878 "Sprudel Salts in the Treatment of Gall Stones" M. Goldsmith

British Medical Journal 1:1144, 1895 "Treatment of Gall Stones by Large Doses of Olive Oil" W.H. Stephenson

British Medical Journal 2:244,414, 1920 "Treatment of Gall Stones by Infusion of Parsley" H.C. Kidd

British Medical Journal 2:293, 1920 "Gall Stones and Infusions" C. Dukes

Canadian Medical Journal 2:293, 1866 "Case of Supposed Poisoning by *Coptis trifolia*" W.J. Anderson

Gut 20:312, 1979 "Rowachol- A Possible Therapy for Cholesterol Gallstones" J. Doran et al.

Journal of Laboratory and Clinical Medicine 27:897, 1942 "Clinical and Laboratory Investigations on the Extract of the European Mountain Ash Berry" G.Y. Shinowara et al.

Lancet 2:722, 1887 "Discussion on Biliary Calculus at the Mexican Academy"

Medical Fortnightly 29:281, 1906 "The Treatment of Gallstones with Cholagen" C.D. Aaron

Medical News 55:573, 1899 "A Suggestion as to the Action of Olive or Cotton Seed Oil in Gallstone Colic" D. Stewart

Medical Review 17:36, 1914 "Treatment of Gall-Stones by Ipecacuanha" T.H. Delany

Medical Standard 6:106, 1889 "*Dioscorea villosa* – Wild Yam" J.V. Shoemaker

Munchener Medizinische Wocherschrift 83:610, 1936 "Radish Therapy of Gallstones and Other Spastic Syndromes" S. Schoenborn

New Orleans Medical and Surgical Journal 35:676, 1883 "Gallstones Successfully Treated with Olive Oil" F. Loeber

Nutrition Reviews 16:25, 1958 "Diet and Gallstones"

Pharmaceutische Zentralhalle 73:260, 1932 "Chollefrey, A New Gallstone Remedy" B. Rossman

Rontgenpraxis 12:286, 1940 "The Juice of Red Pepper and the Gall Bladder Reflex" L. Berkesey

Rumanian Medical Review 7:#4/54, 1963 "Sparteine Sulfate in the Treatment of Atonia of the Gall Bladder" S. Pop et al.

Scientific American 136:392, 1927 "Gallstones, Kidney Stones and Diet" M. Fishbein

Therapeutic Gazette 14:46, 1890 "The Treatment of Hepatic Jaundice by Hypodermic Injections of Pilocarpine"

Therapie 15:1040, 1960 "Protective Effect of *Tiliae alburnum* Against Pain" C. Debray et al.

Ugeskrift fur Laeger 83:82, 1921 "Oil of Peppermint for Relief of Gallstones" A. Boggild

48 DIURETIC HERBS

Acta Scholae Medicinalis in Gifu 11:129,138, 1963 "Diuretic Action of Crude Drugs" K. Tsurumi

Alkaloid Clinic 11:945, 1904 "A Southern Diuretic" T.S. White

American Journal of Medical Science 238:287, 1959 "The Use of L-Lysine Monohydrochloride in the Treatment of Mercurial Resistant Edema" D. Brailovsky et al.

Angiologica 9:375, 1972 "Vitamin P and Lymphatics" M. Foldi

Archiv fur Experimentelle Pathologie 186:565,574,584,592, 1937 & 190:406,522, 1938 "Diuretic Properties of Juniper berries, Levisticum roots, Ononis roots, Birch Leaves, Licorice, Horsetail and Ratten" H. Vollmer et al.

Archives International de Pharmacodynamie 133:127, 1961 "The Antiedema Properties of Aesculin" R.J. Girerd et al.

British Medical Journal 2:492, 1934 "Pineapple Juice in Edema" B. Maegraith

Bulletins et Memoires de la Societe Medicale des Hopitaux.173,1942 "The Remarkable Action of Nicotinamide on Infantile Hydrocephaelis" H. Gounelle et al.

Deutsche Medizinische Wochenschrift 53:1299, 1927 "Indian Kidney Tea Koemis Koetjing *Orthosiphon stamineus*" A. Gurber

Georgia Journal of Medicine and Surgery 4:207, 1899 "*Sambucus* in Parenchymatous Nephritis" J.W. Daniel

Indian Journal of Physiology and Pharmacology 30:91, 1986 "Diuretic Effect of *Aerva lanata*" M. Udupihille

Journal of Allergy 13:173, 1941 "Cerebral Allergic Edema" W.R. Crowe

Journal of Nutrition 47:361, 1952 "The Importance of Choline in the Prevention of Nutritional Edema in Rats Fed Low Protein Diets" H.D. Alexander et al.

Journal of the American Medical Association 14:557, 1890 "*Sambucus nigra* as a Diuretic" M.G. Lemoine

Munchener Medizinische Wochenschrift 64:862, 1917 "Asparagus in Kidney Problems" M. Von Stabsarzt

North Carolina Medical Journal 5:219, 1880 "*Vaccinium crassifolium* var. *repens*" E.A. Anderson

Prevention 24:June/109, 1972 "Kidney Bean Pods and Your Kidney" H.A. Ramm (see also 25:Jan/29, 1972 & 25:Mar/18,1973 & 26:April/184, 1974

Presse Medicale 34:18, 1926 "A Study of the Diuretic Action of *Pyrola umbellata*" H. Busquet

Proceedings of the National Academy of Science 8:39, 1922 "A Study of the Effects of *Curcurbita pepo* Seeds on Kidney Excretion" B. Masurovsky

Quarterly Journal of Crude Drug Research 1:59, 1961 "*Orthosiphon stamineus*" E.F. Steinmetz

Society of Experimental Biology and Medicine, Proceedings 76:349, 1951 "Vitamin B$_{12}$, a Factor in Prevention of Hydrocephalus in Infant Rats" B.L. O'Delli et al.

Therapeutic Gazette 7:140, 1883 "Sourwood *Oxydendron*" F. Clendenen

Therapeutic Gazette 23:589, 1899 "A Preliminary Note on the Use of Asparagus as a Diuretic" H.A. Hare

49 KIDNEY REGENERATION

American Journal of Medical Science 58:47, 1869 "On the Therapeutic Action of *Sambucus canadensis* in Albuminuria" R. McNutt

American Journal of Medicine 48:671, 1970 "On the Pathogenesis of Uremia" P.E. Teschan

Annuaire de Therapeutique 130,1866 "*Clematis* Seeds in Albuminuria" Dr. Sauveur

Archiv fur Experimentelle Pathologie und Pharmakologie 166:56, 1932 "The Effect of Renotret (Sarsaparilla extract) on Experimental Uranium Nephritis" F. Schneider

Chemical and Pharmacological Bulletin 32:4506, 1984 "Effect of Orally Administered Rhubarb Extract in Rats with Chronic Renal Failure" T. Yokozawa

Chemical and Pharmacological Bulletin 36:316, 1988 "Isolation of the Active Component Having the Uremia-Preventive Effect from *Salviae miltiorhizae* Radix Extract" T. Yokozawa et al.

Deutsche Medizinische Wochenscrift 61:377, 1935 "Clinical Research on an *Orthosiphon stamineus* Preparation" H. Rutenbeck

European Journal of Pharmacology 120:171, 1986 "Effects of Saikosaponin-d on Aminonucleoside Nephrosis in Rats" A. Abe et al.

Japanese Journal of Pharmacology 32:823, 1982 "Immunopharmacological Studies of the Aqueous Extract of *Cinnamomun cassia*" H. Nagai

Journal of Pharmacy and Experimental Therapy 48:1, 1933 "A Study of the Effects of Agave Concentrate in the Treatment of Nephrites in Animals" H. Jones

Journal of Pharmacy and Experimental Therapy 75:11, 1942 "The Stimulating Influence of Sodium Citrate on Cellular Regeneration and Repair in the Kidney Injured by Uranium Acetate" G.L. Donnelly et al.

Journal of Research in Indian Medicine 7:#3/28, 1972 "Studies on the Indian Indigenous Herb *Boerhavia diffusa*" R.H. Singh et al.

Journal of the Indian Medical Profession 18:8256, 1972 "A Preliminary Report on Phytochemical and Clinical Trials of *Tinospora cordifolia* in Six Uremia Patients" A.S. Gupta et al.

Journal of the Royal Society of Medicine 73:514, 1980 "The Story of Nephrology" D. Black

Klinische Wochenschr 12:1696, 1933 "The Effect of a Sarsaparilla Preparation in Chronic Nephritis with Reference to the Uric Acid Content of the Blood and Urine" F. Humpert

Lakeland Ledger [Florida newspaper] May 26/10,1963 "Florida's Magic Plants" J. Wellenkamp

Medecine Tropicale 11:869, 1951 "Hepatoreal Diuretics, *Vicia faba* Hulls" J. Balansard

Pacific Science Congress: Proceedings 4A:203, 1953 "*Smilax* Roots and Uremia" A.M. Ernst

Science 208:473, 1980 "Dialysis After Nearly a Decade" G.B. Kolata

Therapeutic Gazette 35:163, 1911 "Notes on Magueys and Maguey Sap or Aquamiel, a Therapeutic Agent of High Value" C.S. Dolley

Urologic and Cutaneous Review 50:679, 1946 "Three Cases of Acute Nephritis Treated with Vitamin E" W.E. Shute

Voenno-Meditsinskii Zhurnal 76:307, 1898 "The Cure of Bright's Disease with Icelandic Moss" A.P. Morozoff

50 KIDNEY STONES

American Journal of Clinical Nutrition 14:240, 1964 "Oral Magnesium Administration in the Treatment of Renal Calculus Formation" H.E. Sauberlich et al.

American Journal of Clinical Nutrition 45:115, 1987 "The Effect of Pumpkin Seeds on Oxalcrystalluria and Urinary Composition of Children in Hyperendemic Urea" V.S. Suphakarn et al.

American Journal of Clinical Nutrition 53:935, 1991 "Vitamin B_6 Deficiency and Renal Function and Structure in Chronically Uremic Rats" M. Wolfson et al.

Boston Medical and Surgical Journal 19:393, 1838 "Pedate Violet" O. Partridge

British Journal of Urology 58:529, 1986 "Rice Bran Treatment for Calcium Stone Formers with Idiopathic Hypercalciuria" E. Ebisuno et al.

British Journal of Urology 71:143, 1993 "Effect of *Desmodium styracifolium* Triterpenoid on Calcium Oxalate Renal Stones" H. Hirayama et al.

British Medical Journal 1:Supplement #268,1904 "Infusion of Birch Leaves as a Solvent of Renal Calculi"

British Medical Journal 1:1544, 1965 "Herbal Cure for Renal Calculi"

Chinese Medical Journal 50:847, 1936 "Notes on the History and Treatment of Urinary Calculi in China" B.E. Read

Drug and Cosmetic Industry 72:42, 1953 "Urinary Stones" M.A. Lesser

Indian Drugs 21:224, 1984 "Herbal Drugs for Urinary Stones – Literature Appraisal" T. Mukerjee et al.

Journal of Alternative and Comparative Medicine 6:Mar/5, 1988 "Secret of the Nile Herb Cure for Stones" G. Dale

Journal of Nutrition 73:308, 1961 "Dietary Magnesium, Calcium and Vitamin B_6 in Experimental Nephropathies in Rats" S.N. Gershoff et al.

Journal of Urology 30:639, 1933 "The Relationship of Vitamin A and Vitamin D to Urinary Calculus Formation" A.R. Bliss et al.

Journal of Urology 112:509, 1974 "Magnesium Oxide-pyridoxine therapy for Recurrent Calcium Oxalate Calculi" E.L. Prient et al.

Journal of Urology 139:240, 1988 "Alkali Action on the Urinary Crystallization of Calcium Salts..." G.M. Preminger

Medical Repository 10:405, 1807 "Important Experiments on Stone and Gravel in the Urinary Passages of Men" T. Egan

Medicine and Surgery 22:Oct/9, 1982 "Study on Indigenous Drug Sitivana *Celosia argentea*" S.D. Dubey et al.

New England Journal of Medicine 213:1007, 1935 "Experimental and Clinical Observations on Urinary Calculi" C.C. Higgins

Pharmaceutical Journal 33:105, 1873 "Note on the reputed Value of *Polygonum aviculare* for Stone" J.R. Jackson

Shikoku Acta Medica 26:283, 1970 "Pharmacological studies on *Quercus stenophylla*" Y. Kawakami

Shikoku Acta Medica 31:149, 1975 "Effect of the Extract of *Uncaria kawakamii* of Formosa Origin in Dissolving Artificial Bladder Calculi" M. Kuramoto et al.

South African Medical Journal 58:652, 1980 "A History of Urinary Stone" M. Modlin

Therapeutic Gazette 5:195,354, 1881 "*Actinomeris helianthoides*" I.J.M. Gross

Zentrablatt fur Urologie 38:1, 1944 "The Operation of Madder on Bladder Stones" J. Keller et al.

51 HYPOGLYCEMIA

Biochemical Journal 41:151, 1947 "The Mechanism of Phloridizine Glucosuria" B. Shapiro

Deutsche Medizinische Wochenschrift 61:377, 1935 "Clinical Tests with *Orthosiphon stamineus*" H. Rutenbeck

Hormones and Metabolic Research 8:379, 1976 "Effects of Lithium on Inducible Enzymes of Rat Liver" G.W. Grier et al.

Indian Medical Gazette 86:42, 1951 "Effect of Rutin on Blood Sugar Levels of Rabbits" H.B. Swift et al.

Journal of Pharmacy and Experimental Therapy 41:83, 1931 "Glycogen Storage in the White Rat When Fed the Roots of *Arctium lappa*" J.C. Krantz Jr. et al.

Journal of Pharmacy and Experimental Therapy 43:295, 1931 "The Mechanism Produced by Guanidine and Carbon Tetrachloride Poisoning and its Relief by Calcium Medication" A.S. Minot

Journal of Pharmacy and Experimental Therapy 55:206, 1935 "The Effect of Zinc Salts on the Action of Insulin" D.A. Scott

Journal of the American Medical Association 83:729, 1924 "Hyperinsulinism and Dysinsulinism" S. Harris

Medical Journal of Australia 2:942, 1965 "Did Winnie the Pooh Have Spontaneous Functional Hypoglycaemia?" J.E. Gault

Northwest Medicine 45:923, 1946 "Diagnosis of Hypoglycemia Neurosis with Minnesota Multiphasic Personality Inventory" T.W. Houk et al.

Trends in Biochemical Sciences 4:124, 1979 "Alanine as a Glucogenic Carrier" K. Snell

52   DIABETES DIETS

American Journal of Digestive Diseases 15:109, 1948 "The Use of High Protein Diets in the Treatment of Diabetes Mellitus" D. Adlersberg

American Journal of Medical Science 175:376, 1928 "Treatment of Diabetes with an Acid-alcoholic Extract of Plants Rich in Vitamin B" C. Mills

Annals of Internal Medicine 35:1028, 1951 "The Use of Vitamin B_{12} in the Management of Neurolgic Manifestation of Diabetes" S.M. Sancetta et al.

Archiv Fur Geschichte der Medizin 25:1, 1932 "Diabetes Mellitis in Ancient Hindu Medicine" R. Muller

British Medical Journal 281:578, 1980 "Exceptionally Low Blood Glucose Response of Dried Beans" D.J. Jenkins et al.

Diabetologia 5:379, 1969 "Hypoglycemic Effect of the Salt Bush *Atriplex halimus* – A Feeding Source of the Sand Rat" Z. Aharonson et al.

European Journal of Clinical Nutrition 42:51, 1988 "Glucose-Lowering Effect of Fenugreek in Non-Insulin Dependent Diabetics" Z. Madar et al.

Indian Journal of Medical Research 45:23, 1957 "Effect of Treatment with Vitamin E and Vitamin K and in Combination with Estrogen" S.K. Mukherjee et al.

Indian Journal of Medical Research 48:720, 1960 "Investigation in the Use of Jasad Bhasma, an Ayurvedic Preparation of Zinc in the treatment of Diabetes Mellitus" R.V. Sathe et al.

Journal of Biological Chemistry 262:6658, 1987 "Oral Administration of Vanadate Normalizes Blood Glucose Levels" J. Mayerovitch et al.

Journal of Chronic Disease 23:123, 1970 "Chromium Deficiency as a Factor in Atherosclerosis" H.A. Schroeder et al.

Journal of Nutritional Medicine 1:217, 1990 "Vitamin B_3 in the Treatment of Diabetes Mellitus" J.P. Cleary

Journal of the American Diabetic Association 6:1, 1930 "The History of the Treatment of Diabetes by Diet" F.N. Allan

Journal of the American Medical Association 185:166, 1963 "Psychological Factors Associated with the Onset of Diabetes Mellitus" P.F. Slawson et al.

Journal of the Indian Medical Association 42:517, 1964 "Oral Manganese Chloride as a Hypoglycemic Agent" M.P. Mehrotra

Lancet 2:1348, 1962 "Manganese Induced Hypoglycemia" A.H. Rubenstein et al.

Medical History 13:190, 1969 "On the Term Diabetes in the Works of Aretaeus and Galen" F. Henschin

Medical Record 27:542, 1885 "Buckwheat Flour in Diabetes" Dr. Alvord

Metabolism 36:51, 1987 "Effects of Supplemental Chromium on Patients with Symptoms of Reactive Hypoglycemia" R.A. Anderson

New York State Journal of Medicine 41:2145, 1941 "Thiamin Chloride in the Treatment of Diabetic Acidosis" J.R. Scott

Post-Graduate 19:408, 1904 "The Oats Cure in Severe Cases of Diabetes Mellitus" C. Von Noordin

Quarterly Journal of Medicine 4:277, 1935 "A Comparison of Various Diets in the Treatment of Diabetes Mellitus" E.M. Watson

Revue de Theraptique Medico-Chirurgicale 81:79, 1914 "Sugar Diabetes and Its Treatment with the Diet of the Ancient Arab Writers" A. Robin

53 DIABETIC TEAS

Annals of Nutrition and Metabolism 28:37, 1984 "Effects of Fenugreek Seeds on Endocrine Pancreatic Secretions in Dogs" G. Ribes et al.

Antiseptic 64:907, 1967 "Role of Saptarangi *Casearia esculenta* in the Treatment of Madhu Meta (Diabetes Mellitus)" R. Nautiyal

British Medical Journal 1:1044, 1980 "Treatment of Diabetes Mellitus with *Coccinia indica*" A.K. Azadkhan et al.

Canadian Medical Association Journal 39:32, 1938 "A Hypoglycemic Substance from the Roots of Devil's Club" R.G. Large et al.

Chicago Medical Times 35:520, 1902 "Specific *Chionanthus* in the Treatment of Diabetes Mellitus" A.P. Hauss

C.R. Societe de Biologie 123:1155, 1936 "Hypoglycemic Action of *Rehmannia glutinosa, Alisma plantago, Scrophularia oldhamii, Atractylis ovata* and *Lycium chinense*" King Li Pin et al.

Far East Medical Journal 6:353, 1970 "The Antidiabetic Action of the Herb *Orthosiphon stamineus*" J.S. Cheah et al.

Fitoterapia 56:190, 1985 "Use of *Annona squamosa* and *Piper nigrum* Against Diabetes" A. Atique et al.

Indian Journal of Pharmacy 7:60, 1945 "*Tephrosa villosa*: A Plant Useful in the Treatment of Diabetes" H. Singh

Journal of the Egyptian Medical Association 48:Sup/153, 1965 "Antidiabetic Properties of *Salix* Leaves" A. Sharef

Journal of the Pakistan Medical Association 32:106, 1982 "Trial of *Momordica charantia* Powder in Patients with Maturity Onset Diabetes" M.S. Akhtara

Journal of the Philippine Medical Association 20:395, 1940 "On the Hypoglycemic Effect of a Decoction of *Lagerstroemia speciosa* Leaves" F. Garcia

Malayan Nature Journal 18:73, 1964 "Dr. Quack's Tea Leaves" K.M. Kochummen

Medical Anthropology 11:255, 1989 "Ethnobotanical Treatment of Diabetes in Baja California Norte" M. Winkelman

Planta Medica 11:159, 1963 "Studies on the Antidiabetic Activity of Some Drugs" A.A. Sharif et al.

Therapeutic Gazette 26:616, 1902 "Eucalypts in the Treatment of Diabetes"

Therapie der Gegenwart 105:266, 1966 "A Trial of *Harungana madagascariensis* in Diabetes" G. Franke

Zeitschrift fur Die Gesamte Experimentelle Medizin 35:1, 1927 "Bean Pod Tea in Diabetes" E. Kaufman

Arden, Harven *Wisdomkeepers: Meetings With Native American Spiritual Elders* Hillsboro, Oregon: Beyond Words Publishing, 1990

54 HERBAL DIABETIC CURES

Annales Pharmaceutique Francaises 31:321, 1973 "On the Composition of *Poterium spinosum*" A. Pourrat et al.

Archives Intenationales de Pharmacodynamie 161:306, 1961 "Hypoglycemic Effect of *Poterium spinosum*" J. Mishinsky et al.

Chemical Abstracts 22:988, 1928 "*Phyllanthus sellowianus* on Blood Sugar Concentration" G. Gonalonset al.

Current Science 56:139, 1987 "Pinitol- A New Anti-diabetic Compound from the Leaves of *Bougainvillea spectabilis*" D.D. Joshi et al.

Eclectic Medical Journal 38:57, 1978 "*Lycopus virginicus*" F.L. Gerald

Indian Drugs 18:184, 1981 "L-epicatechin- A Novel Anti-Diabetic Drug" B.K. Chakravarthy et al.

Journal of Ethnopharmacology 30:295, 1990 "Antidiabetic Effect of a Leaf Extract from *Gymnema sylvestre* in Non-insulin Diabetes Mellitus Patients" K. Baskaran et al.

Journal of Tropical Medicine and Hygiene 39:46, 1936 "Calcium Metasilicate Drogel and Silicon Colloid Dioxide for the Treatment of Sugar in the Urine and Blood" A.S. de Hermany

Lancet 2:759, 1981 "Pancreatic Beta-Cell Regeneration in Rats by (-)-Epicatechin" B.K. Chakravarthy et al.

New York Medical Journal 87:929, 1907 & 89:1147, 1909 "Chimaphila in Diabetes" S.G. Soules

World Health 26:Nov/28, 1977 "Plants That Heal" O. Ampofo

55 PANCREATIC ENZYMES

American Druggist Circular 4:65, 1860 "*Lycopus europaeus*"

American Journal of Physiology 184:449, 1956 "Changes in Pancreatic Enzymes Brought About by Amino Acid Addition to the Diet" D.F. Magee et al.

Archives of Biochemistry 19:329, 1948 "Inositol, An Active Constituent of Pancreatic Alpha Amylase" R.L. Lane et al.

Arzneimittelforschung 21:101,271,421,1971 "Studies in Experimental Animals On Determining the Digestion Regulating Properties of *Harungana madagascariensis*" V.T. Kemeny

Cell and Tissue Research 192:277, 1978 "Catharanthine: A Novel Stimulator of Pancreatic Enzyme Release" J.A. Williams

Deutsche Apotheker Zeitung 106:1053, 1966 "The Botany, Chemistry and Therapeutic Use of *Harungana madagascariensis*" J. Fisel et al.

Journal of Nutrition 87:297, 1965 "Dietary Regulation of Pancreatic Enzymes: Synthesis, Secretion and Inclination in the Rat" J. Snook

Journal of Pediatrics 15:763, 1939 "Cystic Fibrosis of the Pancreas, Vitamin A Deficiency and Bronchiectasis" D. Anderson

Manufacturing Chemist 45:June/25 & Sept/41, 1974 "Effect of Compound 561 on Pancreatic Secretion" A Slovak et al.

Medical Record 150:276, 1939 "The Pancreatic Enzymes and Food Allergy" A.W. Oelgoetz et al.

Medizinische Monatsschrift 29:173, 1975 "The Effect of *Chelidonium, Curcuma,* Absinth and *Carduus marianus* on Biliary and Pancreatic Secretion in Hepatopathies" J.C. Baumann

Nutrition Today 17:Mar/20, 1982 "The Pancreas" D. Enloe

Semaine Medecine 14:190, 1894 "Jurebeba Extract as a Stomachic" A. Michaelis

56 GOITER

British Medical Journal 2:995, 1938 "Early Use of Iodine for Goiter" J.C.L.

Canadian Medical Association Journal 96:995, 1938 "Even the Gods had Goiter" G.D. Hart

Eclectic Medical Journal 72:208, 1912 *"Iris versicolor"*

Journal of Experimental Medicine 57:121, 1933 "The Occurrence of Antigoiterous Substances in Plants" D. Marine et al.

Medical Life 32:53, 1925 "History of Iodine Therapy" J.F. Gudernatsch

Scientific American 224:June/92, 1971 "Endemic Goiter" R.B. Gillie

Yale Journal of Biology and Medicine 51:441, 1978 "Goiter in Tibetan Medicine" G.N. Burrow et al.

Merke, Franz *History and Iconography of Endemic Goiter and Cretinism* Boston: MTP Press, 1984

57 GRAVES' DISEASE

American Journal of Psychiatry 103:831, 1947 "Phobia as a Symptom in Hyperthyroidism" B.J. Ficarra et al.

Arzneimittelforschung 44:41, 1994 "Endocrine Effects of *Lycopus europaeus* Following Oral Application" H. Winterhoff et al.

British Medical Journal 1:Epitome #263,1902 *"Hydrastis canadensis"* W. Cuthbertson

British Medical Journal 1:443, 1925 "The Thyroid and Manganese Treatment in Various Diseases" H.W. Nott

Endocrinology 116:1687, 1985 "Extracts and Auto-oxidized Constituents of Certain Plants Inhibiting the Receptor Binding and the Biological Activity of Graves' Immunoglobulins" M. Auf et al.

Farmatsevticheskii Zhurnal 30:#2/58, 1975 *"Potentilla alba,* An Effective Agent for Treating Thyroid Problems" G.K. Smek et al.

FEBS Letters 150:137, 1982 "Forskolin Stimulates Adenylate Cyclase and Iodine Metabolism in Thyroid" J. Van Sande et al.

Folia Medica 12:188, 1970 "Action of the Alkaloids of *Genista rumelica*" P. Peicev et al.

Journal of Clinical Endocrinology 7:574, 1947 "Use of Massive Doses of Vitamin A in the Treatment of Hyperthyroidism" S. Simkins

Journal of Ophthalmology, Otology and Laryngology 17:94, 1911 *"Lycopus virginicus* as a Remedy of Exophthalmic Goiter: Report of the Cure in a Few Cases" E.J. George et al.

Lancet 2:425, 1919 "The Relationship of Graves' Disease to Diabetes" R.T. Williamson

Medical Interpreter 8:#48, 1926 "Graves Goiter Treatment" M. Loeper et al.

Medical Life 32:35, 1925 "Historic Data on Exophthalmic Goiter" I. Bram

Nature 176:165, 1955 "Protective Action of Vitamin B_{12} in the Hyperthyroid Rat" P. Fatterpaker et al.

Prevention 33:Sept/18, 1981 "Thyroid Symptoms Relieved" J. Woods

Revue de Botanique Appliquee et d'Agriculture Tropicale 19:564, 1939 "On *Pseudocinchona africana,* Its Chemical Composition and Use in Therapy" R. Raymond-Hamet

Wiener Klinische Wochenschrift 54:433, 1941 "The Therapy of Thyrotoxicosis with Magnesium glutamate" H. Puhl

Zeitschrift fur Vitaminforschung 16:322, 1945 "Pantothenic Acid and The Thyroid Gland" E. Glandzmann et al.

Index

✫ ✫ ✫

Resource Guide

Earthpulse Press
P. O. Box 201393
Anchorage, Alaska   99520 USA

Natural Earth: The English Standard Reference on Herbal Substances Volume I: The Herbal Center of Healing

By Gary Lockhart

Earthpulse Press is pleased to bring forward this series – the most complete herbal reference of its kind in the English language. An understandable desk reference on the subject of herbal substances has been needed for years. These books have been compiled for both the trained health practitioner and the lay person as a single reference source. The author has also paid special attention to the collection of bibliographical information at the end of each volume.

This is the largest collection of information on herbal substances since Li Shi Chien published the *Pents'ao* in 1596. The "Great Herbal" has been the Chinese standard of scholarship and information for over four centuries. *Natural Earth: The English Standard Reference on Herbal Substances* may well prove to be the English equivalent.

This encyclopedic work by Gary Lockhart is based on over twenty years of research in traditional healing substances. The author and chronicler of *Natural Earth* has incorporated material from not only scientific literature but also from traditional sources. The tales and science presented in the pages of each volume bring to life a subject which transcends the ages. From ancient traditional herbs – to a modern pharmacology – the subject is explored and presented for ease of reference and understandability. Sourcing documents from the Library of Congress, Stanford and over 40 other research and University libraries the author has organized the most useful set of reference materials assembled to date.

Gary Lockhart presents his work through history, stories and analysis. He breaks each book into sections – dealing with a specific disease or disorder. Through the history of use, he traces each herb and discloses some of the greatest mysteries of healing.

Other Titles Offered by Earthpulse Press

1. **Secrets of the Soil,** by Christopher Bird and Peter Tompkins, is the most important book ever published on new ideas for more production agriculture. Faster growing rates and greater yields without using petrochemical based fertilizers is revealed in this incredible work. The book is of great use to home gardeners and commercial growers alike, an important book for all private collections. Available shipped in the U.S. at $22.95 or internationally for $27.95. Real;easing June 1998.

2. **The Secret Lives of Plants**, by Peter Tompkins and Christopher Bird is a classic on plants and early work in sound stimulation of plant growth. This product is shipped air mail in the U.S. at $19.00 or internationally for $24.00.

3. **Living Energies,** by Callum Coats. This inspiring book could help unravel Nature's mysteries, rewrite science textbooks, revolutionize politics – and safeguard Earth's future. This book is 320 pgs., has 72 photographs, 36 charts and tables and 321 line illustrations. Available shipped in the U.S. at $22.95 or internationally for $27.95.

4. **Towards a New Alchemy: The Millennium Science** is book about the Neurophone™ and other inventions of Dr. Patrick and Dr. Gael Crystal Flanagan. This book will awaken readers to areas of new science which will change the way we live. The book is $17.95 Air Mail in the U.S. or $19.95 internationally.

5. **Earthpulse Flashpoints** is a Microbook series edited by Dr. Nick Begich. Microbooks cover four major areas: government, frontier health sciences, earth science, and new technologies. The goal of the publication is to get hard-to-find information into the hands of individuals on their road to self empowerment and self discovery. For six issues send $24.95 in the U.S. and $30.95 internationally.

6. **The Coming Energy Revolution** was written by <u>Angels Don't Play this HAARP: Advances in Tesla Technology</u> co-author Jeane Manning. The book is about some of the more interesting new energy systems just on the horizon which could revolutionize the production and uses of energy. The book is $15.95 Air Mail in the U.S. or $17.95 internationally.

7. **Scorched Earth: The Military's Assault on the Environment,** by William Thomas is a detailed account of how the military has exposed Americans and people around the world to toxic risks they never disclosed. Every page contains well footnoted evidence of how our lives have been negatively affected by the lack of concern for the impact of military technology. The book is $19.95 Air Mail in the U.S. or $21.95 Air Mail internationally.

8. **Angels Don't Play this HAARP: Advances in Tesla Technology** is a book about non-lethal weapons, mind control, weather warfare and the government's plan to control the environment or maybe even destroy it in the name of national defense. The book is $17.95 Air Mail in the U.S. or $19.95 internationally.

9. **Bringing the War Home**, by William Thomas is a controversial book which explores and challenges the ideas surrounding the events in the Gulf War. Through careful research, and a new perspective, the author describes the problems leading to the conflict and the startling results. The U.S. government's cover-up and military personnel's exposer to biological weapons is detailed in the most incredible ever written on the subject. But it doesn't stop there, in the 448 pages of this book a cure of some of the diseases is put forward. The book is $22.95 shipped airmail in the U.S. or $27.95 internationally.

**24 Hours a Day
VISA or Master Card Accepted
Voice Mail Ordering: 1-888-690-1277
or 1-907-249-9111
http://www.earthpulse.com**

A free catalog of all of our products and books is available on request.

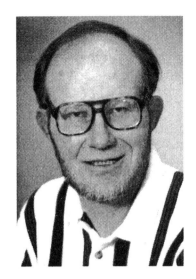

About the Author

Gary Lockhart grew up on an Iowa farm, where he learned the common and botanical names of some of the herbs in this book, from the back of weed killer cans. He developed an interest in nature and weather observations from the remarks of farmers in his childhood. He has written books on weather folklore and the use of plants to predict the weather.

He graduated from the State University of Iowa and worked as a chemist, process engineer and laboratory director in the paper and pulp field. When he returned to Seattle from Alaska, he began work on 12 books covering all aspects of alternative medicine. This project took more than 35,000 hours and resulted in visits to major libraries all over the United States and Canada.

Gary found that large amounts of material on the use of plants and alternative medicine can be found in the old medical and scientific literature. Since there is little indexing, the observations are almost unknown. Doctors have found herbs that cure migraines, failing hearts, cancer, leukemia, asthma and many other disorders, but their observations have received no publicity and gather dust in the basement of libraries. His interests include saving heritage seeds and organic farming. He has a strong belief that the future of medicine involves learning and applying the lessons of the past. He has taught classes and led tours on the identification and use of herbs.